Spiritual Interventions in Child and Adolescent Psychotherapy

Spiritual Interventions in Child and Adolescent Psychotherapy

Edited by

Donald F. Walker and William L. Hathaway

American Psychological Association • Washington, DC

Published by
American Psychological Association
750 First Street, NE
Washington, DC 20002
www.apa.org

To order
APA Order Department
P.O. Box 92984
Washington, DC 20090-2984
Tel: (800) 374-2721; Direct: (202) 336-5510
Fax: (202) 336-5502; TDD/TTY: (202) 336-6123
Online: www.apa.org/pubs/books
E-mail: order@apa.org

In the U.K., Europe, Africa, and the Middle East, copies may be ordered from
American Psychological Association
3 Henrietta Street
Covent Garden, London
WC2E 8LU England

Typeset in Goudy by Circle Graphics, Inc., Columbia, MD

Printer: Edwards Brothers, Ann Arbor, MI
Cover Designer: Mercury Publishing Services, Rockville, MD
Cover illustration by Chrissy S., age 5, courtesy of The Global Children's Art Gallery (http://naturalchild.org/).

Library of Congress Cataloging-in-Publication Data

Spiritual interventions in child and adolescent psychotherapy / edited by Donald F. Walker and William L. Hathaway.
p. cm.
ISBN 978-1-4338-1218-7—ISBN 1-4338-1218-5 1. Adolescent psychotherapy. 2. Spirituality. 3. Psychotherapy—Moral and ethical aspects. 4. Counseling—Moral and ethical aspects. I. Walker, Donald F. (Donald Franklin) II. Hathaway, William L. (William Lloyd)

RJ503.S68 2013
618.92'8914—dc23

2012014366

British Library Cataloguing-in-Publication Data
A CIP record is available from the British Library.

Printed in the United States of America
First Edition

DOI: 10.1037/13947-000

This book is dedicated to my Aunt Meredith and my Uncle Wilfred—my second set of parents. You taught me to "hunt bears" in your living room when I was a child and always saved a seat for me at church when I was a teenager. Your gentle grace, dignity, and love will live on in your nieces and nephews for generations to come.

—Don

For my wife, Viva, our now adult children, Josh and Christina, and their families that include our four granddaughters, all seemingly moving too fast through their own childhoods. Any value in my contributions to this work is indebted to my friends and teachers in the psychology of religion, Ken Pargament, and in clinical child psychology, Russ Barkley: mentors par excellence in both profession and life.

—Bill

CONTENTS

CONTRIBUTORS

Sameera Ahmed, PhD, Director, The Family and Youth Institute; Assistant Professor, Department of Psychiatry and Behavioral Neuroscience, Wayne State University, Detroit, MI

Anisah Bagasra, PhD, Instructor, Department of Psychology, Claflin University, Orangeburg, SC

Heather Bermudez, MA, Doctoral Student, Clinical Psychology, Regent University, Virginia Beach, VA

Joshua Childers, PsyD, Adjunct Assistant Professor, Department of Psychology, Regent University, Virginia Beach, VA

Frederick A. DiBlasio, PhD, Professor, School of Social Work, University of Maryland, Baltimore

William Doverspike, PhD, Independent Practice, Atlanta, GA

Lisa Grimes, Doctoral Student, Clinical Psychology, Bowling Green State University, Bowling Green, OH

William L. Hathaway, PhD, Dean, School of Psychology and Counseling, Regent University, Virginia Beach, VA

David J. Jennings II, MS, Doctoral Student, Counseling Psychology, Virginia Commonwealth University, Richmond

Pamela Ebstyne King, PhD, Assistant Professor, Marriage and Family Studies, Fuller Theological Seminary, Pasadena, CA

Katherine Kusner, Doctoral Student, Clinical Psychology, Bowling Green State University, Bowling Green, OH

Michelle LeRoy, Doctoral Student, Clinical Psychology, Bowling Green State University, Bowling Green, OH

Vickey Maclin, PsyD, Assistant Professor, Department of Clinical Psychology, Regent University, Virginia Beach, VA

Annette Mahoney, PhD, Professor, Department of Psychology, Bowling Green State University, Bowling Green, OH

Kerry McGregor, MA, Doctoral Student, Clinical Psychology, Regent University, Virginia Beach, VA

Avidan Milevsky, PhD, Department of Psychology, Kutztown University of Pennsylvania, Kutztown

Lisa Miller, PhD, Associate Professor and Director of Clinical Psychology, Teachers College, Columbia University, New York, NY

Glen Moriarty, PsyD, Associate Professor, Department of Clinical Psychology, Regent University, Virginia Beach, VA

Lynn Olson, PhD, Adjunct Professor, Department of Clinical Psychology, Regent University, Virginia Beach, VA

Emily Padgett, MA, Doctoral Student, Clinical Psychology, Bowling Green State University, Bowling Green, OH

David Peter Quagliana, PhD, Assistant Director, Lee University Counseling Center, Cleveland, TN

Heather Lewis Quagliana, PhD, Assistant Professor of Psychology, Department of Behavioral and Social Sciences; Executive Director, Play Therapy Center, Lee University, Cleveland, TN

Steven A. Rogers, PhD, Associate Professor, Department of Psychology, Westmont College, Santa Barbara, CA

LeAnne Steen, PhD, Associate Professor and Chair, Department of Counseling, Loyola University New Orleans, New Orleans, LA

Linda Mans Wagener, PhD, Adjunct Professor, Department of Psychology, Fuller Theological Seminary, Pasadena, CA

Donald F. Walker, PhD, Assistant Professor and Director, Child Trauma Institute, Regent University, Virginia Beach, VA

Jacqueline D. Woolley, PhD, Professor, Department of Psychology, University of Texas at Austin

Everett L. Worthington Jr., PhD, Professor, Department of Psychology, Virginia Commonwealth University, Richmond

ACKNOWLEDGMENTS

The editors gratefully acknowledge the help and support of Susan Reynolds, senior acquisitions editor at the American Psychological Association (APA), in supporting and overseeing the production of this book. We also wish to thank the editorial staff at APA, as well as the anonymous reviewers whose comments greatly enhanced the book.

Spiritual Interventions in Child and Adolescent Psychotherapy

INTRODUCTION

DONALD F. WALKER

In many ways, my interest in writing about and applying spiritual interventions in child and adolescent psychotherapy stems from my own experience, first as a doctoral student, later as a psychotherapist in private practice, and finally as a supervisor in a university setting. I have seen firsthand the power of spirituality and religion to be problematic or helpful in resolving client issues.

My first practicum rotation was in an explicitly Christian outpatient private practice in Southern California. There, one of my first referrals was an African American child whose Christian mother, when calling to set up the initial appointment, apparently told the office staff that she thought her son was suffering from demon possession. I did not work in the central office and, as a result, received the referral via phone message, with little elaboration other than an inquiry about whether I did work around demon possession. Desperate for practicum hours, and full of the bravado that comes with a 1st-year spring semester of six practice sessions, I swallowed hard and called the client.

DOI: 10.1037/13947-001
Spiritual Interventions in Child and Adolescent Psychotherapy, D. F. Walker and W. L. Hathaway (Editors)

Several assessment sessions later, I confirmed my suspicion that the child was not, in fact, demon possessed but had been playing some violent video games (one of which was Diablo, or the Spanish word for *devil*). My client was also engaging in some problematic behavior at home and at school that responded somewhat well to behavioral interventions implemented by his mother, who was a single parent working hard to raise my client, with several other children at home. However, his mother was consistently tougher on him and more controlling of him than I thought she needed to be. Several months into psychotherapy, I attempted to help her apply the Bible to her parenting style by quoting Ephesians 6:4, which instructs parents to "not exasperate your children." She promptly cancelled the next session and the one after that. Luckily, I was able to repair the working alliance by calling her and apologizing, and she returned for psychotherapy. We worked together for most of my practicum rotation, and the family terminated psychotherapy successfully after more than 6 months of working together.

In the process of working with this family, I learned several valuable lessons about using spiritual interventions in psychotherapy. First, as Mahoney and her colleagues discuss later in Chapter 3, the ways in which people live out their religion are not always psychologically or spiritually healthy. In this particular case, my client's mother's attempt to live out her faith led her to overinterpret the spiritual meaning of her son's choice of video games. As a result, she may have been more inclined to selectively interpret scriptural passages that supported her interpretation of the meaning of the video game to her son's spirituality. Therefore, the use of scripture with this particular parent may have been contraindicated to begin with.

Second, although I believe that my assessment of her parenting practice as ineffectual was accurate, I failed to consider how offended she would be at my challenge to her parenting approach to her son when I used scripture to support it. In retrospect, I should have realized the weight that my words carried when a reference to a sacred passage from her faith was used to support my therapeutic challenge to her parenting.

Because of the significance that highly religious parents place on sacred writings, before directly challenging her parenting approach with the full weight of the Christian Bible, I should have more explicitly explored the meaning of her current parenting practices with her and then explored (rather than directly challenged with a specific reference) her understanding of various scriptural references related to parenting in the Bible. Had I opened up the conversation related to her parenting in this way, she would probably have responded less defensively. Afterward, she might have been more receptive to reflecting on the discrepancy between her stated parenting goals (raising her child in her faith using parenting practices that were compatible with her faith) and her parenting practices.

I never made the same combination of mistakes with a religious parent again. Indeed, after learning from my mistakes, I eventually went on to write a protocol for using scripture in the context of empirically supported parenting programs with conservative Christian parents that is presented later in this volume (Chapter 7).

Several years and clinical rotations later, I worked in an outpatient children's community mental health center in Canton, Ohio, for my predoctoral internship. Early in the internship year, I noticed that I had multiple clients with spiritual issues that seemed to be relevant to their presenting problems. For example, more than a few parents brought in children with behavioral problems and openly discussed their discouragement that their youths were not behaving in a manner consistent with their religious upbringing. Such parents often discussed their specific parenting practices in light of the teachings of their spiritual tradition. These parents also often made reference to specific spiritual practices, such as reading sacred texts or prayer, in their attempts to cope with their children's behavior and to raise them. In a related vein, these parents also often turned to their churches for social support and treated church members as extended family.

Furthermore, several youths who were diagnosed with oppositional defiant disorder or conduct disorder invariably ended up discussing issues of forgiveness with their parents at some point in their treatment, even if they could not identify what they were seeking from their parents as forgiveness. In addition, I noticed that some children who experienced traumatic grief after loved ones died talked with God about missing them. Little did they know that in bringing their discussions with God into the psychotherapy room with me, they were raising issues related to the use of prayer in psychotherapy. Finally, one boy who had molested several younger children struggled with wondering whether God could forgive him.

I cautiously brought these issues up in supervision. I was a little hesitant to do so because I wanted to be sensitive to the setting that I was working in, and I also wanted to avoid a perception that I was imposing my religious values on my clients. Somewhat to my surprise, my supervisor supported my case conceptualizations of my clients. He told me that we were in the Bible Belt and that many of my clients would think about their lives in religious terms and bring up religious or spiritual issues. Throughout the internship year, he helped me address these spiritual concerns in a way that was also considerate of our milieu as a community mental health center. Later in the year, I learned that he was Jewish and that our considerations of client religion and spirituality were being conducted in a cross-religious dyad in supervision.

These experiences highlight the diversity of ways in which spirituality is manifested in child and adolescent psychotherapy. They show the potential of spiritually oriented interventions to assist or, if unskillfully applied, to hinder the therapeutic process. Accordingly, although increasing numbers of mental health practitioners recognize the value of addressing spirituality in therapy, guidance is needed to ensure that spirituality is effectively blended with evidence-based techniques.

Such guidance is particularly needed for child and adolescent psychotherapy. As my previous experiences make clear, children and their family dynamics present unique challenges to therapists interested in applying spiritual interventions. Perhaps foremost of these challenges is the need to address ethical concerns, such as obtaining parental consent and child assent. Additionally, the family and developmental contexts of children and adolescents present unique challenges. In some cases, the child's or parent's spirituality can be problematic rather than a resource. Indeed, spirituality may or may not be relevant to the presenting problem and case conceptualization. Given these challenges, careful assessment is critical.

This book demonstrates how to provide spiritual interventions for child and adolescent clients and their families with a range of presenting problems. Ethics, assessment, and family and developmental contexts serve as a framework, and various types of interventions are represented within this framework, such as prayer, forgiveness, the use of sacred texts, and God images. The interventions can be applied in both explicitly religious and decidedly secular settings and with clients of varying belief systems. The book specifically addresses Christianity, Judaism, Islam, and a more general spirituality based on a guiding universe. Each chapter includes illustrative case studies.

The book is driven by two larger, separate, yet converging forces: advances in the fields of child psychotherapy and advances in the psychology of religion and spirituality. Regarding the former, much of the field of child and adolescent psychotherapy has become increasingly dominated by evidence-based practices for presenting problems as diverse as oppositional behavior, anxiety, depression, and childhood abuse, among others (e.g., Cohen, Mannarino, & Deblinger, 2006; Weisz & Kazdin, 2010). Regarding the latter, researchers have been developing empirically supported spiritual interventions involving forgiveness, prayer, and sacred texts, among others, for mental health problems such as anger, anxiety, and depression (see, e.g., Aten, McMinn, & Worthington, 2011). I view the ideas discussed in this book as a springboard for the convergence of these two cutting-edge areas of practice and clinical research. Although the spiritual interventions that are discussed for children and teens in this book are only beginning to gain empirical support, the authors' clinical experience has shown that these approaches work. The remainder of this introduction provides background information about spiritual interventions and explains how this book is organized.

TERMINOLOGY

Psychotherapists typically differentiate spirituality from religion on the basis that spirituality is more personal, experiential, affective, and transcendent (Richards & Bergin, 2005). Conversely, religion is more often thought of as something that is rooted in doctrine, institutional, and conducted corporately (Pargament, 1999; Richards & Bergin, 2005). I personally view spirituality and religion as interrelated and complementary, in that many people practice their personal spirituality in the context of organized religion. However, many people practice their spirituality outside of organized religion. Throughout the book, the authors focus on client *spirituality* in an attempt to be considerate of numerous psychotherapists who view this term as more inclusive than the term *religion* or *religiousness*. However, instances in which client religiousness should be carefully considered in case conceptualization and treatment are also noted.

TYPES OF SPIRITUAL INTERVENTIONS

Aten et al. (2011) provided a helpful heuristic for categorizing approaches to spiritual interventions in counseling and psychotherapy. Using categories previously defined by Worthington (1986) and reviewed by Post and Wade (2009), Aten et al. suggested that spiritual interventions can be classified as belonging to one of three groups. The first group consists of secular interventions that can be used for the purpose of strengthening the faith of a religiously committed client. This type of intervention has no explicit spiritual content, but the purpose in applying the intervention could meet a spiritual goal. For example, in working with the mother of the child client whom I described earlier, I could have used parent–child interaction therapy (PCIT; Eyberg & Bussing, 2010) to assist the parent in modifying the child's behavior. PCIT could be used for what could be perceived as a spiritual purpose on the part of the parent (e.g., teaching the child to behave in way congruent with the parent's faith). However, without explicitly modifying secular PCIT to include spiritual content in the delivery of PCIT, it would remain a secular intervention to meet a spiritual goal.

The second set of spiritual interventions includes secular techniques that have been modified to include explicitly religious and spiritual content. An example of this kind of spiritual intervention would include PCIT modified to include spiritual content such as references to sacred writings from the client's spiritual and religious background. Chapter 7 provides an example of this kind of spiritual intervention when the authors suggest specific references to sacred writings that can be used to support the use of selective attention as an intervention in contrast to the parental use of corporal punishment.

Finally, a third kind of spiritually oriented intervention involves actions or behaviors taken exclusively from religious and spiritual practice. For example, Chapter 8 presents a case study in which a psychotherapist helped a child express her grief through the use of prayer.

I find these categories helpful in organizing approaches to religious and spiritual interventions. Like Aten et al. (2011), the authors in this book emphasize the second and third categories described by Worthington (1986). It is important to note, however, that some spiritual interventions could belong to more than one category, depending on their use. For example, in considering prayer, Walker et al. (Chapter 8) present two case studies in which the clients' psychotherapists asked their clients to use prayer in the context of secular cognitive–behavioral treatments for anxiety.

Tan's (1996) conceptualization for addressing spiritual and religious issues in psychotherapy is also extremely valuable. Tan suggested that all spiritual interventions could be theoretically conceptualized as occurring along a continuum ranging from implicit to explicit intervention. According to Tan, psychotherapists operate from the implicit end of the continuum when they demonstrate respect for clients' religious and spiritual beliefs and values but do not openly incorporate spiritually oriented interventions in psychotherapy. At the explicit end of the continuum, psychotherapists openly incorporate spiritual interventions such as prayer and reference to sacred texts in psychotherapy. These diverse approaches to using spiritual interventions represent endpoints on a continuum rather than discrete categories.

Tan (1996) suggested that a psychotherapist's approach to using spiritual interventions will be determined by factors such as the site at which the psychotherapist is working, the relevance of the client's personal religion and spirituality to the presenting problem, the degree to which the client or (in the case of children) the parents wish to discuss religious and spiritual issues, and the psychotherapist's level of comfort using spiritual interventions. Tan's categorization is a useful heuristic with which to organize the different spiritual interventions presented in this book.

It is my contention that spiritual interventions are just as appropriate for children as for adults when applied with therapeutic sensitivity to clients. Although the authors in this book present a variety of spiritual interventions, I personally prefer spiritual interventions that involve adapting secular treatment protocols to include spiritual content. This approach makes sense to me for several reasons. First, this appears to be the most practical way to assist a majority of child and adolescent psychotherapists to fulfill the ethical mandate to treat client spirituality and religion with respect. It is probably not practical for the vast majority of child psychotherapists to try to become fluent in spiritual interventions that are taken purely from spiritual practice per se. However, many, if not most, clinicians treating children and teens are proficient in at least one, if not more, secular empirically supported treatments for children. Asking practitioners to assess clients' spirituality and to be willing to incorporate spirituality into treatments they are already familiar with seems far easier than asking them to learn completely new treatment protocols dependent exclusively on spiritual content.

Spiritual interventions that are taken exclusively from spiritual practice (e.g., prayer, consideration of God images, forgiveness) can be sensitively applied to clients' presenting problems without psychotherapists' imposition of their own spiritual beliefs and values. However, spiritual interventions such as these typically require more thoughtfulness in case conceptualization and clinical application on the part of psychotherapists. These types of spiritual interventions are more easily delivered in explicit, rather than implicit, fashion and, as such, need to be carefully thought out when delivered in public practice settings. I consider these issues in more detail in the next section.

SPIRITUAL INTERVENTIONS IN DIVERSE CLINICAL SETTINGS

The treatments presented in this book can be applied in a variety of practice settings. My own clinical experience has been that when working in public settings such as community mental health centers or children's hospitals, I have tended to apply spiritual interventions in a more implicit than explicit manner. Consistent with my discussion of my own predoctoral internship experience, psychotherapists in public settings are well advised to discuss clinic policy related to sensitive discussion of client spirituality with their clinic directors before initiating the discussion with clients. My particular predoctoral internship site was very open to considering client spiritual issues, but the directors there also had a limit. For example, when considering client requests to pray, we were discouraged from praying together in session and particularly discouraged from initiating prayer together. Although I listened to several child clients in session talk to God about their problems, the clinic director would have been concerned had such discussions not been relevant to the child's presenting problem (typically traumatic grief) or if I had initiated the discussion without assessing the relevance of the client's spirituality to his or her presenting problem beforehand. Furthermore, concern would have been expressed if, on opening a session, I had offered to pray with the clients and their parents together about their grief. As another example, although I was supported by my supervisor in addressing client spiritual issues when appropriate, I was told that another staff member had previously been instructed to take down explicitly religious imagery displayed in his or her office.

Conversely, such open expressions of shared faith are expected in explicitly spiritual private practice settings. In such settings, clients (in this case, children's parents) may expect their psychotherapists to openly and explicitly engage in spiritual interventions and may express disappointment if they do not receive spiritual interventions as part of their treatment.

Psychotherapists working in school settings potentially face both sets of challenges, depending on the nature (public vs. private) of the schools they are working in. Across school settings, I would argue that psychotherapists should always initially assess and consider in case conceptualization the relevance of a client's spirituality, even if on later reflection, spirituality is not particularly relevant to a particular child's presenting problem. In public school settings, psychotherapists have typically been encouraged to avoid using spiritual interventions (Richards & Bergin, 2005). I concur with the general idea that it would be inappropriate to engage in a spiritual intervention such as referring to a sacred text or praying with a client in the actual public school setting in an explicit fashion. However, I would also suggest that there may be times when a client's personal spirituality is part of his or her presenting problem. When this is the case, psychotherapists should be prepared to address those spiritual issues as much as is feasible given the public nature of the setting.

For example, consider a child who reported to the psychotherapist that his or her parent had repeatedly beaten the child with an object and had done so because the parent needed to "beat the sin" out of the child and that the Bible told the parent to do so. Such a disclosure would undoubtedly warrant a child abuse report. In my opinion, it would be cruel to not also address the spiritual nature of the abuse in this situation. Using Tan's (1996) explicit–implicit continuum as a guide, in a public school setting I would advise against opening up a Bible and collaboratively looking up Biblical passages that speak to God's love for people in an attempt to challenge the seeming religious backing of the abuse from the Bible. Openly referring to specific passages in this instance would represent an explicit spiritual intervention.

However, this child's psychotherapist could, from a more implicit perspective, reflect back to this hypothetical client that he or she thought that the Bible talked about God's love for people. The psychotherapist in this hypothetical scenario could also indicate to the client that he or she was personally unaware of any Biblical passages that supported abusing children. The psychotherapist could also recommend that the child client consult with a religious leader from his or her church (or even from multiple churches) or extended family members about the Bible's teachings with respect to corporal punishment and abuse.

The challenge in addressing client spirituality is multifaceted. I would suggest that cultural sensitivity toward spiritual issues means that therapists must be willing to engage clients in discussion of such issues. Applying the ethical mandate to treat spirituality with cultural sensitivity means being willing to engage clients in discussion of such issues and to not avoid them. However, at the same time, psychotherapists must work diligently to avoid imposing their personal spiritual beliefs on clients. Sensitive application of spiritual interventions involves considering the client's presenting problem, the clinical setting, and the role of personal spirituality in the client's life. Throughout this book, the authors attempt to address these competing challenges.

STRUCTURE OF THIS BOOK

The first four chapters of this book provide a foundation and context for the use of spiritually oriented interventions with children and adolescents. In Chapter 1, Hathaway addresses ethical issues involved in using spiritually oriented interventions with children and teens. Some psychotherapists may wonder whether it is appropriate to use spiritually oriented interventions with children and adolescents and, if so, how to gain parental informed consent and child assent to do so. Hathaway discusses these considerations, as well as ethical principles and practice guidelines that inform decisions to use spiritually oriented interventions in therapy. Particular attention will be paid to situations involving discrepancies in the expression of parental and child spirituality or between a therapist and client.

In Chapter 2, Hathaway and Childers describe how to assess the potential role of religion and spirituality as a resource for change within treatment, as well as the potential effects of a child's disorder on his or her religious and spiritual functioning. For example, a child's ability to participate in organized religious activities is undoubtedly affected by the severity of hyperactive or inattentive symptoms associated with attention-deficit/hyperactivity disorder. However, parental spirituality may be a resource that can be drawn on in parenting interventions for childhood attention deficit/hyperactivity disorder. In addition, specific measures that can be used in treatment to assess for religious and spiritual domains are reviewed. Finally, Hathaway and Childers also discuss the use of assessment information to tailor specific spiritually oriented interventions to various child and adolescent presenting issues.

In Chapter 3, Mahoney, LeRoy, Kusner, Padgett, and Grimes consider forms of parental spirituality that can impede or enhance treatment. They address problematic parental spirituality, such as maladaptive parenting practices and religious perfectionism. For example, some religious parents may use unnecessarily harsh methods of discipline or hold unreasonable expectations about personal conduct. In addition, Mahoney et al. also consider parental religious and spiritual resources for change within psychotherapy.

In Chapter 4, Quagliana, King, Quagliana, and Wagener reflect on the use of spiritually oriented interventions in developmental context. They review developmental theories from different perspectives and consider the appropriateness of various spiritually oriented interventions at different developmental stages. For example, both a child and a teen who have suffered physical or sexual abuse undoubtedly struggle with maintaining an image of a loving God, but their understanding of God is different because of their age. A variety of spiritually oriented interventions at different developmental stages are considered in this chapter.

The next six chapters describe the use of spiritual interventions from different theoretical and spiritual perspectives. In Chapter 5, Rogers, Steen, and McGregor describe the use of acceptance as a spiritually oriented intervention. Acceptance is central to interpersonal relationships and is considered a core element of some psychotherapeutic approaches. They describe acceptance as a spiritual approach to psychotherapy built on a belief in the innate ability of children to strive toward personal and spiritual growth and a deep and abiding belief in the child's ability to be. Ways in which acceptance functions therapeutically are discussed. In addition, personal attributes of the psychotherapist that foster acceptance in therapy are also reviewed.

In Chapter 6, Miller discusses spiritual awareness in psychotherapy. Spiritual awareness has been described as a process in which the client is helped to grow more attuned to the universe or the divine and to evolve along a spiritual path. In using this approach, psychotherapists help clients listen for direction, with a whole and open heart, from the universe or one's personal creator. The psychotherapist becomes a guide on this journey, and as such the therapist's own spiritual voyage is an important resource for therapy. The theoretical and philosophical underpinnings of this approach, informed by Jung and Rogers, are described.

In Chapter 7, Walker, Ahmed, Milevsky, Quagliana, and Bagasra examine the use of sacred writings as a spiritual intervention. Every world religion has a way of life that is communicated through a sacred text. For religiously committed children and their families, reference to passages from sacred texts may be helpful in conceptualizing and treating presenting problems. For example, both empirically supported parenting programs and most major world religions prescribe specific parenting practices. Moreover, some have suggested that narratives found in sacred texts can be helpful in resolving the trauma of physical and sexual abuse.

In Chapter 8, Walker, Doverspike, Ahmed, Milevsky, and Woolley consider the use of prayer as an intervention in psychotherapy. Although prayer is a central element of every major world religion, it may be a controversial practice when considered in the context of child and adolescent psychotherapy. Walker et al. discuss the appropriateness of prayer as an intervention in psychotherapy with children and teens. Ethical principles that should be considered before using prayer, as well as theoretical and empirical research regarding the use of prayer with children and adolescents, are reviewed. The use of prayer with clients of different ages, with different presenting problems, and in different therapeutic contexts is described.

In Chapter 9, Olson, Maclin, Moriarty, and Bermudez discuss ways to address children's God images in psychotherapy. They examine the role of one's God image in a determining a child's view of him- or herself and in relating to others. Sources of distortion in one's God image are discussed. In addition, therapeutic practices to correct distorted or maladaptive God images are described. The use of God images across different therapeutic approaches is also reviewed.

In Chapter 10, DiBlasio, Worthington, and Jennings discuss the use of forgiveness in psychotherapy with children and teens. Forgiveness and reconciliation are inherently spiritual practices that serve to heal broken relationships. In the context of psychotherapy, forgiveness has been described as a process that reduces negative emotions such as anger and fosters positive emotions or a renewed relationship with an offending party. The adaptation of empirically supported treatment protocols to promote forgiveness for use with children and families is reviewed.

In the Afterword, Walker and Hathaway conclude the book by reflecting on the future of spiritually oriented interventions in child and adolescent psychotherapy. We focus our reflections on clinical practice, training, and research in this area.

CONCLUSION

Although work in applying the growing body of knowledge about the psychology of religion and spirituality to treatment of children and adolescents is in its infancy, I feel in some ways like a proud father watching a baby learning to walk in the presence of his or her surrounding family. The approaches described in this book are in the early stages of empirical investigation. However, randomized clinical trials are only one form of empirical evidence needed for the development of an evidence base for practice. Indeed, a recent presidential task force of the American Psychological Association (2006) acknowledged that clinical case studies are a valid type of evidence for evidence-based practice. Much of the clinical applications described in this book are well grounded in theory, have been tested in varying degrees in empirical research, and are supported by clinical experience. Thus, the clinical experiences that are described by each of the chapter authors serve as an evidence base for the utility of each of these approaches, broadly defined.

As the field matures, I look forward to the day when work applying spiritually oriented interventions to child and adolescent psychotherapy takes off running with additional empirical support, including randomized clinical trials. Until then, it is my sincerest hope that this book will be an aid to you in conducting psychotherapy, assessment, and supervision with religiously committed children, teens, and their families.

REFERENCES

American Psychological Association. (2006). *APA presidential task force on evidence-based practice*. Washington, DC: Author.

Aten, J. D., McMinn, M. R., & Worthington, E. L., Jr. (2011). (Eds.). *Spiritually oriented interventions in counseling and psychotherapy*. Washington, DC: American Psychological Association.

Cohen, J. A., Mannarino, A. P., & Deblinger, E. (2006). *Treating trauma and traumatic grief in children and adolescents*. New York, NY: Guilford Press.

Eyberg, S., & Bussing, R. (2010). Parent-child interaction therapy for preschool children with conduct problems. In M. Murrihy, A. Kidman, & T. Ollendick (Eds.), *Clinical handbook of assessing and treating conduct problems in youth* (pp. 139–162). New York, NY: Springer. doi:10.1007/978-1-4419-6297-3_6

Pargament, K. I. (1999). The psychology of religion and spirituality? Yes and no. *International Journal for the Psychology of Religion*, 9, 3–16. doi:10.1207/s15327582ijpr0901_2

Post, B. C., & Wade, N. G. (2009). Religion and spirituality in psychotherapy: A practice friendly review of research. *Journal of Clinical Psychology*, 65, 131–146. doi:10.1002/jclp.20563

Richards, P. S., & Bergin, A. E. (2005). *A spiritual strategy for counseling and psychotherapy* (2nd ed.). Washington, DC: American Psychological Association. doi:10.1037/11214-000

Tan, S. Y. (1996). Religion in clinical practice: Implicit and explicit integration. In E. P. Shafranske (Ed.), *Religion and the clinical practice of psychology* (pp. 365–387). Washington, DC: American Psychological Association. doi:10.1037/10199-013

Weisz, J. R., & Kazdin, A. E. (2010). (Eds.). *Evidence-based psychotherapies for children and adolescents* (2nd ed.). New York, NY: Guilford Press.

Worthington, E. L., Jr. (1986). Religious counseling: A review of published empirical research. *Journal of Counseling & Development*, 64, 421–431. doi:10.1002/j.1556-6676.1986.tb01153.x

I

FOUNDATIONS AND CONTEXT

1

ETHICS, RELIGIOUS ISSUES, AND CLINICAL CHILD PSYCHOLOGY

WILLIAM L. HATHAWAY

Katrina, a 14-year-old girl of Russian descent, was brought in for treatment by her parents because they were contemplating a divorce. Her parents said they wanted to make sure that Katrina was doing okay. They felt she had been avoiding them. She was now spending quite a bit of time going to her friend's church and other religious activities. Neither Katrina nor her family had been very active in organized religion in the past. Katrina's religious participation picked up after she started attending a Young Life religious club that met at her school when invited by a friend several months earlier. Her parents were concerned about how religious she was becoming and how this seemed to be pulling her away from them.

The family had previously been infrequent attendees at an Episcopal church. Katrina's friend attended a nondenominational evangelical church. Her parents did not object to her attending the church but were concerned that it was quite conservative and wondered

DOI: 10.1037/13947-002
Spiritual Interventions in Child and Adolescent Psychotherapy, D. F. Walker and W. L. Hathaway (Editors)

whether something might be wrong with her given how religious she had recently become. Was this normal? Was her religious involvement just a way to stay away from home? Katrina was now engaging in personal Bible reading and praying on a daily basis and was going to youth group and other religious events at her friend's church two or three times a week. Katrina said that she was not trying to avoid her parents but explained to becoming very involved in the youth group. She relayed that she started thinking more about religious things after she heard her friends at the Young Life meetings talk about how much God was doing in their lives. She did not think she was trying to avoid her family but explained that her newfound faith was helping her handle things in her life better. Katrina was sad that her parents were having problems and prayed regularly for them to work things out. She had been very worried about what might happen to her family, and although she was still concerned, she was finding comfort from turning the situation over to God.

After Katrina described the role her new faith was playing in her life, the room became quiet. Her parents and Katrina collectively looked at her psychotherapist, clearly seeking direction about where to go next in the discussion. The psychotherapist had a decision to make. What should be made of the presenting issue brought in by the family? Was it a clinical topic? Was it perhaps just a religious issue? Was it perhaps both? What would be an ethical way to move forward in the session? If the religious issues remained central to the case presentation, should a referral be made to a religious professional? Would the psychotherapist have sufficient self-awareness to prevent his or her own attitudes about the religious issues from adversely biasing the clinical response? Would the psychotherapist be competent to intervene if it seemed that the treatment goal should accommodate explicit religious foci? Thus, the decision at the outset of treatment was not merely a strategic one but also an ethical one.

In this chapter, I discuss ways in which the American Psychological Association's (APA's) "Ethical Principles of Psychologists and Code of Conduct" (APA, 2010a; hereinafter referred to as the APA Ethics Code) pertains to the practice of child and adolescent psychotherapy with spiritually oriented children, teens, and families. I begin by providing a rationale detailing the relevance of spiritual concerns related to ethical practice with children. I then discuss the application of ethics in clinical practice with children and teens. Throughout this discussion, I present a series of case studies illustrating ways in which various aspects of the APA Ethics Code may be relevant to presenting issues related to client spirituality. I then discuss ways to resolve ethical concerns related to spiritual issues when working with children and teens.

RATIONALE FOR CONSIDERING ETHICS RELATED TO SPIRITUALITY WITH CHILDREN AND TEENS

An exploration of ethical concerns in a clinical child practice niche that accommodates religious spiritual issues may be esoteric yet should not be. Detailed explorations of ethical issues in dealing with children reflect a subspecialty within professional ethics. A cursory review of textbooks on clinical child psychology will find only rare pages dedicated explicitly to ethics (viz., Mash & Barkley, 2006). Ollendick and Schroeder's (2003) wide-ranging *Encyclopedia of Clinical Child and Pediatric Psychology* has very few of its 748 pages devoted to ethical issues. As of early 2011, 22,999 articles were retrieved in a PsycINFO search on the keyword phrase *professional ethics*, but only 989 remained after adding the term *child*. Many articles in this smaller set appeared to be focused on general topics in practice with only incidental attention being given to ethical issues in child therapy.

Focused discussion on professional ethical concerns with religion was also relatively infrequent, with only 344 hits arising from a search on *professional ethics* and *religion*. Including the overlapping category of *child* resulted in just nine articles, none of which explicitly focused on a discussion of ethical concerns in this practice niche. A cursory exploration of the smaller but growing literature within the clinical psychology of religion and spirituality similarly provided only rare discussions of the ethical issues involved in dealing with religious and spiritual themes in clinical child practice. In this sense, the focus of this chapter is indeed somewhat esoteric.

Yet from another perspective, the topic is potentially quite broad. Psychological exploration of religious issues among children and adolescents is one of the oldest topics explored by the "new psychology." Starbuck's (1899) *The Psychology of Religion* provided an empirical exploration of religious development in children and adolescents. The developmental psychology of religion has recently experienced a resurgence (Roehlkepartain, King, Wagener, & Benson, 2006). At the turn of the millennium in North America, all but about 5% of married couples and parents acknowledged a religious affiliation (Mahoney, Pargament, Swank, & Tarakeshwar, 2001). Given the high likelihood that religious or spiritual factors may be part of the "ethnoreligious" context of clinical child practice, there is reason to suppose that religious and spiritual factors are either actually or potentially a ubiquitous issue in clinical child practice despite the sparse attention they receive in the literature (Sattler, 1998).

Ethical considerations in attempting to explicitly engage the religious and spiritual domain in clinical child practice can be clustered into two group: those that arise from the same ethical principles and standards that are always present in practice and those that arise from the unique considerations of the delimited treatment population. Standard ethical considerations from the APA (2010a) Ethics Code for clinical practice with religious and spiritual issues have been addressed elsewhere (Hathaway, 2011; Hathaway & Ripley, 2009; Richards & Bergin, 2005). These discussions noted the particular salience of ethical considerations such as avoiding bias and prejudice, respect for the client's autonomy, avoiding conflictual dual relationships, doing no harm, and practicing within the bounds of competence. All of these sorts of standard ethical considerations are relevant to the clinical child case as well. Additional concerns arising from the clinical child practice regarding confidentiality issues, the child as having special vulnerabilities, developmental considerations, and the systemic complexities of the legal status of a minor are also pertinent.

ETHICAL CONSIDERATIONS IN PRACTICE

The APA Ethics Code delineates aspirational principles and enforceable standards that can guide clinical practice in working with children and adolescents. The principles and standards pertain broadly in all practice contexts but must be concretely applied to appropriately connect with the specific contours of the concrete clinical situation through a careful ethical decision-making process. Because children and adolescents often have reduced self-determination from a legal standpoint and are less able developmentally to protect their own interests the younger they are, it is vital that clinicians take special care to protect the child's well-being. As Rae (2003b) stated,

> Because of the special vulnerabilities of children and the complexities involved in coordinating with schools, health care facilities, and families, psychological services for children, adolescents, and families require an exceptionally high standard of ethical behavior. The APA Ethics Code is written broadly to apply to psychologists with varied roles in many different professional contexts. The ethical guidelines are written primarily with adults in mind and, as a result, they may not always apply to the special needs of children. In this regard, "special needs" of children might include not only the child, but also other family members as well during assessment, intervention or research. Legal standards for minors are very different than those for adults. . . . The psychologist must aspire to maintain the highest legal and ethical practices in working with children and families. (p. 214)

Principled Conduct

The APA Ethics Code outlines aspirational principles that undergird and shape the specific expectations presented in its standards. A list of the princi-

EXHIBIT 1.1
American Psychological Association's (2010a)
"Ethical Principles of Psychologists and Code of Conduct"

General Principles
Principle A: Beneficence and Nonmaleficence
Principle B: Fidelity and Responsibility
Principle C: Integrity
Principle D: Justice
Principle E: Respect for People's Rights and Dignity

Ethical Standards
1. Resolving Ethical Issues
2. Competence
3. Human Relations
4. Privacy and Confidentiality
5. Advertising and Other Public Statements
6. Record Keeping and Fees
7. Education and Training
8. Research and Publication
9. Assessment
10. Therapy

ples and standards from the APA Ethics Code is presented in Exhibit 1.1. The principles function as normative anchors that direct the motivational goals and purposes of the ethical practitioner. At the end of the case example, Katrina's therapist could go in many directions. Regardless of the direction taken next, however, the decision should be motivated by a desire to promote the well-being of Katrina and her parents and by a concern to do no harm. APA's first principle of Beneficence and Nonmaleficence indicates that the next step in the therapy should be taken carefully with due guard against destructive biases or other unhelpful factors influencing the treatment in a noxious or nonproductive direction.

The therapist will likely need to get more information about the family to make a decision about what to do with the religiously themed presenting problem. It might be tempting for a clinician who is not personally religious to view Katrina's religious change in a way that discounts its significance. Doing so could lead the therapist to move too quickly away from the religiously focused themes brought into the session by the family, viewing them instead as superficial features of nonreligious issues deemed to be more important by the therapist. Therapists who are dismissive of religion may see such adolescent spiritual explorations and involvements as being relatively uninteresting apart from their potential role as symptomatic indicators of insecurity or other nonreligious concerns. In fact, adolescence is a frequently observed critical window in religious identity formation that can have a lifelong impact (Roehlkepartain et al., 2006). Although many adolescents adopt the faith tradition and identity of their parents, some develop in independent ways, and still others function as spiritual leaders, occasionally drawing their families to new forms or levels of religiousness (Boyatzis, Dollahite, & Marks, 2006).

An equally problematic temptation could arise if Katrina's therapist was religious and consequently assumed that the religious and spiritual issues were the most salient topic to make the focus of treatment. The American Psychiatric Association (1989) issued guidelines cautioning psychiatrists against imposing their religious views on clients. Similarly, Principle E of the APA (2010a) Ethics Code, Respect for People's Rights and Dignity, calls for psychologists to work to eliminate biases on the basis of a range of factors, including religion. It is possible that other issues would be more salient to the welfare of Katrina or her family than the religious-themed initial presenting problem provided by the family. Beginning therapists quickly learn that a client's first presentation of a problem may not adequately convey what really motivated the client to seek treatment. A religious therapist who failed to complete an adequate assessment or who chose to persist with the religious focus only because of the therapist's own valuing of religion would be making an ethical misstep analogous to the error of neglecting the domain out of irreligious bias.

Principle B, Fidelity and Responsibility, enjoins psychologists to build a relationship of trust with clients. A variety of things are conceptualized as relevant to this principle, from acting in a professional manner to engaging in appropriate consultation or collaboration with other professionals to better serve the client's interests. If Katrina's therapist was unfamiliar with adolescent religious development or the sorts of religious groups with which she was becoming involved, he or she would have been well served to consult with a colleague better able to assess their psychosocial significance. If the therapist did not know about the religious group or its nature or did not have sufficient competence to work with the religious concerns, and if those concerns continued to be relevant to the treatment, both Principle C (Integrity) and Principle D (Justice) would call for the therapist to be honest in presenting his or her ability to work with the issue.

Some Relevant Standards

This peripatetic discussion of principled practice has already suggested some specific patterns of conduct that ethical therapy may display in Katrina's case. Although all of the APA standards may be applicable in clinical child psychology, the practice-oriented standards relating to competent practice, the nature of the professional relationship, client privacy and confidentiality, and assessment and therapy are particularly relevant to the interface of clinical child psychology ethics and practice with religious and spiritual issues.

Practicing Within the Boundaries of Competence

Standard 2.01 of the APA Ethics Code requires psychologists to practice within their limits of competence "based on their education, training, supervised experience, consultation, study, or professional experience" (APA, 2010a, p. 5). If Katrina's therapist did not possess the competence to address the religion-focused themes with which the family presented, he or she would need to seek out appropriate consultation or other training or make a referral to a suitably qualified individual. Now, what type of training or consultation would be appropriate in this case? I have elsewhere argued that clinical work with religious and spiritual issues is a practice niche that possesses features of a clinical proficiency or specialty (Hathaway, 2008). Although it is not a formalized proficiency or specialty, there is specialized knowledge and a growing body of specialty interventions that have been shown to be relevant to the practice niche. At present, there is no compelling evidence that one needs to use religious and spiritual techniques to practice competently with even religiously concerned clients (see Aten, McMinn, & Worthington, 2011). Yet, such explicitly religious or spiritual treatment approaches may be valued and preferred by some clients. The research has suggested that the accommodation of religious and spiritual interventions with standard treatments has promising benefits for the therapy, possibly by facilitating treatment completion and adherence by motivating religious clients to more highly value the treatment or by adding incremental benefit to treatment outcomes (Tan & Johnson, 2005; Worthington & Sandage, 2002).

Even if such religiously accommodative approaches were not shown to produce better outcomes for clients who would otherwise have persisted in treatment, the current evidence indicates that they do not reduce treatment effectiveness. Given that religious clients often seek out therapists who self-identify as Christian, spiritually oriented, or other such religious or spiritual modifiers, it is quite possible that religious clients may be less likely to enter treatment or persist without explicit accommodation of a compatible spiritual dimension in therapy. This would understandably have an impact on treatment outcome, but only if the lack of treatment benefit for treatment refusers or dropouts was factored into the data. I have encountered numerous case anecdotes to suggest this issue may be prevalent, particularly in large, conventionally religious communities that tend to distrust the secular mental health professions. So construed, developing a religiously or spiritually accommodative practice competency is also a matter of further developing one's multicultural and relational competencies (Bartoli, 2007; Moore-Thomas & Day-Vines, 2008).

How does one obtain such competency? In some cases, psychologists have obtained specific advanced training in religious or spiritual interventions. Such training is increasingly available through continuing education workshops, training tapes, professional texts such as this one, or even through organized training programs at a doctoral, internship, or postdoctoral level. The Association of Psychology Postdoctoral Internship Centers' online internship and postdoctoral fellowship directory (http://www.appic.org/Directory) now allows its users to specify sites that have an emphasis on religion or spirituality.

Although no authoritative entity sets broadly embraced standards for religious and spiritual practice competence at present, the body of exemplar guidance materials in these areas is growing. Additionally, a working committee from the Society for the Psychology of Religion and Spirituality (APA Division 36) has formulated preliminary practice guidelines for the appropriate use of religious and spiritual interventions that have been presented elsewhere (Hathaway, 2011). As a general point of guidance, appropriate use of religious and spiritual interventions in professional practice is appropriate clinical use, which means that a religious or spiritual technique or relational focus should be incorporated into practice to achieve a clinical outcome and should be carried out in a manner respectful of the client's religious or spiritual values and beliefs.

Still, religious and spiritual competence in treatment is not only about one's ability to use religious and spiritual interventions such as the therapeutic use of prayer. Appropriate evaluation of the clinical significance of religious content in therapy may require a greater contextual understanding of the relevant religious or spiritual forms of life than the therapist possesses. In such cases, consultation with a psychologically informed religious professional or a mental health professional with particular competence in working with religious and spiritual issues is advised (McMinn, Aikins, & Lish, 2003).

In some cases, it is advisable to supplement one's expertise by formally collaborating with a religious professional or other member of a religious community. McMinn et al. (2003) described both general and advanced forms of competency in collaborating with clergy. In Katrina's case, most practitioners would be unlikely to need to go beyond consultation. Other cases, however, may present more challenging scenarios in which formal collaboration with members of religious communities may be needed. Therapists who treat clients with religious scrupulosity may find it quite difficult to get such clients to accept the need to alter their religious compulsions. In such cases, collaborative involvement of a religious professional who is viewed as having credible religious authority by the client is sometimes necessary. Consider the following case:

> Tony, a Catholic 15-year-old, was seen at a prominent clinic specializing in the treatment of anxiety disorders. Tony had developed obsessive–compulsive disorder over the past year. He was distraught because of reoccurring "blasphemous thoughts about cursing God" and fears that

he was going to hell because he could not keep the thoughts from coming into his head. This pattern did not appear to have been precipitated by any specific life event. He was using a variety of religious practices to try to ward off his fears of damnation, including repeatedly saying the Hail Mary to such an extent that he was not able to do other activities, including completing homework. The therapist explained the nature of obsessive–compulsive disorder to Tony and his parents, but Tony did not want to do anything to reduce his compulsive religious behaviors because of his fears of possible adverse spiritual consequences. The therapist asked the family whether he could have a Catholic priest with whom he had worked on such cases participate in some of the sessions. Tony and his parents agreed. The priest was able to successfully challenge Tony's beliefs about the spiritual necessity of the compulsions, and he agreed to cooperate with the course of treatment, including response prevention, that the therapist then continued. By the end of the treatment, Tony's compulsive religious behaviors had stopped, and he reported being free of the obsessive thoughts and fears that had plagued him previously. He continued to be active in his faith community but now reported feeling good about God. His parents noted that his school performance had improved, and there were no other concerning behaviors evident at home.

Tony's case indicates the potential importance of cooperative competencies. Cooperation with other professionals for the benefit of the client is specifically enjoined by APA Ethics Code Standard 3.09 but is done only infrequently with religious professionals in practice. Numerous practical and ethical complexities have to be navigated to engage in this sort of advanced collaboration. Issues of confidentiality need to be adequately addressed, for instance. Although many religious professionals value confidentiality, it may not be a binding ethical obligation for them. In such a case, the situation is somewhat analogous to the special challenges for confidentiality arising within group therapy from group members' access to one another's shared information. Issues of client privacy are a similar concern. By inviting a member of the client's religious community, or at least perhaps of his or her faith tradition, into the session, some loss of privacy occurs. Appropriate steps should be taken to safeguard the client's privacy and to ensure informed consent is obtained from the client and his or her parents.

Avoiding Multiple Relationships, Conflicts of Interest, and Unfair Discrimination

APA Ethics Code Standards 3.01, 3.05, and 3.06 direct psychologists to practice in a manner that avoids unfair discrimination, multiple relationships, and conflicts of interest, respectively. These standards could be separately unpacked in clinical child practice with religious or spiritual issues, but I address them together here because of their relevance to ethical concerns in child custody work. APA's (2010b) recently updated "Guidelines for Child Custody Evaluations in Family Law Proceedings" provides two extensions of these standards for the specific practice of child custody evaluation.

Guideline 6 states that "psychologists strive to engage in culturally informed, nondiscriminatory evaluation practices" (APA, 2010b, p. 865). The guideline calls for psychologists engaged in child custody evaluations to be "aware of their own biases, and those of others," regarding a variety of possible factors that could influence the evaluation, including religion (p. 865). Guideline 7 calls child custody evaluators to avoid conflicts of interest and multiple relationships. The guideline illustrates an inappropriate multiple relationship for a child custody evaluation with the example of performing such an evaluation on a child who had previously been a therapy client. However, any type of multiple relationship that "could reasonably be expected to result in (a) impaired impartiality, competence, or effectiveness or (b) exposure of the person or organization with whom the professional relationship exists to harm or exploitation" (p. 865) is in view.

I (Hathaway & Ripley, 2009) described a composite case of a child custody evaluation that was based on real cases on which I have consulted around issues of bias, conflicts of interest, and multiple relationships. Because the case is particularly relevant to the current exploration of clinical child psychology ethics and religion and spirituality, I reproduce it here.

> Dr. Bob, a psychologist in a rural Midwest location, was asked to do a custody evaluation of Mr. Smith's 8-year-old daughter. Mr. Smith is an active member of a conservative Baptist church where his daughter has also been active in the youth group since they moved to the region 2 years ago. Mr. Smith and his wife are now going through a divorce, and both parents are contesting for custody. His daughter has visited her mother periodically since the separation. Mrs. Smith has relocated to the Northeast where she grew up before the couple met at a Midwestern college. In a report to the court, Dr. Bob indicated that although both parents appear to have certain strengths, it would be better for the daughter to be raised by her father. He reasoned this because the daughter expressed religious faith and the mother was an agnostic. He asserted that, all things being equal, it is better to have a child raised in a home that is faith congruent. Mrs. Smith felt that the court was being hostile toward her because of her agnosticism. Dr. Bob and the family court judge both attended a church in the same denomination as Mr. Smith. (Hathaway & Ripley, 2009, p. 38)

The psychologist in this case reflected apparent bias that may have prejudiced his recommendation by asserting that the mother's agnosticism alone was an adequate consideration for a custody recommendation. Unless

Dr. Bob could demonstrate on the basis of appropriate professional evidence that parental agnosticism for a child with a professed religion predicts poorer child-rearing outcomes, such a judgment would be the result of ethically inappropriate considerations. No adequate research evidence exists for such a claim, to my knowledge, and clinical anecdotes are readily adducible showing healthy adjustment of children raised by agnostic parents. So what was the basis for Dr. Bob's judgment? Recall that Dr. Bob and the presiding family court judge shared the same faith, and indeed the same faith community, as the father and daughter in the custody dispute. This is strong prima facie evidence of unfair discrimination, a conflict of interest, and a problematic multiple relationship.

A psychologist could use a number of strategies to guard against these ethical missteps. The cleanest and most straightforward solution would simply have been to decline the custody evaluation (APA, 2010b). But let us suppose that the shared church relationship did not exist, rather only a shared faith background, thus avoiding multiple relationships. The psychologist could have collaborated with a colleague who represented a nonreligious worldview. He could also have engaged in a literature review to see whether there was empirical information pertaining to the child-rearing outcomes of children being raised by parents who do not share their religious views. Such strategies would be important first efforts at protecting against unfair discrimination.

Informed Consent and Assent

APA Ethics Code Standards 3.10, 9.03, and 10.1 direct psychologists to obtain informed consent from their clients for professional services including assessment and therapy except for those cases in which services are mandated by law without such consent. However, in the case of a child, the client is typically unable to give consent as a matter of law. The prerogative for such consent is the parents' or other legal guardian's. In such cases, the APA Ethics Code states that assent should still be sought from the client:

> For persons who are legally incapable of giving informed consent, psychologists nevertheless (1) provide an appropriate explanation, (2) seek the individual's assent, (3) consider such persons' preferences and best interests, and (4) obtain appropriate permission from a legally authorized person, if such substitute consent is permitted or required by law. When consent by a legally authorized person is not permitted or required by law, psychologists take reasonable steps to protect the individual's rights and welfare. (APA, 2010a, p. 6)

The amount of detailed explanation given to, and degree of informed assent expected from, children should depend on their level of development.

Explanations of assessment, treatment, or other professional services should be expressed in a developmentally appropriate manner. Thus, in a standard treatment scenario with children, the psychologist will adequately explain the clinical service to be provided to the child's parents or other legal guardian and obtain informed consent from the parents for the service. As Richards and Bergin (2005) recommended, "When working with children and adolescents, therapists should . . . obtain written consent from parents before using spiritual interventions" (p. 204). The psychologist will also offer an explanation of what service is to be provided to the child or teen. This latter explanation must be expressed in a manner suitable to the child's or teen's cognitive level. Once it is evident that appropriate explanation has been received and understood by the youth, the psychologist should then seek the client's assent to treatment.

What might a developmentally sensitive way to obtain client assent look like? Consider cognitive–behavioral therapy for anxiety, adapted to incorporate verses from sacred texts. With a child who is 8 years old, a psychotherapist might say something like this:

> It looks like you have a lot of worries that have been bothering you, and I'd like to help you with this. I think it would be helpful to you, and your mom has agreed, to learn how to deal with the worries. Some of the things we can do are (a) practice relaxing your body so that you feel calm, (b) practice deep breathing to help you feel calm, and (c) take a look at the thoughts you have and the things you say to yourself when you feel worried. Then, I'll help you change the things you say to yourself so that you feel calm and not worried. I also think it will help you to pray for help with your worries when you are practicing relaxing, so that you can feel God helping you. What do you think about this plan?

With a teenager, the language in this explanation could be altered to refer more explicitly to anxiety rather than referring to anxiety as *worries* and to refer to relaxation training as *relaxation training* rather than *practice relaxing*.

APA Ethics Code Standard 10.01b further states,

> When obtaining informed consent for treatment for which generally recognized techniques and procedures have not been established, psychologists inform their clients/patients of the developing nature of the treatment, the potential risks involved, alternative treatments that may be available, and the voluntary nature of their participation. (APA, 2010a, p. 13)

Although some empirical data have supported the benign nature of religious-congruent therapy, stand-alone religious or spiritual treatments have not yet reached the level that constitutes standardized, well-established treatments. Thus, careful explanation of the procedures to be used is called for if clinical practice is to incorporate religious or spiritual techniques.

As Stark et al. (2006) noted, "It is also important for the client to provide informed assent to treatment, as well as to understand the limited legal rights of minors in treatment, to the extent that the child can do so" (p. 391). For children age 14 and older, a discussion with a similar level of detail offered to the parents is often appropriate. Because cognitive maturity is less developed, more simplified descriptions are indicated.

Privacy and Confidentiality

APA Ethics Code Standard 4 addresses issues related to protecting the privacy of the confidential information received from the client. Rae (2003a) pointed out that confidentiality issues are complicated in clinical child cases because it is typically the parents or legal guardians who hold the legal privilege to the information obtained by the clinician. Thus, with a few exceptions that vary across jurisdictions, parents or legal guardians can request and obtain any information shared in the course of practice. It is the parent as the holder of the privilege who must grant release for information to be shared with a third party, not the child client.

The APA Ethics Code Standard 4.02 requires psychologists to discuss the limits of confidentiality with their clients "including, to the extent feasible, persons who are legally incapable of giving informed consent" (APA, 2010a, p. 7). If a therapeutic relationship is to be developed and maintained, it is generally important that clients understand to what extent they can expect the information they share in the treatment to remain private. Rae (2003a) noted that young children do not typically expect privacy in their personal matters because their parents are typically aware of even very personal aspects of their daily lives. However, as they move into the teenage years, young people frequently develop an expectation of privacy. Such expectations may arise from teens' ability to keep the parents uninformed about personal aspects of their lives. They can also arise from family norms that promise a certain level of privacy to youths. Yet these common sources of privacy expectation do not alter the fact that the parent is the holder of the legal privilege and can request access to the information shared in therapy at any point.

It is thus important to convey to young people the various limitations of confidentiality, not only those arising from mandatory reporting situations but also those arising from the parent's privilege as well. In practice, the adverse impact of the parent's privilege on child disclosure and participation in treatment can often be minimized by negotiating in advance with the parent what sorts of information will be reported and what sort will be kept private. In such cases, it is still vital to not overpromise. There is no guarantee that the parent may not change his or her mind. Yet a clinician can make a strong case to the parent that a young person is unlikely to fully participate or benefit from treatment unless he or she has a reasonable expectation of privacy. Consequently, it will be important for the parent to respect the private nature of the individual sessions with a youth to maximize the likelihood of treatment success.

Consider the following case.

> Justin was a 12-year-old boy who was tall for his age and already moving into puberty. His parents sent him to a private religious school in a southern state so that he could avoid bad peer influences. He was a bright student who had done well in elementary school. His grades dropped in sixth grade, and his parents decided to send him to the private school midway through the year. When he returned to school for seventh grade, he had changed his dress and appearance. He now dressed daily in all-black clothes and typically wore black nail polish. He described himself as a Goth and became more withdrawn. His parents tried to alter his behavior using different strategies but said that nothing was working and that they did not know what was going on with him. During the first session, the psychologist met with the client and his parents. The limits of confidentiality were discussed, and the parents agreed to respect the privacy of any individual sessions that would follow with the assurance that any information indicating a threat to his or anyone else's safety would be discussed. After several individual sessions, Justin began to describe doubts he was struggling with about God. He said he had a lot of questions about his family's church. He reported beginning to have those doubts at the end of fifth grade but also that he had not attempted to share them with anyone. He denied any self-destructive ideas or intent. However, he was discouraged because he did not feel that he could talk openly about his spiritual struggles with the people at his church or his family because they would not understand. He explained that he dressed differently because he did not feel a part of his peers at the private religious school, who did not seem to be struggling with the same doubts. Because therapy created a place in which Justin felt safe in exploring these issues, he was able to talk through them. Over several months, he became less withdrawn at school, was more engaged at home, and improved in his grades. Toward the end of treatment, Justin was willing to talk to a youth pastor, and then his parents, about some of his spiritual doubts. Shortly before termination, he reported his discouragement had gone away, but he remained inquisitive and no longer felt that he needed to keep his questions private.

Justin's issues were driven by private doubts he did not feel safe in expressing. By establishing a trusting relationship with the parents, the therapist was able to carve out a sufficiently private space for Justin to begin to open up about his personal doubts. This safe and accepting context helped him constructively work through those private struggles and to reengage with his parents and faith community. Yet the therapist was careful not to overpromise. Justin understood that his parents had the right to ask what was being conveyed in treatment. During one session early in the treatment, Justin brought this up. The therapist acknowledged Justin's concern and assured him that he would let him know if his parents changed their minds about respecting the privacy of the sessions but that there had been no indication that they were planning to do this. This ethical management of the confidentiality and privacy issues in the case of a minor who was not the holder of the privilege vindicated the parents' trust in the treatment. It allowed the therapy to be effective and produced changes that they deemed beneficial.

Justin's personal doubts seemed to him to be something no one else would understand. They led to a spiritual crisis that adversely affected his life adjustment. Spiritual doubts have been shown to have a positive relationship to stress and depression among college students (Hood, Hill, & Spilka, 2009). Popular culture frequently thinks of the college years as the peak time for spiritual doubt. However, in a study of spiritual doubt in a comprehensive parochial school system, Kooistra and Pargament (1999) found that many youths reported first experiencing doubts just before adolescence, but at this age they were more likely to keep it private.

TOXIC FAITH AND RELIGIOUSLY ACCOMMODATIVE CHILD INTERVENTIONS

The recent flurry of publications on the culture wars between the new atheists and religionists has recapitulated claims made popular in Soviet culture that religious instruction of children is a form of child abuse (e.g., Dawkins, 2006). The notion is expressed in several varied forms that share a common idea that religious perspectives teach a false view of the world and commit their adherents to reason-impairing habits of the mind (see, e.g., Dennett, 2006; Harris, 2006). Consequently, some people have argued that instruction of vulnerable children is a type of abuse (Hitchens, 2007). For example, in response to a question about the Catholic priest sex abuse scandals, Dawkins (2006) wrote, as "horrible as sexual abuse no doubt was the damage was arguably less than the long-term psychological damage inflicted by bringing up a child Catholic in the first place" (p. 317). It would of course be inappropriate in a psychological text to try to settle the validity of theological claims or atheist counterclaims, at least about the questions such as whether God exists or whether there is sufficient rational warrant to believe in God. Yet notice that Dawkins made a psychological claim about religious child rearing, specifically with regard to Catholicism, intending in his broader argument to implicate all religion as a psychologically noxious phenomenon.

Such claims have sometimes found their way into the psychological literature. In a 1970 article for Mensa, Albert Ellis famously described religion as the primary thing responsible for mental illness because of its facilitation of irrational beliefs. These types of claims also surface on various APA e-mail lists when issues of religion are raised. Now, if Ellis (1970) and Dawkins (2006) were right, then the APA Ethics Code principle of doing no harm should obligate practitioners to avoid any accommodation of religion or spirituality in clinical work with children (or adults, for that matter).

Another argument that is sometimes used to object to religious instruction is that religious child rearing is viewed as equivalent to brainwashing. The process of religious socialization involves an imposition of parental religious beliefs on children that override their autonomy. According to this argument, even if religion is not argued to be psychologically noxious on such an account, religious indoctrination is still hostile to the child's right of self-determination and should thus be opposed as a violation of the APA Ethics Code principles and standards enjoining psychologists to respect client autonomy.

The problem with these types of claims is that they are not supported by the empirical evidence. The developmental psychologists Boyatzis (2005) and his colleagues (Boyatzis et al., 2006) summarized the research by stating that "family spirituality and religiosity are linked with many desirable outcomes and inversely linked with negative outcomes in children and youth" (Boyatzis et al., 2006, p. 297). As with the religious-instruction-is-noxious claim, the religious-instruction-violates-autonomy claim is not supported by the available research. Research on religious spiritual development has not shown a simplistic model of parent-to-child religious transmission. Although parents do frequently appear successful in transmitting their faith to their offspring, primarily through the vehicle of embedded religious routines, children also develop in religious trajectories that are independent of their parents (Boyatzis, 2005; Boyatzis et al., 2006). Similarly, this same mixed pattern of worldview transmission and independence is observed in secular families who disavow religious perspectives (Boyatzis, 2005). Finally, the latter argument further begs the question in asserting that the right to self-determine religious and spiritual activity belongs to the child and not the parent. This point is contested in Western domestic and international law, with some precedents supporting the right of the state to intervene against parental religious wishes in some cases but not others (Witte & Nichols, 2011). Even if a strong parent-rights view is assumed, such rights are tied to the child's minority status. When children reach the age of majority, they may self-determine their own religious and spiritual practices from that point forward, even under strong parent-rights interpretations of religious liberty. In such a view, it would not deprive a child of autonomy to accommodate religious and spiritual issues in practice at parental request because the child would in fact not yet possess this autonomy.

Yet an analogous discussion could be made here with regard to what was previously introduced with regards to informed consent versus informed assent. Children may not possess autonomy as a legal prerogative, but they will likely develop greater capacities associated with psychological self-determination as they move through adolescence. Adopting a clinical posture that solicits parental support of the child's responsible exercise of growing psychological autonomy even in religious and spiritual matters may be advisable.

McCullough and Willoughby (2009) reviewed much of the data on the positive outcomes of religiousness and hypothesized that they are the result of religion's facilitation of self-regulation processes. If McCullough and Willoughby's work on religion as a self-regulation promotion pathway is correct, it would seem particularly at odds with both versions of the religious-instruction-as-child-abuse claim. Regardless of why such observed benefits are associated with religiousness, it is sufficient for the current purposes to simply point out that Dawkins's (2006) claim about the noxious outcomes of religious child rearing is far from established.

Although religious instruction of children may be benign or at least not noxious as a general factor, there are clearly toxic forms of religious influence. As Wagener and Malony (2006) noted, "for a minority, particularly those who are vulnerable owing to psychopathology, family or cultural disintegration, or trauma, their religious and spiritual development may become pathological, leading to harm to self or others" (p. 140). Psychologists should not accommodate toxic forms of religion or spirituality in their practice given the cardinal principle to do no harm. To make this distinction, a psychologist must be capable of identifying when religion and spirituality might be toxic and when they might be valuable. In Chapter 2 of this volume, I and Joshua Childers argue that psychologists can be capable of making such distinctions and provide further guidance for doing so. In Chapter 3, Mahoney, LeRoy, Kusner, Padgett, and Grimes provide further direction in differentiating between toxic and healthy forms of spirituality. They also present case studies demonstrating therapeutic responses to toxic forms of faith that avoid alienating clients practicing maladaptive forms of religion.

Because some forms of religion and spirituality can be psychologically harmful, it does not follow that psychologists should avoid any accommodation of this domain in clinical practice with children. The same basic problem arises with all major life domains. Social influences and occupational experiences, for instance, can be either benign or deleterious. This does not mean psychologists should avoid promoting healthy sociality or occupational adjustment (Hathaway, 2003).

Some psychologists may choose to ignore the religious and spiritual dimension of their clients' lives simply because they are either irreligious or agnostic and do not know what to make of religion. At best, they may suspect religion is a useful fiction or protective illusion. Consequently, such religion-dismissive psychologists may feel that ignoring the domain may at best cost the client some wishful thinking. In contrast, they may feel that entertaining religious and spiritual concerns may promote an illusory belief system. Whether this motivational pattern or another underlies clinical neglect of religious or spiritual issues in practice, the common result is being dismissive of a significant, if not the primary, orienting system in many of their clients' lives. Such a pattern of practice so hostile to a client's major diversity features would clearly be inconsistent with the aspirations outlined in the APA Ethics Code.

ETHICAL ROLES IN THE CLINICAL CHILD PSYCHOLOGY OF RELIGION

Ethical clinical child psychologists will be appropriately and competently accommodative of religious or spiritual concerns in practice. This justifies explicit and intentional engagement of client-valued religious or spiritual issues. It does not support therapist-imposed spiritual interventions that are alien to the client's worldview. The practice guideline committee for APA's Division 36 has identified five key treatment principles that have shaped its formulation of preliminary guidelines for clinical work with religious or spiritual issues (Hathaway, 2011). Table 1.1 summarizes examples of relevant applications to clinical child work with religious and spiritual issues. These treatment principles were primarily derived from reflections on the implications of the APA Ethics Code for practice in clinical psychology of religion. Their extension to clinical child psychology is straightforward and has been illustrated throughout this chapter.

As the Division 36 (Society for the Psychology of Spirituality and Religion) practice principles and the APA Ethics Code both indicate, one should practice within the bounds of competence. Although it is on the rise, formal training in the clinical psychology of religion has been relatively infrequent in APA-accredited internships (Russell & Yarhouse, 2006) and in APA-accredited doctoral programs (Brawer, Handal, Fabricatore, Roberts, & Wajda-Johnston,

TABLE 1.1
APA Division 36 (Society for the Psychology of Spirituality and Religion) Practice Guideline Principles

Principle	Example of application to clinical child practice
Awareness	Engage in self-exploration around his/her own religious and spiritual development and how this might impact one's work with children and/or families of the same or diverse religious/spiritual backgrounds.
Respect	Recognize and appropriately accommodate the religious issues and forms of life of children and their family.
Routine assessment focus	Make clinically relevant religious/spiritual assessment a standard part of clinical evaluation beginning with general probes and following up with more detailed assessment as needed.
Clinically congruent roles	All incorporations of religion/spirituality in practice must be done for clinically relevant reasons and in a manner congruent with one's professional roles.
Competence	Limit one's efforts at incorporating religious/spiritual practice into clinical child practice to one's range of competence/pursue additional training as needed to be sufficiently competent to accommodate likely religious/spiritual issues in one's treatment population.

Note. Adapted from *Spiritually Oriented Interventions for Counseling and Psychotherapy* (p. 74) by J. D. Aten, M. R. McMinn, and E. L. Worthington Jr. (Eds.), 2011, Washington, DC: American Psychological Association. Copyright 2011 by the American Psychological Association.

2002). Despite a mushrooming increase in training opportunities, it is still likely that most practicing clinical child psychologists will not have received any formal systematic training in the area. APA Ethics Code Standard 2.01 directs psychologists to practice within the parameters of their existing competencies. This does not mean, though, that psychologists should be content to remain relatively untrained in areas that are highly salient to their clients when relevant training becomes available. As APA Ethics Standard 2.03 notes, "Psychologists undertake ongoing efforts to develop and maintain their competence" (APA, 2010a, p. 5). The pursuit of competence in addressing religious and spiritual issues with children or teenagers in child practice reflects a pioneering and relatively uncultivated niche. The following case illustrates why it is time for clinicians to aspire to this outcome.

> Samuel was a friendly 9-year-old Jewish boy. He was brought into a child specialty clinic by his parents for an attention-deficit/hyperactivity disorder reassessment and consultation. He had been previously diagnosed with moderate to severe attention-deficit/hyperactivity disorder. The family had been taught behavioral management techniques for him, and

he had been placed on methylphenidate. He continued to be disruptive at school and home, was now a grade behind because he had failed subjects mostly because of uncompleted work, and had great difficulty in social settings because of his impulsive behaviors. Despite these challenges, the family went through the reevaluation as though it was a routine event, showing very little affect. Toward the end of the assessment, a simple probe was given. Was religion or spirituality a part of the family's life in any way? At that point, the parents paused, looking somewhat surprised, and then displayed the first visible signs of emotional distress they had shown during the entire evaluation. Samuel's father cleared his throat and then said simply, "We used to go to temple." The clinician followed up: "Can you tell me more about that and what led to the change in your participation?" The parents, now sitting up and leaning forward, proceeded to describe how they were both Jewish and that their religion was very important to them, but they had to stop attending temple because their son was too disruptive there. Now tearful, they explained that they had finally decided after a particularly bad day that they would have to wait until he was old enough for them to go without him. The clinician next asked, "Have you ever attempted to work on managing the behavioral problems arising at temple in treatment?" The parents looked surprised again and said no. It had never come up. They were never asked about their religious or spiritual concerns, nor did they think to volunteer them because "we didn't think we were supposed to talk about that with counselors."

Samuel's case is but one of several I have encountered in which clients have relayed a similar story. Mental health professionals have so neglected and distanced themselves from the religious and spiritual domain that even when such issues are among the most salient and distressing concerns facing clients, they will, I suspect, often not bring them up with professionals unprompted. This is an unfortunate situation that can be remedied if psychologists embrace the principles and standards of the APA Ethics Code as they apply to religious and spiritual issues with children, teens, and their families.

REFERENCES

American Psychiatric Association. (1989). *Guidelines regarding possible conflict between psychiatrists' religious commitments and psychiatric practice.* Washington, DC: Author.

American Psychological Association. (2010a). *Ethical principles of psychologists and code of conduct* (2002, amended June 1, 2010). Retrieved from http://www.apa.org/ethics/code/index.aspx

American Psychological Association. (2010b). Guidelines for child custody evaluations in family law proceedings. *American Psychologist, 65*, 863–867. doi:10.1037/a0021250

Aten, J. D., McMinn, M. R., & Worthington, E. L., Jr. (Eds.). (2011). *Spirituality oriented interventions for counseling and psychotherapy*. Washington, DC: American Psychological Association. doi:10.1037/12313-003

Bartoli, E. (2007). Religious and spiritual issues in psychotherapy practice: Training the trainer. *Psychotherapy: Theory, Research, Practice, Training, 44*, 54–65. doi:10.1037/0033-3204.44.1.54

Boyatzis, C. J. (2005). Religious and spiritual development in children. In R. F. Paloutzian & C. L. Park (Eds.), *Handbook of the psychology of religion & spirituality* (pp. 123–143). New York, NY: Guilford Press.

Boyatzis, C. J., Dollahite, D. C., & Marks, L. D. (2006). The family as a context for religious and spiritual development in children and youth. In E. C. Roehlkepartain, P. E. King, L. Wagener, & P. Benson (Eds.), *The handbook of spiritual development in childhood and adolescence* (pp. 297–309). Thousand Oaks, CA: Sage.

Brawer, P. A., Handal, P. J., Fabricatore, A. N., Roberts, R., & Wajda-Johnston, V. A. (2002). Training and education in religion/spirituality within APA-accredited clinical psychology programs. *Professional Psychology: Research and Practice, 33*, 203–206. doi:10.1037/0735-7028.33.2.203

Dawkins, R. (2006). *The God delusion*. Boston, MA: Houghton Mifflin.

Dennett, D. C. (2006). *Breaking the spell: Religion as a natural phenomenon*. New York, NY: Viking.

Ellis, A. (1970). The case against religion. *Mensa Bulletin, 38*, 5–6.

Harris, S. (2006). *Letter to a Christian nation*. New York, NY: Knopf.

Hathaway, W. L. (2003). Clinically significant religious impairment. *Mental Health, Religion & Culture, 6*, 113–129.

Hathaway, W. L. (2008). Clinical practice with religious/spiritual issues: Niche, proficiency or specialty. *Journal of Psychology and Theology, 36*, 16–25.

Hathaway, W. L. (2011). Ethical guidelines for using spiritually oriented interventions. In J. D. Aten, M. R. McMinn, & E. L. Worthington, Jr. (Eds.), *Spirituality oriented interventions for counseling and psychotherapy* (pp. 65–81). Washington, DC: American Psychological Association. doi:10.1037/12313-003

Hathaway, W. L., & Ripley, J. S. (2009). Ethical concerns around spirituality and religion in clinical practice. In J. D. Aten & M. M. Leach (Eds.), *Spirituality and the therapeutic process: A comprehensive resource from intake to termination* (pp. 25–52). Washington, DC: American Psychological Association. doi:10.1037/11853-002

Hitchens, C. (2007). *God is not great: How religion poisons everything*. Lebanon, IN: Hatchette.

Hood, R. W., Hill, P. C., & Spilka, B. (Eds.). (2009). *The psychology of religion: An empirical approach* (4th ed.). London, England: Guilford Press.

Kooistra, W., & Pargament, K. (1999). Religious doubting in parochial school adolescents. *Journal of Psychology and Theology, 27*, 33–42.

Mahoney, A., Pargament, K. I., Swank, A., & Tarakeshwar, N. (2001). Religion in the home in the 1980s and 1990s: A meta-analytic review and conceptual analysis of religion. *Journal of Family Psychology, 15*, 559–596. doi:10.1037/0893-3200.15.4.559

Mash, E. J., & Barkley, R. A. (Eds.). (2006). *Treatment of childhood disorders* (3rd ed.). New York, NY: Guilford Press.

McCullough, M. E., & Willoughby, B. L. B. (2009). Religion, self-regulation, and self-control: Associations, explanations, and implications. *Psychological Bulletin, 135*, 69–93. doi:10.1037/a0014213

McMinn, M. R., Aikins, D. C., & Lish, R. A. (2003). Basic and advanced competence in collaborating with clergy. *Professional Psychology: Research and Practice, 34*, 197–202. doi:10.1037/0735-7028.34.2.197

Moore-Thomas, C., & Day-Vines, N. L. (2008). Culturally competent counseling for religious and spiritual African American adolescents. *Professional School Counseling, 11*, 159–165. doi:10.5330/PSC.n.2010-11.159

Ollendick, T. H., & Schroeder, C. S. (Eds.). (2003). *Encyclopedia of clinical child and pediatric psychology*. New York, NY: Kluwer Academic. doi:10.1007/978-1-4615-0107-7

Rae, W. (2003a). Confidentiality and privilege. In T. H. Ollendick & C. S. Schroeder (Eds.), *Encyclopedia of clinical child and pediatric psychology* (pp. 132–134). New York, NY: Kluwer Academic.

Rae, W. (2003b). Ethical issues. In T. H. Ollendick & C. S. Schroeder (Eds.), *Encyclopedia of clinical child and pediatric psychology* (pp. 213–215). New York, NY: Kluwer Academic.

Richards, P. S., & Bergin, A. E. (2005). *A spiritual strategy for counseling and psychotherapy* (2nd ed.). Washington, DC: American Psychological Association. doi:10.1037/11214-000

Roehlkepartain, E. C., King, P. E., Wagener, L., & Benson, P. (Eds.). (2006). *The handbook of spiritual development in childhood and adolescence*. Thousand Oaks, CA: Sage.

Russell, S. R., & Yarhouse, M. A. (2006). Religion/spirituality within APA-accredited psychology predoctoral internships. *Professional Psychology: Research and Practice, 37*, 430–436. doi:10.1037/0735-7028.37.4.430

Sattler, J. M. (1998). *Clinical and forensic interviewing of children and families: Guidelines for the mental health, education, pediatric, and child maltreatment fields*. San Diego, CA: Jerome M. Sattler.

Starbuck, E. D. (1899). *The psychology of religion*. New York, NY: Scribner.

Stark, K. D., Sander, J., Hauser, M., Simpson, J., Schnoebelen, S., Glenn, R., & Molnar, J. (2006). Depressive disorders during childhood and adolescence. In E. J. Mash & R. A. Barkley (Eds.), *Treatment of childhood disorders* (3rd ed., pp. 336–407). New York, NY: Guilford Press.

Tan, S.-Y., & Johnson, W. B. (2005). Spiritually oriented cognitive behavioral therapy. In L. Sperry & E. Shafranske (Eds.), *Spiritually oriented psychotherapy* (pp. 77–103). Washington, DC: American Psychological Association. doi:10.1037/10886-004

Wagener, L., & Malony, H. N. (2006). Spiritual and religious pathology in children and adolescence. In E. C. Roehlkepartain, P. E. King, L. Wagener, & P. Benson (Eds.), *The handbook of spiritual development in childhood and adolescence* (pp. 137–149). Thousand Oaks, CA: Sage.

Witte, J., Jr., & Nichols, J. A. (2011). *Religion and the constitutional experiment* (3rd ed.). Boulder, CO: Westview Press.

Worthington, E., Jr., & Sandage, S. (2002). Religion and spirituality. In J. C. Norcross (Ed.), *Psychotherapy relationships that work: Therapist contributions and responsiveness to patients* (pp. 383–399). New York, NY: Oxford University.

2

ASSESSMENT OF RELIGIOUS AND SPIRITUAL ISSUES IN CLINICAL CHILD PSYCHOLOGY

WILLIAM L. HATHAWAY AND JOSHUA CHILDERS

The resurgence of the psychology of religion in the mid-20th century happened in large part because of the adoption of a measurement paradigm (Gorsuch, 1984). The development of paper-and-pencil scales, mostly self-report, that attempted to measure everything from vaguely defined global measures of religiousness to fine-grained parsings of various aspects of religious and spiritual functioning promulgated for decades was largely inspired by the productive contribution of Allport's (1950) intrinsic religious orientation research (Hill & Hood, 1999). Simultaneously, measurement and conceptualization efforts in the sociology of religion and the field of religious studies debated whether religiousness should be conceptualized as a unidimensional or multidimensional construct.

Despite the stimulation the measurement tradition has given to psychology of religion, there have been few areas in which knowledge has accumulated from the systematic use of the measures that have been developed,

DOI: 10.1037/13947-003
Spiritual Interventions in Child and Adolescent Psychotherapy, D. F. Walker and W. L. Hathaway (Editors)

in part because researchers tended to introduce new instruments to address niche questions rather than build on measures already introduced into the field. Psychology of religion and spirituality measures were rarely used; nor were clinical applications (Richards & Bergin, 2005). When researchers studied the relationship between religiousness and clinical variables such as depression or substance use, they tended to use simplistic measures of both variables. Although this generated some interesting data about the connection between religion and mental health, it rarely influenced the clinical assessment process itself (Hathaway, Scott, & Garver, 2004).

Still, the literature on the clinical assessment of religious and spiritual issues is growing, and some plausible suggestions can be made on the basis of standard assessment considerations that can help inform a more intentional assessment of the domain in clinical child practice. A committee from the American Psychological Association's Society for the Psychology of Religion and Spirituality (Division 36) has promulgated preliminary guidelines for the assessment of religious and spiritual issues in clinical practice (Hathaway & Ripley, 2009). These assessment guidelines can be found in Exhibit 2.1. A review of the guidelines shows that much of what they contain is a straightforward application of the professional ethical principles and multicultural considerations that are explored more fully in Chapter 1 of this volume. For instance, Guideline A-3 calls for psychologists to "routinely incorporate brief screening questions to assess for the presence of clinically salient religious/spiritual client concerns." Guidelines A-4 and A-5 indicate when more extensive assessment of religious or spiritual functioning is appropriate and for what purpose. Although the guidelines do not specify the form more extensive assessment should take, they do emphasize that such evaluation should be done with caution to avoid stereotypic judgments, insensitivity to individual differences, and a failure to understand religious or spiritual functioning in light of the client's religious or spiritual cultural norms.

In this chapter, we discuss ways to assess the relevance of children's spirituality to their presenting problems. We begin by reviewing previously published general guidelines for assessing client spirituality and religiousness. We then discuss developmentally sensitive assessment probes related to spirituality for use with children and teens. Afterward, we present assessment strategies for in-depth assessment of client spirituality and case conceptualization related to clients' presenting problems. Next, we discuss the Faith Situations Questionnaire (FSQ), an exemplar measure for assessing impairment in spiritual and religious functioning among children who have been diagnosed with attention-deficit/hyperactivity disorder (ADHD). We conclude with a case study illustrating the process of assessing functional impairment in spiritual functioning among children.

EXHIBIT 2.1
American Psychological Association Division 36 Preliminary Guidelines for Assessment of Religious and Spiritual Issues

A-1. Psychologists are mindful that religion/spirituality is a vital and important aspect of many clients' lives.

A-2. Psychologists are attentive to indications that clients have religious/spiritual concerns and take steps to convey to the client that expressing such concerns is appropriate if present.

A-3. Psychologists are encouraged to routinely incorporate brief screening questions to assess for the presence of clinically salient religious/spiritual client concerns.

A-4. The need for more extensive spiritual assessments is suggested when clients indicate that religious/spiritual factors are personally and clinically salient to their presenting concern.

A-5. Spiritual assessment is most helpful when aimed at gaining an understanding of the clinically relevant dimensions of the client's religious/spiritual life. Such assessment should be directed towards the following goals:
(a) determining how normative the client's religious/spiritual life is for the client's religious reference group;
(b) exploring whether clinical problems are adversely impacting religious/spiritual functioning; and
(c) evaluating how aspects of the client's religion/spirituality might constitute either constraints on treatment or productive resources for coping.

A-6. Psychologists are sensitive to biases that arise from religious/spiritual factors in the way in which clients complete psychological tests.

A-7. Psychologists are cautious to avoid interpreting client reports of attitudes or behaviors that are normative for a client's religious community as indicative of pathology.

A-8. Psychologists strive to be attentive to individual differences in religion/spirituality and avoid stereotypic inferences based on the client's identification with a spiritual tradition.

Note. Adapted from *Spirituality and the Therapeutic Process: A Comprehensive Resource From Intake to Termination* (pp. 46–49) by J. D. Aten and M. M. Leach (Eds.), 2009, Washington, DC: American Psychological Association. Copyright 2009 by the American Psychological Association.

GENERAL GUIDANCE

Let us first briefly survey the general guidance regarding assessment in the clinical psychology of religion and spirituality and then move on to consider how such assessment may be profitably used in clinical child practice. Several clinical psychologists of religion have recommended using general screening questions as a routine part of assessment (Hathaway et al., 2004; Richards & Bergin, 2005). For instance, Richards and Bergin (2005) stated that "a religious-spiritual assessment should be embedded in a multilevel, multisystemic assessment strategy" (p. 234). They explained that such a strategy requires two levels of assessment. In the first, general screening questions, such as whether the client believes in God or considers faith important, are asked as part of the general assessment along with inquiry into other standard domains (e.g., social, occupational, behavioral, physical). If the client answers yes to this generic ecumenical probe, designed to be broadly relevant to many faith traditions, then a more detailed assessment of the clinically relevant areas of the client's religious and spiritual functioning occurs.

What clinical reasons would psychologists and other mental health professionals have to engage in routine screening and assessment of client religious functioning? Richards and Bergin (2005) delineated several:

- enhanced clinician empathy for the client produced by better appreciation of the client's worldview;
- evaluating whether the client's religious and spiritual functioning might be having a protective or maladaptive impact on the presenting problem;
- determining whether the client's religiousness or spirituality could be a constructive resource to help the client "better cope, heal, and grow" (p. 221);
- determining whether and which spiritual interventions may be appropriately incorporated into the treatment; and
- identifying any spiritual struggles that should properly be addressed in therapy.

Pargament and Krumrei (2009) pointed out that "spiritual assessment should be grounded in a clear understanding of spirituality, including how it works, how it may be a part of clients' problems, and how it may be a part of their solutions" (p. 93). They recommended a framework for spiritual assessment that focuses on the role of spirituality for the client, the location of the client within his or her spiritual journey, a delineation of the content of the client's spirituality (i.e., what the client holds sacred, how the client expresses his or her spirituality), identifying the context of client spirituality, assessing its impact on functioning, and determining the appropriate place of spirituality in treatment.

The *Diagnostic and Statistical Manual of Mental Disorders* (4th ed.; *DSM–IV;* American Psychiatric Association, 1994) introduced the notion of a religious or spiritual problem V code to describe religious or spiritual struggles that could be a focus of treatment. Although this offered some ability within the influential psychiatric nosology for clinicians to identify a spiritual treatment focus, the V-code label encourages neglect of the spiritual domain by mainstream practitioners for at least two reasons. First, treatment for V-code diagnoses are not typically compensated by third-party payers. Second, because the V-code identifies the religious or spiritual problem as a separate focal point for treatment, clinicians who are not predisposed to find such a consideration clinically relevant may simply neglect religious or spiritual issues.

In contrast, Hathaway (2003) previously argued that religious and spiritual functioning is a significant adaptive domain that should routinely be assessed as part of a general assessment for all clients analogous to social or occupational functioning. Approximately half of the *DSM–IV* diagnoses require that a threshold level of symptoms must also evidence clinically significant impairment before a diagnosis of disorder is warranted. The *DSM–IV* does not delineate what constitutes such impairment in a definitive way but offers examples such as impaired social, occupational, or other adaptive functioning. Hathaway summarized the data on the adaptive implications of religious or spiritual functioning that support its inclusion among the major life domains that can be adversely affected by psychopathology. Because religious and spiritual functioning is still ubiquitous in human cultures and reported as salient by a majority of the population in many cultures, including those of North America, it follows that clinicians should routinely assess whether psychological difficulty adversely affects this domain.

Religious and spiritual functioning may be a contributor to the client's difficulties or a coping resource to help overcome them. Yet, it is also possible that depression or externalizing disorders may result in a clinically significant religious impairment. For example, clients who are depressed might report that they feel more distant from God and less motivated to engage in personally meaningful spiritual practices, such as prayer or reading sacred writings. For highly religious clients, such adverse impact on their spiritual functioning may be the most salient problem they report arising from their psychological difficulties. One of us (William L. Hathaway) has had clients report this to be the case while simultaneously acknowledging that concerns had gone unaddressed in prior psychological evaluations or treatments, often being quickly ignored or overlooked by the clinician when raised by the client.

DEVELOPMENTALLY APPROPRIATE SCREENING ASSESSMENTS AND PROBES

When religious and spiritual functioning are assessed in clinical practice, the most common assessment method is the clinical interview. Consistent with Richards and Bergin's (2005) Level 1 assessment recommendation, clinicians exploring the domain will typically ask probe questions using common religious concepts and phrases such as, "Do you believe in God?" or "Is your faith important to you?" Pargament and Krumrei's (2009) enjoinder to have a clear understanding of spirituality has an added significance when one considers assessment of religious or spiritual functioning with children and adolescents. The probe questions frequently used by clinicians to assess religiousness with adults may be ill suited to the psychologically relevant screening of child spiritual functioning.

A qualitative investigation of parent–adolescent conversations about religiousness found that both parents and teens reported more positive perception of conversations that were prompted by the youths than of those that were initiated by parents (Dollahite & Thatcher, 2008):

> Parents and adolescents reported that when religious conversation was focused on the adolescent child's needs and interests, the adolescents were engaged, interested, and enjoyed discussing religion. In contrast, when the conversations were tailored more to the parents' desires and needs, the adolescents were more likely to be disengaged and uninterested. (p. 625)

Examples of what the researchers called *parent-centered religious conversations* included parents talking too much about religion, parents engaging in unsolicited religious talk, and parents making religious demands of the child without explanation. It is plausible that these same features would characterize problematic explorations by a clinician of youths' religious and spiritual functioning in the context of treatment. Given the unpleasant nature of parent-centered religious conversations, it is perhaps fortunate that researchers have found most parent–child communications about religion to be more transactional or child centered (Boyatzis & Janicki, 2003; Dollahite & Thatcher, 2008).

As with the clinical assessment of any domain, the ideal engagement of a child client would be a reflective clarification of a theme or topic spontaneously introduced by the child. In some cases, this may occur. For example, elementary-school-age children have drawn pictures with religious content, such a deceased relative observing a family from a cloud that the child described as heaven or drawings of figures labeled as God, an angel, or a demon. In interviews, children will sometimes describe significant experiences or problems tied to a religious context, such as a spiritual experience at a religious summer camp or youth group or a problem arising within a spiritual situation.

One 16-year-old with conduct problems relayed the following story to Hathaway. He had stopped going to church by middle school but felt drawn back to his faith after some difficult life experiences, so he visited a local church in his community. The experience did not turn out quite as he expected because the minister attempted to forcibly cut his longer-than-usual hair. By this point, the teen was large enough to successfully fend off the minister's efforts, but the experience left him perplexed. He still wanted to reconnect to his earlier childhood faith but was not sure how to do this. In this case, this was perhaps more of a pastoral than a clinical issue. Yet, the attempt to reengage with religion represented this young person's desire to move his life in a more adaptive direction. A healthier religious environment would likely have been a potent resource in addressing his conduct issues. Because the teen brought up the experience and spiritual journey, encouraging the conversation and then reconnecting it back to the clinical focus would have been facilitative of a spiritually sensitive treatment strategy.

It is not uncommon for the child or adolescent client to be passive or resistant in a clinical session, particularly during the initial evaluation. In such cases, clinicians will often find it necessary to engage the youth to obtain information on virtually any domain, not just the youth's potential religious or spiritual issues. Barry and Pickard (2008) noted that the assessment of child clinical functioning is complicated by the tendency for diagnostic and clinical nomenclature to be tied to adult presentations. Although a growing body of developmentally appropriate assessment methods for children and teens is emerging, much work has to be done in this regard. It is often necessary to obtain critical diagnostic information from key informants for child clients, although the occasionally psychologically precocious young child may be quite competent in his or her own self-report.

A challenge arises in assessing child religious and spiritual functioning from key informant responses. Such discussions may be well suited for reports of the child's public religious behaviors such as frequency of church attendance, saying grace at meals, and apparent focus during religious service. However, there is some reason to think that these discussions may be unreliable as sources of information about private religious struggles facing youths, particularly those in preadolescence. Kooistra and Pargament (1999) found that religious doubt was reported as frequently first arising in preadolescence despite the fact that it was not typically expressed to others in this period. Summarizing data from 30 years of research on religious doubt, Puffer et al. (2008) noted that such religious doubt is associated with greater depression, stress, anxiety, and other problematic outcomes. It is predicted by harsh parental discipline, low religious commitment, and family environments with disengagement and low cohesion. Using an identity formation model, Puffer et al. differentiated healthy and unhealthy roles for doubt in the formation of child religious identity. It is plausible that problematic family environments may both provide direct impetus to painful spiritual struggles among children and fail to provide support for their constructive resolution. Consequently, a competent clinical probe of child and adolescent religious functioning will need to consider multiple sources of information and use clinical acumen in exploring underreported issues that may be relevant to the client's pattern of adjustment.

Exhibit 2.2 contains interview-based clinical probes William L. Hathaway has used to explore clinically relevant religious or spiritual issues with children

EXHIBIT 2.2
Interview Probes for Parents on Religious and Spiritual Functioning

Generic Family Religiousness Probes
Is faith or spirituality important for your family?
Are you active in a faith community?
Does religion play a role in your family life?
Are there any differences in your family on religious issues?

Child Probes Related to Early Childhood
Can you tell me about your Sunday school class?
Are there any questions you would like to ask God if you could?
What do you like best about going to . . . (church, temple, etc.)?
Is there anything you don't like about going to . . . (church, temple, etc.)?

Child Probes Related to Middle Childhood
Do you have many friends at your . . . (church, temple, etc.)?
Are there any things that are problems for you about . . . (church, temple, etc.)?
Can you describe anything you think God was trying to teach you?

Adolescent Probes
How important is God to you?
Do you feel as close to God now as you have in the past?
Do you have any doubts about your religious beliefs that have been a concern for you?
Have you made any decisions about God in your personal life?

or adolescents. The probes represent an attempt to engage this domain in developmentally sensitive ways. They are admittedly most appropriate for children raised in an Abrahamic faith tradition. Most of these probe questions are closed-ended. Although closed-ended questions can elicit a terse, one-word response (i.e., yes or no) from a client, they also function as icebreakers, making it clear that religious or spiritual topics are appropriate for discussion. They have resulted in spontaneous follow-up comments by clients regarding salient religious and spiritual issues. In several cases, clients had greater affect around religious and spiritual topics than around those they initially reported in the presenting problem description. Some clients who had been in lengthy courses of treatment were surprised to be addressing religious concerns because they did not think they were supposed to be addressed with a mental health professional despite the fact that they were direct sequelae of the clinical problem. For instance, parents have reported great distress over being alienated from their religious services because of their child's disruptive behavior arising from conduct problems or ADHD.

The list of probe questions is not intended to be comprehensive. As with any interview-based approach to assessment, useful probe questions often have to be adapted to the particular client with whom the psychotherapist is in dialogue and frequently make use of phrases or concepts drawn from client's own discourse. We typically obtain most background information regarding a child client from an interview of the parents or caregivers before the child interview. If religion is identified as a salient family variable in the parent interview on a probe question, we would try to briefly gather additional information about the religious identification, nature, and frequency of organized religious activities involving the child and whether there are presenting issues related to religion or spirituality. If religion and spirituality are not viewed as salient by the family, we would not typically make this a focus in the child interview. However, even in such cases we would remain attentive to religious or spiritual issues spontaneously reported by the child.

Because young children frequently have no influence over whether they are involved in organized religious activities, the probe questions we have used in early childhood have explored their experience of this involvement. Is it a positive thing for them? What do they like and dislike about it? Such questions often provide additional data about the child's social adjustment and family dynamics. In conflictual families, struggles related to behavior in a religious context are common. Parents often feel pressure to be on their best behavior in such settings and respond with elevated concern to child misbehavior, making faith situations a potential flashpoint for family tension. In middle childhood, social involvement at church continues to be a salient issue for children. Some families participate in religious organizations that have few children who are the same age as their children. Others are active in organizations in which many children who attend are also a part of the child's life in other contexts such as team sports, Cub Scouts, or school. In some cases, children will have a separate peer group in the religious setting than in other ones. These social network complexities can create competing peer influences or provide additional social resources for youths.

In early childhood, it is not uncommon for children to have specially tailored alternatives, such as children's church. By middle childhood, though, many children are expected to attend adult services with their parents and older siblings, which can present a heightened opportunity for conflict. One adult client with ADHD recounted some struggles with his faith and described what it was like for him growing up in his church. He said at first he enjoyed it, but when he was told he had to come to the regular service with his parents, the problems started. He became restless during the service, often shifting in his seat and flipping through the Bibles or hymnals in a noisy way. His parents decided to manage this by placing him between them in the pew with his father's arm resting on the back of the pew behind his head. If he started to get restless, his father would quietly but painfully thump the back of his head with a thumb. He quickly associated church services with pain, not just a possibly boring sermon.

Middle childhood is also a time when children may report personal religious experiences. Although they usually think of their own faith tradition in light of their family's faith, these individual faith experiences may start to give rise to a personal faith trajectory that can diverge from that of their family. By preadolescence, spiritual doubts are not uncommon (Kooistra & Pargament, 1999). These doubts may not signal a loss or weakening of faith but could reflect a shift from one set of beliefs to another type of religious or spiritual belief.

One of the earliest areas of research in the psychology of religion was the exploration of conversion experience. Starbuck (1899) studied religious development and found adolescence to be the modal age of religious conversion. This finding has remained relatively stable since, although not all religious traditions fit the religious conversion motif. In adolescence, it is not unusual for young people to reach religious decisions of various sorts. Adolescence is also a time of identity formation in spirituality and religion, just as it is other domains (Puffer et al., 2008). By later adolescence, clinical interviews may profitably engage the teen regarding more abstract religious notions such as, "Do you feel as close to God now as you have in the past?"

ADVANCED CLINICAL CHILD ASSESSMENT OF RELIGIOUS AND SPIRITUAL ISSUES

This section is titled somewhat insincerely because very few assessment tools have been developed that would allow for more than a cursory clinically relevant assessment of child religious or spiritual functioning. Various attempts have been made to use religious and spiritual assessment tools developed within the psychology of religion to assess religious or spiritual functioning with adults (Plante, 2009; Richards & Bergin, 2005). Plante (2009) summarized the potential relevance for clinical practice of the Brief Multidimensional Measure of Religiousness/Spirituality (Fetzer Institute, 1999), Santa Clara Strength of Religious Faith Questionnaire (Plante & Boccaccini, 1997), Duke University Religious Index (Koenig, Meador, & Parkerson, 1997), Religious Commitment Inventory—10 (Worthington et al., 2003), and the Religious Coping Inventory (Pargament, Koenig, & Perez, 2000). Yet these measures have not been developed with a child population in mind, and despite their usefulness for clinically relevant research, none of these measures have become widely used assessment tools in general clinical practice even for adults. Thus, two significant challenges are present with any attempt to deploy psychology of religion research measures for clinical use with children and adolescents. Such measures have rarely been constructed in a developmentally appropriate way for preadolescent respondents. Additionally, they have not been validated or designed for clinical use. As Richards and Bergin (2005) noted,

> Because most religious and spiritual measures have not been adequately validated in clinical situations, therapists should use them only after carefully examining them and personally verifying their suitability for their clients. Even then, therapists should interpret these measures tentatively. Normative data are so limited for most of these measures that sharing normative comparisons with clients should be avoided. At most, these measures should be used only to give therapists some tentative insights into their clients and perhaps as a tool to help clients engage in exploration and self-discovery. (p. 241)

What appropriate clinical functions would a more engaged assessment of religious and spiritual issues in a child population potentially serve? They can be an aid in diagnostic assessment, clinical formulation, treatment planning, and outcome assessment. For this domain of clinical assessment to reach its potential, clinical tools need to be developed and normed specifically with these purposes in mind. Such tools would be more likely to become commonly used in mainstream practice if they conformed with standard assessment tools, methods, and relevant constructs in specific clinical problem areas.

Diagnostic Assessment

If the argument is accepted that clinically significant religious impairment can fulfill the impairment criterion for disorders that require such impairment, then establishing that such impairment has occurred can be used as confirmatory evidence for a disorder (Hathaway, 2003). Similarly, some disorders may have symptoms that present as religious behaviors, cognitions, or experiences. It might be necessary to sort out whether religious content represents a delusional process or perhaps an unconventional or subcultural religious perspective that does not represent a disturbed thought process. Koenig (2011) noted that religious delusions are common among people with psychosis and are associated with problematic clinical outcomes. He summarized the earlier suggestions of Pierre (2001) regarding differentiation of normal and delusional or hallucinatory religious content. Is a delusional belief a reflection of conformity to a subculture that is collectively embracing a delusional belief structure? If so, it may not reflect a psychotic process per se but rather a conformity dynamic. Is there evidence that the apparently delusional belief arose in conjunction with neurological lesions that can produce such states (e.g., temporal lobe lesions)? How might religious professionals view such ideation, particularly those familiar with the client's faith background? How normative is the belief for the person's own faith convention? Does the religious belief impair the person's ability to function in normal life domains such as social or occupational functioning?

The importance of familiarity with the client's faith convention or of collaboration with helpful informants who are familiar with that faith convention is particularly important when religious ideation or practices are unfamiliar to a clinician or alien to his or her background. For instance, mental health professionals have frequently assumed that speaking in tongues (a spiritual practice frequently reported by Pentecostal Christians, among other faith traditions) is a sign of psychological disturbance. Yet research has not supported this link despite this widespread belief among professionals.

Clinical Formulation

Establishing a diagnosis is part of developing a clinical formulation, but articulating a formulation is a larger issue than merely establishing a diagnosis. It also involves a more comprehensive set of considerations, such as delineation of a hypothesized etiology, maintaining and mitigating factors, and a tailored prognosis (Eells, 2010). Mabe, Dell, and Josephson (2011) proposed a research agenda for the fifth edition of the *Diagnostic and Statistical Manual of Mental Disorders* engaging the role of religion and spirituality in specific areas of clinical concern on the basis of their review of research on religion and child mental health. They proposed wording changes to statements in the text revision of the *DSM–IV* (American Psychiatric Association, 2000) in sections on childhood disorders, conduct disorder, substance-related disorders, mood disorders, and culture-bound syndrome to guide this agenda with regard to children and adolescents. The wording additions are presented in Exhibit 2.3. The data suggest that personal, parental, and familial religion may be an important protective factor, coping resource, complication, or adjustment constraint in the etiology and maintenance of disorders that can manifest in childhood. As Mabe et al.'s proposals suggest, it is likely that religious and spiritual considerations should be a routine part of any clinical formulation when religion and spirituality are present in the child's background (Boyatzis, 2005; Boyatzis, Dollahite, & Marks, 2006).

Treatment Planning and Outcome Assessment

Maruish (2002) provided a concise description of the role and importance of assessment in establishment of treatment goals and monitoring of treatment progress. If a client reports a clinically significant impairment, it is natural to conclude that measurement of such impairment would allow the establishment of a clinically relevant spiritual treatment goal and an indicator to monitor treatment progress. Unfortunately, the relatively under-

EXHIBIT 2.3
Mabe, Dell, and Josephson's (2011) Proposed Child Spirituality Additions to the *Diagnostic and Statistical Manual of Mental Disorders* (4th ed., text rev.)

Ethnic and Cultural Consideration Section of Introduction
"In childhood and adolescence, culturally shaped parental expectations of child behavior are influenced by the spiritual perspectives of faith traditions and communicated through family relationships" (p. 138).

Disorders First Diagnosed in Infancy, Childhood, or Adolescence—Specific Culture, Age, and Gender Features
"This section also includes familial aspects of cultural significance (e.g., religious/spiritual) that place children at risk for, or protect from, disorder" (p. 138).

Conduct Disorder—Specific Culture, Age, and Gender Features
"The early onset of risk behaviors (e.g., sexual behavior, drinking, illegal substance use) are strongly affected by family spiritual precepts" (p. 138).

Substance-Related-Disorder—Specific Culture, Age, and Gender Features
"Parental and family influences moderate early adolescence substance abuse, and these influences are broad ranging (e.g., spiritual beliefs)" (p. 138).

Mood Disorder—Specific Culture, Age, and Gender Features
"The predisposition to Depression may be influenced by a specific aspect of culture, namely religious and spiritual context" (p. 139).

Glossary of Culture-Bound Syndromes
"Parent behavior and decisions regarding childrearing may be directly influenced and promoted by religion and spirituality" (p. 139).

developed nature of clinical tools for the assessment of religious and spiritual functioning would allow this to occur only in a crude or face-valid method such as having a person rate how close he or she feels to God on a 0–10 scale (analogous to the use of subjective units of distress) or tracking frequency of particular religious activities (e.g., church attendance, daily Bible reading, prayer). One religious assessment tool has been developed for the specific clinical purpose of treatment planning and outcome assessment with a child population. In the next section, we describe this instrument and its use with a clinical case to illustrate the potential for other such tools in this domain.

Faith Situations Questionnaire

The Faith Situations Questionnaire (FSQ) is a key informant rating scale that assesses 19 potential problem situations for children in Judeo-Christian religious and spiritual contexts, both in the home and in other settings. Hathaway, Douglas, and Grabowski (2003) presented clinical norms for an instrument for childhood behavior problems manifested in a religious or spiritual situation. The instrument is reprinted in Figure 2.1 and may be reproduced for clinical use. The FSQ was constructed to follow the structure and scoring of Barkley's (2005; Barkley & Edelbrock, 1987) Home and

FSQ

Child's Name: ____________________________ **Date FSQ Completed**: ____________________________

Child's Gender: ______Male ______Female **Child's Date of Birth**: ____________________________

Person Completing Form: _____Mother ______Father ______Step-Mother _____Step-Father

_____Other (Please specify: ______________________________)

Where do you attend religious services?: ____

How frequently does your child participate in religious services?

____More than once a week ____One time per week ____Two to three times per month

____One time per month ____One to two times per year ____ We don't attend

Instructions: Does your child present any problems with compliance to instructions, commands, or rules for you in any of these situations? If so, please circle the word Yes and then circle a number beside that situation that describes how severe the problem is for you. If your child is not a problem in a situation, circle No and go on to the next situation on the form.

Situations	Yes/No		If yes, how severe? Mild								Severe
During family devotions fsq1	Yes	No	1	2	3	4	5	6	7	8	9
While a blessing is being given at mealtime fsq2	Yes	No	1	2	3	4	5	6	7	8	9
When saying prayers fsq3	Yes	No	1	2	3	4	5	6	7	8	9
During personal devotion time, religious study or Bible reading fsq4	Yes	No	1	2	3	4	5	6	7	8	9
When preparing to go to a religious service fsq5	Yes	No	1	2	3	4	5	6	7	8	9
On the way to the service fsq6	Yes	No	1	2	3	4	5	6	7	8	9
While entering the service fsq7	Yes	No	1	2	3	4	5	6	7	8	9
During the seated portions of the service fsq8	Yes	No	1	2	3	4	5	6	7	8	9
When handling materials during the service (bulletin, hymnal, Siddur) fsq9	Yes	No	1	2	3	4	5	6	7	8	9
At quiet times during the service fsq10	Yes	No	1	2	3	4	5	6	7	8	9
During the offertory or communion fsq11	Yes	No	1	2	3	4	5	6	7	8	9

Figure 2.1. Faith Situations Questionnaire. This instrument may be copied for clinical use. From "Faith Situations Questionnaire: Childhood Normative Data," by W. L. Hathaway, D. Douglas, and K. Grabowski, 2003, *Journal of Psychology & Christianity, 22,* pp. 153–154. Copyright 2003 by the Christian Association for Psychological Studies. Reprinted with permission.

FSQ (Continued)

Situations	Yes/No		If yes, how severe? Mild								Severe
While the congregation is participating, such as through responsive readings or singing fsq12	Yes	No	1	2	3	4	5	6	7	8	9
During the sermon fsq13	Yes	No	1	2	3	4	5	6	7	8	9
While leaving worship for other activities fsq14	Yes	No	1	2	3	4	5	6	7	8	9
As the child is leaving the service fsq15	Yes	No	1	2	3	4	5	6	7	8	9
During the child's message fsq16	Yes	No	1	2	3	4	5	6	7	8	9
During a religious instruction class, such as Sunday school, catechism or Hebrew school fsq17	Yes	No	1	2	3	4	5	6	7	8	9
While participating in youth program recreational activities fsq18	Yes	No	1	2	3	4	5	6	7	8	9
During moral instruction fsq19	Yes	No	1	2	3	4	5	6	7	8	9
OTHER [Please write-in]											
______________________	Yes	No	1	2	3	4	5	6	7	8	9
______________________	Yes	No	1	2	3	4	5	6	7	8	9

Please write any comments which you wish to pass on about faith activities or situations which are a problem for your child:

Please do not write below this line

A: ________FSQ+ (Number of Yes Responses, FSQ1-FSQ19)

B: ________FSQT (Total of Severity Ratings, FSQ1-FSQ19)

Figure 2.1. (Continued)

School Situations Questionnaires (HSQ–SSQ). The HSQ and SSQ were designed to measure the prevalence and intensity of common behavioral problems arising from externalizing disorders such as ADHD that adversely affect children's self-regulation ability. FSQ raters, typically parents or custodians, are asked to rate whether each of the situations is a problem for the child. If rated as a problem, a follow-up rating of its severity is then requested using a 9-point Likert rating scale ranging from 1 (*mild*) to 9 (*severe*). Two scores are derived from the ratings: a total number of situations described as problematic and a mean severity score obtained by dividing the sum of the severity ratings for situations rated as problematic divided by the number of those situations. Additionally, individual item ratings can be explored ordinally for treatment planning purposes to strategically target the problem situations in order of severity.

The FSQ was normed on a sample of 249 children ranging in age from 5 to 12 years. The sample was stratified to mimic the relative percentage of Roman Catholics, high- and low-church Protestants, Pentecostals, and "other" in the U.S. population. An effort was also made to approximate the relative gender and race prevalence in the 2000 U.S. Census. The sample consisted of children who were rated in the normative study and was 51.8% female and 62.2% Caucasian, 29.7% African American, 3.6% Hispanic or Latino, 0.4% Native American, 2.0% other, and 2.0% with no ethnic identity reported. Thus, Hispanics and Native Americans were underrepresented in the sample. In terms of religious affiliation, 31.3% of the children rated were Roman Catholic; 6.4%, high-church Protestant; 34.9%, low-church Protestant; 18.1%, Pentecostal; and 8.8%, other; one respondent reported no affiliation (0.5%). Nearly three quarters of the ratings were completed by mothers, and approximately the same percentage of the children rated were from homes in which the parents are married.

The FSQ average severity rating score had a Cronbach's alpha of .92 in the normative sample. The FSQ mean severity and total problem scores were significantly correlated at a moderate level with inattention, hyperactivity, oppositional defiant behavior severity ratings on the Disruptive Behavior Rating Scale, and the total number of ADHD and oppositional defiant disorder (ODD) positive symptom ratings on this measure (i.e., rated as "often" displayed by the rated children). A hierarchical regression predicted *DSM–IV* disruptive behavior disorder symptom clusters from the HSQ and FSQ total problem scores. The FSQ was found to account for modest but significant unique variance from that accounted for by the HSQ alone in total ADHD, inattention, hyperactivity–impulsivity, and oppositional defiant symptom severity ratings. Eighteen children in the normative sample were rated as often or very often displaying six or more of both the inattentive and the hyperactive–impulsive symptoms of ADHD. A comparison of the ratings for these positive screening cases of ADHD with the ratings of the rest of the sample that did not reach the threshold level showed significantly higher total problem situations and mean problem severity on the FSQ for the ADHD-positive group. Fourteen children were reported to be on medication for ADHD in the pooled sample. These children were found to have higher problem mean severity but not higher total number of problems on the FSQ.

In terms of the most commonly acknowledged problematic situations by age,

> the four most frequently acknowledged faith problem situations in order were "During the seated portions of the service" (40.2%), "When preparing to go a religious service" (34.1%), "During the sermon" (33.3%) and "At quiet times during the service" (30.5%). The least frequently acknowledged problematic faith situation continued to be "During the child's message" (6.4%). (Hathaway et al., 2003, p. 146)

Consequently, the data from the normative validation of the FSQ support its reliability and validity as an assessment tool for behavioral difficulties in conventional Judeo–Christian religious settings. In terms of the disruptive behavior disorders, the FSQ could be useful for establishing yet another domain of clinically significant impairment arising from ADHD or ODD symptoms, for instance. Following a common clinical convention, we recommended a cutoff score of 5 to indicate clinical significance that is 1.5 standard deviations above the mean for the total normative sample. Cutoff scores could be used to identify problems that should be of particular clinical focus. These cutoffs are crude and represent one of Jacobson and Truax's (1991) proposed approaches to outcome assessment. At present, no test–retest reliability data are available for the FSQ. The addition of test–retest reliability data would allow the calculation of the reliable change index for the measure, another tool for outcome assessment in individual therapy cases in which a measure is given pretreatment and then at subsequent points during treatment (Jacobson & Truax, 1991; Wise, 2004). Derivation of a reliable change index would allow assessment of whether change occurs on a measure over the course of treatment that is less than what would be expected by chance in 5% of cases. Still, even as a crude outcome measure, the FSQ shows promise, as is reflected in the following case example from Childers (2005).

THE CASE OF TIMMY

As part of a dissertation project, Childers (2005) conducted a religiously accommodated form of parent training with a family using the FSQ as an assessment and outcome instrument. Timmy, a 9-year-old Caucasian boy, was brought to a campus training clinic by his parents for behavioral problems at home, school, and church. His parents complained that he was disruptive wherever they took him, talking constantly and doing things on impulse. During his preschool years, the family had given him the nickname Ricochet Rabbit because of his behavior. His parents stated that from a very early age, he would do impulsive things as though he lacked the ability to think ahead. They described situations such as the time as a preschooler when he cut the screen out of his bedroom window and threw his toys out seemingly just on impulse.

On rating scales and during a semistructured interview, Timmy's parents both rated him as frequently displaying all of the nine inattentive and all of the nine overactive–impulsive symptoms of ADHD. They also stated that he frequently displayed seven of the eight symptoms of ODD with the exception of frequently losing his temper. The overactive, inattentive, and impulsive behaviors had reportedly been present at a problematic level for Timmy since his earlier years. He would "talk incessantly," babbling even as a baby before he could make meaningful words.

At the time of the evaluation, Timmy resided with his biological mother and adoptive father. His mother's and biological father's relationship had been short and ended before he was born with no contact between him and the biological father. Timmy's mother and her husband were married when Timmy was 2 years old and have an 8-year-old son together. None of the presenting problems were described as an issue for his brother. The year before the evaluation, Timmy was adopted by his stepfather, who is referred to in the family simply as Timmy's father. Timmy was described as an extraverted child who makes friends quickly but has some trouble because of his immaturity and impulsivity in maintaining relationships. He likes to play sports but frequently has to run extra laps or face other discipline because of inappropriate behavior.

Timmy was enrolled in a private preschool for a few months before kindergarten but had numerous problems with aggression toward his peers, including pushing and biting them. In elementary school, he was described by his teachers as challenging and difficult to handle. It was not uncommon for his mother to get multiple calls a week from the school about his aggressive behavior or his disruptiveness in class because he could not sit still. His parents took him for a psychological evaluation at the end of kindergarten, and he was diagnosed with ADHD. However, they decided not to start psychological treatment or medication for him at that time because they wanted to see whether he would grow out of it. There were fewer complaints in first grade. His parents attributed this to a difference in teaching style, with a teacher more accepting of his impulsive behaviors. However, his third-grade teacher noted frequent problems. Consequently, his parents started him on Concerta before he entered fourth grade. At the time of the evaluation, Timmy was in the fourth grade, and the parents stated that they had not been contacted by the school with complaints about his behavior. His grades in school ranged from As to Cs, but he was enrolled in a remedial reading class for problems with reading comprehension.

Although Timmy's school behaviors improved after he was placed on Concerta, the family continued to have problems managing his behaviors at home and at church. The defiant and impulsive behaviors resulted in a constant battle, and his parents did not feel that any of the rewards or consequence-based programs they had tried to implement at home had worked. The family attended a Lutheran church. His mother described Timmy as "not having a conscience" before being placed on the medication because he never seemed to have guilt or remorse for his behavior even when he hurt other people. That had improved somewhat since the medication. Yet he often seemed to be spiritually stunted in comparison with his peers at church, being behind where they seemed to be in learning religious or moral concepts or adopting the values being taught by his faith community. Timmy had been removed from his Sunday school class and the church service on multiple occasions. Before Timmy began the medication, his mother had decided that she would stay home from church rather than bring Timmy if her husband was away for work and could not be there to provide support.

Timmy's family sought treatment for a reevaluation and to learn how to better manage his behaviors, particularly at home and at church. The evaluation corroborated the diagnosis of ADHD, combined type, and ODD. The threshold level of the symptoms of ADHD and ODD had clearly been present since his preschool years and were not better accounted for by other factors. Although the family history suggested some improvement with subsequent medication management, his ADHD and ODD symptoms continued to be of moderate severity.

Timmy's mother rated him as having problematic behavior in six situations on the FSQ, with a mean severity rating of 5 out of 9. This number of problematic situations was sufficient to exceed the recommended cutoff score on the FSQ, indicating that Timmy was displaying a clinically significant number of problems in his religious context. The situations rated as problems for Timmy are presented in Table 2.1. Timmy also displayed a significant level of problems on the HSQ. Ratings on both the HSQ and FSQ were used to inform treatment goals.

The treatment consisted of a 9-week parent training program for defiant children developed by Barkley (1997). The treatment provides psychoeducation about the causes of ADHD and ODD, age-appropriate behavioral management methods, and practical strategies aimed at interrupting and countering defiance cycles that perpetuate oppositional behavior. A major goal of the treatment is to give parents the skills they need to effectively adapt and continue to apply the principles in their child rearing after the treatment has ended.

The standard components of Barkley's (1997) model used in the treatment and each session were applied to the specific home- and church-based problem scenarios identified in the opening assessment. During the first,

TABLE 2.1
Faith Situations Questionnaire Results for Timmy

Problem situation	Evaluation	First session	Termination
During family devotions			2
When preparing to go to a religious service		3	2
On the way to service		2	
While entering the service	3	4	
During the seated portions of the service	6	4	
At quiet times during the seated portions	6	4	
While the congregation is participating in reading or seated		3	
During the sermon		2	
While leaving worship for other activities	5	2	
As the child is leaving the service		2	
During the child's message	5	2	
During Sunday school	5	3	
Number of problem situations	6	11	2
Mean severity	5	2.82	2

Note. Ratings are made on a 9-point scale ranging from 1 (*mild*) to 9 (*severe*). From *Preliminary Exploration of the Faith Situations Questionnaire as an Assessment Instrument,* by J. B. Childers, 2005, unpublished doctoral dissertation, Regent University, Virginia Beach, VA. Reprinted with permission.

fourth, and final sessions, his mother submitted another complete FSQ and HSQ to target changes in the number of problem situations Timmy was displaying as well as their severity. Ratings were also completed 1 month posttreatment. Table 2.1 shows the change in these ratings from the initial evaluation to posttreatment. Note that a greater number of problematic faith situations were noted for Timmy in the first treatment session than had been reported during the evaluation but that the average severity of the problems was rated as less. By the end of treatment, the number of problems dropped dramatically, and the mean severity lessened.

Each week, the principles covered in the program were applied to the specific common and recent problems Timmy was displaying. For instance, in Session 7, the parents were introduced to the "think aloud—think ahead" procedure for anticipating and then reducing misbehavior. By this point in the treatment, Timmy had been placed on a point system. The parents focused on applying the session's lesson to Timmy's disruptive behavior at church. His parents pulled him aside nonconspicuously before entering the church and clearly expressed to him the behavior that was expected in the church. They also provided him with an incentive if he displayed the correct behavior and a response cost for failing to do so. Finally, the parents problem solved an appropriate activity Timmy could engage in during the seated portion of the service that would be less likely to be disruptive than the sorts of things he usually did to occupy himself. This involved giving him some interactive children's materials that the church had available. This sort of targeted application of the parent training program to the specific faith and home situations relayed as problematic on the FSQ and HSQ ratings continued for the duration of the treatment.

CONCLUSION

There is already good reason to routinely screen for clinically relevant religious or spiritual issues in clinical child practice. However, much more work needs to be done to go beyond a cursory engagement with this domain to a more sophisticated clinical practice that fully engages scientific assessment procedures in all aspects of the evaluation process from formulation through treatment planning to outcome assessment. At present, a developmentally sensitive clinical interview will likely continue to be the primary tool for routine screening of religious or spiritual issues in child clients. However, tools such as the FSQ point to the possibility of a more advanced assessment of clinically relevant aspects of child religious and spiritual functioning. Such tools need to be developed by individuals with a combined clinical child practice competency and a psychology of religion competency.

The case of Timmy demonstrates the potential utility of a clinical measure of the religious or spiritual domain for both assessment and treatment planning. The FSQ data provided converging evidence of a significant impairment arising from Timmy's ADHD and ODD symptoms, a requirement indicated for the establishment of the diagnoses. The FSQ also provided a goal-setting tool for treatment planning that allowed for the setting of targeted and situationally delimited treatment objectives in a religious or spiritual context using standard and empirically supported treatment approaches. Finally, the FSQ data also allowed for outcome assessment throughout the process of religious and spiritual indicators in keeping with an evidence-based practice motif. Timmy's case indicates the potential value of developing other clinical tools for the clinical assessment of religion and spirituality in a manner congruent with standard assessment and treatment practices in specific clinical niches.

REFERENCES

Allport, G. W. (1950). *The individual and his religion*. New York, NY: Macmillan.

American Psychiatric Association. (1994). *Diagnostic and statistical manual of mental disorders* (4th ed.). Washington, DC: Author.

American Psychiatric Association. (2000). *Diagnostic and statistical manual of mental disorders* (4th ed., text rev.). Washington, DC: Author.

Barkley, R. A. (1997). *Defiant children: A clinician's manual for assessment and parent training* (2nd ed.). New York, NY: Guilford Press.

Barkley, R. A. (Ed.). (2005). *Attention-deficit hyperactivity disorder: A handbook for diagnosis and treatment* (3rd ed.). New York, NY: Guilford Press.

Barkley, R. A., & Edelbrock, C. (1987). Assessing situational variation in children's behavior problems: The Home and School Situations Questionnaires. In R. Prinz (Ed.), *Advances in behavioral assessment of children and families* (Vol. 3, pp. 157–175). Greenwich, CT: JAI Press.

Barry, C. T., & Pickard, J. D. (2008). Developmental issues. In M. Hersen & D. Reitman (Eds.), *Handbook of psychological assessment, case conceptualization, and treatment: Vol. 2. Children and adolescents* (pp. 76–101). Hoboken, NJ: Wiley.

Boyatzis, C. J. (2005). Religious and spiritual development in children. In R. F. Paloutzian & C. L. Park (Eds.), *Handbook of the psychology of religion & spirituality* (pp. 123–143). New York, NY: Guilford Press.

Boyatzis, C. J., Dollahite, D. C., & Marks, L. D. (2006). The family as a context for religious and spiritual development in children and youth. In E. C. Roehlkepartain, P. E. King, L. Wagener, & P. Benson (Eds.), *The handbook of spiritual development in childhood and adolescence* (pp. 297–309). Thousand Oaks, CA: Sage.

Boyatzis, C. J., & Janicki, D. L. (2003). Parent-adolescent communication about religion: Survey and diary data on unilateral transmission and bidirectional reciprocity styles. *Review of Religious Research, 44,* 252–270. doi:10.2307/3512386

Childers, J. B. (2005). *Preliminary exploration of the Faith Situations Questionnaire as an assessment instrument.* Unpublished doctoral dissertation, Regent University.

Dollahite, D. C., & Thatcher, J. Y. (2008). Talking about religion: How highly religious youth and parents discuss their faith. *Journal of Adolescent Research, 23,* 611–641. doi:10.1177/0743558408322141

Eells, T. D. (Ed.). (2010). *Handbook of psychotherapy case formulation* (2nd ed.). New York, NY: Guilford Press.

Fetzer Institute. (1999). *Multidimensional measure of religiousness/spirituality for use in health research: A report of the Fetzer Institute/National Institute on Aging Working Group.* Kalamazoo, MI: Author.

Gorsuch, R. L. (1984). Measurement: The boon and bane of investigating religion. *American Psychologist, 39,* 228–236. doi:10.1037/0003-066X.39.3.228

Hathaway, W. L. (2003). Clinically significant religious impairment. *Mental Health, Religion & Culture, 6,* 113–129.

Hathaway, W. L., Douglas, D., & Grabowski, K. (2003). Faith Situations Questionnaire: Childhood normative data. *Journal of Psychology and Christianity, 22,* 141–154.

Hathaway, W. L., & Ripley, J. S. (2009). Ethical concerns around spirituality and religion in clinical practice. In J. D. Aten & M. M. Leach (Eds.), *Spirituality and the therapeutic process: A comprehensive resource from intake to termination* (pp. 25–52). Washington, DC: American Psychological Association. doi:10.1037/11853-002

Hathaway, W. L., Scott, S. Y., & Garver, S. A. (2004). Assessing religious/spiritual functioning: A neglected domain in clinical practice? *Professional Psychology: Research and Practice, 35,* 97–104. doi:10.1037/0735-7028.35.1.97

Hill, P. C., & Hood, R. W. (1999). *Measures of religiosity.* Birmingham, AL: Religious Education Press.

Jacobson, N. S., & Truax, P. (1991). Clinical significance: A statistical approach to defining meaningful change in psychotherapy research. *Journal of Consulting and Clinical Psychology, 59,* 12–19. doi:10.1037/0022-006X.59.1.12

Koenig, H. G. (2011). Schizophrenia and other psychotic disorders. In J. R. Peteet, F. G. Lu, & W. E. Narrow (Eds.), *Religious and spiritual issues in psychiatric diagnosis: A research agenda for DSM–V* (pp. 31–51). Washington, DC: American Psychiatric Association.

Koenig, H. G., Meador, K., & Parkerson, G. (1997). Religion Index for Psychiatric Research: A 5-item measure for use in health outcome studies [Letter to the editor]. *American Journal of Psychiatry, 154,* 885–886.

Kooistra, W. P., & Pargament, K. I. (1999). Religious doubting in parochial school adolescents. *Journal of Psychology and Theology, 27,* 33–42.

Mabe, P. A., Dell, M. L., & Josephson, A. M. (2011). Spiritual and religious perspectives on child and adolescent psychopathology. In J. R. Peteet, F. G. Lu, & W. E. Narrow (Eds.), *Religious and spiritual issues in psychiatric diagnosis: A research agenda for DSM-5* (pp. 123–142). Washington, DC: American Psychiatric Association.

Maruish, M. E. (2002). *Essentials of treatment planning.* New York, NY: Wiley.

Pargament, K. I., Koenig, H. G., & Perez, L. (2000). The many methods of religious coping: Initial development and validation of the RCOPE. *Journal of Clinical Psychology, 56,* 519–543. doi:10.1002/(SICI)1097-4679(200004)56:4<519::AID-JCLP6>3.0.CO;2-1

Pargament, K. I., & Krumrei, E. J. (2009). Clinical assessment of clients' spirituality. In J. D. Aten & M. M. Leach (Eds.), *Spirituality and the therapeutic process: A comprehensive resource from intake to termination* (pp. 93–120). Washington, DC: American Psychological Association. doi:10.1037/11853-005

Pierre, J. M. (2001). Faith or delusion: At the crossroads of religion and psychosis. *Journal of Psychiatric Practice, 7,* 163–172. doi:10.1097/00131746-200105000-00004

Plante, T. G. (2009). *Spiritual practices in psychotherapy.* Washington, DC: American Psychological Association. doi:10.1037/11872-000

Plante, T. G., & Boccaccini, B. F. (1997). The Santa Clara Strength of Religious Faith Questionnaire. *Pastoral Psychology, 45,* 375–387. doi:10.1007/BF02230993

Puffer, K. A., Pence, K. G., Graverson, T. M., Wolfe, M., Pate, E., & Clegg, S. (2008). Religious doubt and identity formation: Salient predictors of adolescent religious doubt. *Journal of Psychology and Theology, 36,* 270–284.

Richards, P. S., & Bergin, A. E. (2005). *A spiritual strategy for counseling and psychotherapy* (2nd ed.). Washington, DC: American Psychological Association. doi:10.1037/11214-000

Starbuck, E. D. (1899). *The psychology of religion*. New York, NY: Scribner.

Wise, E. A. (2004). Methods for analyzing psychotherapy outcomes: A review of clinical significance, reliable change, and recommendations for future directions. *Journal of Personality Assessment, 82,* 50–59. doi:10.1207/s15327752jpa8201_10

Worthington, E. L., Jr., Wade, N. G., Hight, T. L., Ripley, J. S., McCullough, M. E., Berry, J. W., . . . O'Connor, L. (2003). The Religious Commitment Inventory—10: Development, refinement, and validation of a brief scale for research and counseling. *Journal of Counseling Psychology, 50,* 84–96. doi:10.1037/0022-0167.50.1.84

3

ADDRESSING PARENTAL SPIRITUALITY AS PART OF THE PROBLEM AND SOLUTION IN FAMILY PSYCHOTHERAPY

ANNETTE MAHONEY, MICHELLE LEROY, KATHERINE KUSNER, EMILY PADGETT, AND LISA GRIMES

> Foolishness is bound up in the heart of a child; the rod of correction will drive it far from him.
>
> —Proverbs 22:15
>
> Do not withhold correction from a child, for if you beat him with a rod, he will not die. You shall beat him with a rod, and deliver his soul from hell.
>
> —Proverbs 23:13–14, New King James Version

For years, critics of corporal punishment have pointed out that parents may lean on Bible passages such as these to justify harsh or physically abusive parenting (Dyslin & Thomsen, 2005). Yet parental spirituality encompasses more than isolated disciplinary beliefs or practices shored up by narrow interpretations of sacred scriptures. Broadly speaking, spirituality can be part of the problem or the solution when dysfunctional parenting occurs within families referred for psychotherapy. Moreover, numerous studies of non–clinic-referred families have shown that greater parental spirituality tends to predict better parenting in national or community samples of married heterosexual people and single mothers (Mahoney, 2010; Mahoney, Pargament, Swank, & Tarakeshwar, 2001). For example, greater importance of religion or spirituality in one's life and religious attendance correlate with greater maternal self-efficacy and positive parenting methods by single, adolescent mothers and with a lower risk of child maltreatment in low-income and minority families (e.g., Carothers, Borkowski, Lefever, & Whitman, 2005). Also, the more par-

DOI: 10.1037/13947-004
Spiritual Interventions in Child and Adolescent Psychotherapy, D. F. Walker and W. L. Hathaway (Editors)

ents attend religious services or say religion is personally important, the less often their adolescents and children display behavioral or emotional problems (e.g., Smith, 2005). Conversely, however, major conflict between parents regarding spiritual matters increases the risk of child adjustment problems (e.g., Bartkowski, Xu, & Levin, 2008), and religious clashes between parents and adolescents are tied to more distance and dissatisfaction in their relationship (e.g., Stokes & Regnerus, 2009). Yet serious intrafamilial disputes about religion are the exception, not the rule. Taken together, available studies have indicated that greater private and public engagement in religion tends to prevent problems in parenting from emerging. Thus, sensationalistic stories in the media about spiritual beliefs fueling child physical abuse obscure scientific evidence that greater religious involvement generally lowers the risk of poor parenting and family crises in the general population (Mahoney, 2010). Nevertheless, because psychotherapists work with clinically distressed families, they are likely to witness parental spirituality gone awry.

The aim of this chapter is to present a conceptual model that helps psychotherapists identify ways in which parental spirituality can reinforce maladaptive parenting as well as foster adaptive changes. Drawing on theory and research about relational spirituality, we focus on parents' relationships with God, family members, and faith communities as three relational contexts within which spirituality may shape parental goals (destinations) and methods (pathways) for better or worse. After we delineate our conceptual model, we illustrate the applicability of our ideas to clinical practice. Specifically, we offer case material and discussion on the following three topics: parental perfectionism and rigidity, religiously based physical maltreatment of children, and parent–adolescent conflict about sexuality and identity individuation. We close with comments about parental attributions about youth psychopathology and resistance to secular mental health interventions.

Before proceeding, we would like readers to know that we were unable to locate published, peer-reviewed studies on the negative or positive role that parental spirituality plays in the lives of families who seek psychotherapy (i.e., clinic-referred samples). Although we located resources to help address spirituality in family psychotherapy (e.g., Onedera, 2008; Walsh, 1999; Weaver, Revilla, & Koenig, 2002), parenting workshops (Howard et al., 2007), family therapy training programs (e.g., Patterson, Hayworth, Turner, & Raskin, 2000), and psychosocial treatments for children with chronic physical illnesses (e.g., Cotton, Yi, & Weekes, in press), we were unable to locate controlled treatment outcome studies on the efficacy or effectiveness of integrating parental spirituality into family-focused psychotherapy, such as incorporating spirituality into parent training programs. Therefore, much of this chapter is based on theory and clinical anecdotal evidence that needs to be empirically tested with clinically distressed samples of families.

Another important caveat is that more than 90% of peer-reviewed studies on faith and family life in the past 30 years involve families from the United States (Mahoney, 2010; Mahoney et al., 2001). Thus, findings speak primarily to Christians from varying denominations because relatively few U.S. families belong to other religious traditions. Here, for example, are percentages of religious affiliation based on a nationally representative sample of adolescents: 75% endorsed a Christian affiliation (52% Protestant, 23% Catholic), 16% reported no religious affiliation, 7% were affiliated with one of the many minority U.S. religions, particularly the Latter-day Saints (2.5%) and Judaism (1.5%), and 2% did not know or disclose an affiliation (Smith, 2005). Although our heuristic model is intended to generalize across families from different religious traditions, the case examples we later use to illustrate our model depict parents with varying Christian backgrounds because these families reflect whom U.S. psychotherapists, such as us, are mostly likely to see. We hope our chapter encourages more research on parental spirituality within families from diverse religious backgrounds who are referred for psychotherapy because of dysfunctional parenting.

OVERVIEW OF THE RELATIONAL SPIRITUALITY FRAMEWORK AND PARENTAL SPIRITUALITY

Key Elements of the Relational Spirituality Framework

Consistent with world religions having developed rituals and doctrines surrounding significant family events from birth to death (Onedera, 2008), scientific studies on faith and family life have covered a wide range of family experiences, such as childbearing, mate selection, parenting strategies, and domestic violence. Mahoney (2010) developed a framework called *relational spirituality* to organize these diverse topics into three general stages of family relationships: (a) discovery—forming and structuring family relationships, (b) maintenance—engaging in processes to sustain family relationships, and (c) transformation—experiencing family difficulties that call for radical change in the structure or processes of family relationships. Within this framework, *spirituality* is defined as the "search for the sacred," a definition that encompasses the discovery, maintenance, and transformation in individuals' approach to the sacred over the life span (see Pargament, 2007; and Pargament & Mahoney, 2009, for elaboration). Thus, the relational spirituality framework emphasizes that people's searches for intimate relationships and for the sacred often overlap, and both pursuits often occur within the context of larger established religious institutions; notably, no other social organization besides religion promotes spirituality as a central goal. Mahoney's relational spirituality framework unpacks the multifaceted interface between spirituality and the three major stages of family relationships by highlighting unique, specific psychospiritual factors that could undermine or enhance relationships in both traditional and nontraditional families.

For the purposes of this chapter, Mahoney's (2010) relational spirituality framework illuminates three key issues for psychotherapists to recognize. First, within and across religious groups, the formation of a nuclear or extended family consisting of married heterosexual individuals with biological children is uniformly upheld as a spiritually desirable goal, whereas conflicting theological stances exist about the morality of other family structures (Mahoney & Krumrei, in press). For instance, parents and adolescents may disagree about whether a same-sex marriage and the adoption or birth of children by single adults or cohabiting couples of any sexual orientation should be spiritually condoned as valid destinations for family life.

A second issue is that spiritually based conflicts about whether people should form nontraditional family bonds make it easy to lose sight of the fact that diverse religious groups agree about the virtues that people should exhibit to maintain the traditional or nontraditional family relationships they do create. For example, widespread theological consensus exists on the spiritual goals of family members giving and receiving love, commitment, sacrifice, honesty, fairness, and forgiveness to and from one another. Ideally, spirituality can inspire parents to display these virtues, although some manifestations of faith may reinforce maladaptive parenting methods. Third, family problems can occur that call for the transformation of the structure or processes underlying family relationships. To date, however, scarce empirical research exists on how spirituality operates within clinic-referred families in which, from the perspective of psychotherapists, parents need to make fundamental changes in their goals and methods of parenting. We elaborate on this latter topic.

Mahoney's (2010) relational spirituality framework also delineates three relational contexts in which psychotherapists can explore ways that spirituality may play positive and negative roles in parenting: relationships with God, family members, and faith communities. In our model for working with spirituality as part of family psychotherapy, we discuss each context separately, and we highlight specific spiritual beliefs or practices that could either reinforce maladaptive parenting or, conversely, motivate parents to change for the better.

Focus on the Transformation of Problematic Parental Destinations and Pathways

Because of the virtual absence of controlled research on specific spiritual beliefs or practices about parenting in clinic-referred families, our heuristic model for working with distressed families draws on extensive literature about individuals turning to spirituality to cope in times of trouble. Specifically, Pargament (1997, 2007) theorized that individuals proactively identify and pursue destinations in life that they appraise as significant. Parents, for example, may strive for certain child-rearing destinations, such as their children being obedient or emotionally close to their parents. Pargament's framework also emphasizes that individuals travel down diverse pathways to reach desired goals. Parents, for instance, may rely on positive or punitive methods of discipline to gain child compliance. Finally, Pargament's model of integrating spirituality into individual psychotherapy emphasizes ways in which spirituality can be part of the problem when dysfunction is evident in the goals or methods that clients pursue and, alternatively, part of the solution when transformation is needed. Similarly, the major focus in our model is for family psychotherapists to consider ways in which spirituality can shape, for better or for worse, the goals that parents believe should be sought in family life and the methods they use to reach their objectives (Mahoney, 2005). We suggest that conflict between parents and their children can be amplified or inhibited on the basis of the extent to which family members disagree or agree regarding spiritual guidelines for the destinations or pathways of parenting. Next, we delineate ways in which parental spirituality may reinforce problematic parental goals and methods or spur change in both dimensions of parenting. Consistent with Mahoney's (2010) relational spirituality framework, we divide our discussion into ways in which parents may draw on a relationship with God, the spiritual nature of a family relationship, and relationships with religious communities to shape their parenting destinations or pathways.

ASSESSING WAYS IN WHICH PARENTAL SPIRITUALITY MAY BE PART OF THE PROBLEM

We now lay out guidelines for assessing various ways in which parental spirituality may be part of the problem for clinic-referred parents, followed by an overview of intervention steps. We then offer three sets of case material to illustrate our approach to intervention more concretely.

Screening for the Relevance of Parental Spirituality

Consistent with Richards and Bergin's (2005) recommendations that psychotherapists routinely screen for the relevance of religion and spirituality with individual clients and then follow up with more detailed questions as needed, we suggest that family psychotherapists habitually open up the topic of spirituality in initial sessions with parents. Hodge (in press) consolidated the following four screening items from work published by leading scientist–practitioners in the psychology of religion and spirituality for therapists to use. The items assess, respectively, the overall importance, affiliation, resources, and problematic role of spirituality:

1. I am wondering how important spirituality or religion is to you.
2. Do you happen to attend religious services in a church or some other type of religious or spiritual community?
3. Are there certain spiritual or religious beliefs and practices that you find particularly helpful in dealing with difficulties?
4. I am wondering whether your present problem has affected you spiritually or religiously.

When parents' responses indicate that spirituality is relevant to their lives, psychotherapists can then assess specific ways in which spirituality may be part of the problem or the solution in parenting.

Assessing Problems in Parenting Across the Three Contexts of Relational Spirituality

Problems in the Parent's Relationship With God or the Divine

In our model, parents' felt connection to God is one spiritual context that may shape their goals and methods of parenting. Research spurred by Baumrind's (1967) widely cited model of parenting styles, along with Maccoby and Martin's (1983) expansion of Baumrind's work, highlights two major parenting goals for psychotherapists to explore: control and warmth or closeness. With regard to parental control, parents may believe that God intends for them to elicit child obedience and conformity to social norms. With regard to warmth, parents may believe that God intends for them to love their children unconditionally and to form close, affectionate bonds that nurture their children's unique individuality. Obviously, these two goals are not mutually exclusive. Specifically, authoritative parenting that involves both ample control and warmth appears to be an optimal parenting style, at least among European American families (Demo & Cox, 2000). Moreover, although conservative Christians are more prone than people affiliated with other groups to say that they value child conformity more, wide variability exists within and across religious groups about this parental goal (Starks & Robinson, 2007). Thus, psychotherapists need to ask directly about the importance that parents place on the goals of achieving control over and closeness to their child. The second key question for psychotherapists to explore is whether parents believe that their connection to God requires that they follow certain pathways to achieve their parenting goals. Parents may embrace a wide range of specific parenting methods to reach their goals that vary in effectiveness in the short and long term.

Parental spirituality can be problematic if parents believe that they must pursue destinations or pathways that intensify negative parenting to have a satisfactory connection with God. With regard to goals, parents may believe that they would violate God's intentions if they abandoned the goal of socializing their children to conform to certain social norms, and they may therefore hold onto excessively high or rigid expectations. Alternatively, some parents may believe that God's highest priority is for their children to feel unconditionally accepted. Thus, parents may avoid or feel ambivalent about upholding high or conventional expectations for their children's performance in or out of the home. With regard to pathways, parents may adopt methods to achieve parenting goals that are counterproductive because they fear disappointing God. Take, for example, the mother of an 8-year-old who discloses in an anxious, guilt-ridden manner, "I know that I should spank my child more often," and then explains that she feels as though she is letting God down by being too lax with discipline. In short, parents may implicitly or explicitly believe that God sanctions certain parenting styles. To change either their parenting goals or methods, parents may risk feeling distant, abandoned, judged negatively, or rejected by God because they are contradicting God's preferences.

Problems in the Spirituality of the Parent–Child Relationship

A second context in our model pertains to family relationships possessing spiritual properties because of the beliefs or behaviors of family members. Cognitively, people often perceive marriage and parenting to be a manifestation of a higher power or imbued with sacred qualities (Mahoney, Pargament, & Hernandez, in press). Behaviorally, family members may engage in shared spiritual rituals or in-depth dialogues about sacred matters that endow the relationship with sacred meaning and deepen their personal sense of spirituality. Even parents who do not feel a strong personal relationship with God or are not heavily involved in organized religious activities may strive to create family relationships that they view as reflective of the presence of a higher power, characterized by sacred qualities (e.g., transcendence, boundlessness, ultimate importance) or marked by spiritual activities. Thus, a major goal of parenting could be to create parent–child relationships that possess a spiritual dimension. Parents may also pursue a wide variety of pathways to preserve and protect the spiritual nature of their parent–child relationships. For example, research has suggested that parents who view parenting as a sacred endeavor may be more motivated to spend time with their children, prioritize parenting over other demanding life tasks, and invest the necessary energy into effective discipline strategies and bonding activities (Mahoney, 2010).

Psychotherapists can explore problems that emerge if parents perceive family difficulties as threatening the spiritual nature of the parent–child bond. Emerging research on the concepts of sacred loss and desecration has suggested that people frequently perceive negative life events (e.g., severe illnesses, divorce) as involving the loss or injury of a sacred aspect of life (e.g., Abu-Raiya, Pargament, Mahoney, & Trevino, 2011). This line of work also indicates that the more people interpret life stressors as damaging to a sacred object, the more emotional distress they experience about the event. People also tend to feel more hostility toward those they hold responsible for harming sacred elements of their lives. Parents could likewise interpret family problems, such as chronic parent–child conflict or child misbehavior, as threatening or violating the existence of a sacred parent–child relationship, and they may react strongly to events that they feel threaten their spiritual oversight of their child's life. One example would be parents who believe that their preschooler's lying is damaging the parents' ability to trust the child, which in turn violates beliefs the parents hold (perhaps implicitly) about how sacred parent–child relationships should function. Paradoxically, parents' heightened anger or fear about events that threaten their divine connection with their child may make them act in irrational or emotional ways that drive a deeper wedge into the relationship. In particular, parents may pull God or spiritual communities into parent–child conflicts in ways that exacerbate tension or distance.

Parents may be more open to corrective education about family dynamics and child development if psychotherapists fully recognize and address, rather than dismiss or minimize, the parents' perception that their children's conduct has grave spiritual implications for the parents' ultimate goals as parents. The psychotherapist can then work to help the parents find alternative routes to reach their desired goals with less resistance from the parents. A father, for example, may overreact to his teenage son's desire for privacy regarding his romantic relationships. In exploring the father's spiritual concerns about this situation, a psychotherapist may discover the father wants to ensure that his son grasps the spiritual significance of fatherhood. Accurately identifying this goal may foster a stronger therapeutic alliance so the father is more receptive to the psychotherapist's input about constructive methods to discuss sexuality with the son.

Problems in the Parent's Relationship With the Spiritual Community

The third context in our model addresses parents' relationships with a faith community. Although higher involvement in a religious community tends to be linked to more positive parenting methods, under certain circumstances spiritual networks may intensify negative manifestations of parental spirituality. A spiritual community may reinforce problematic beliefs or behaviors about the goals a parent pursues to fulfill God's mandates or the methods a parent uses to sustain a sacred bond with a child. For example, a parent may turn to fellow believers for validation that God requires excessively harsh parenting to achieve the goal of child compliance. Also, a spiritual community could intensify parental distress when a parent perceives that he or she will risk rejection by the community by choosing parenting destinations or pathways that clash with those advocated by the faith community. Such struggles with a religious network may trigger confusion or ambivalence about relying on secular resources. For instance, conservative Christian parents who are struggling with their son's disclosure that he is gay may fear being shunned by their church community, which complicates their exploration of alternative viewpoints about human sexuality and whether to accept their child's sexual orientation.

INTERVENING WHEN PARENTAL SPIRITUALITY MAY BE PART OF THE PROBLEM OR SOLUTION

Clarifying the Psychotherapist's Role

The American Psychological Association's (APA's; 2010) "Ethical Principles of Psychologists and Code of Conduct" (APA Ethics Code) states that psychotherapists must attend to cultural barriers and resources in treatment interventions with clients, including their spiritual identities. We highlight here the duty of practitioners to communicate in a transparent manner with clients about their approach toward spirituality in psychotherapy. We assume that psychotherapists can simultaneously present themselves as experts on how parents could respond differently when they or their children exhibit maladaptive functioning while respecting parents' spiritual values. Namely, psychotherapists can engage in collaborative dialogues with parents that elicit parental disclosure about ways in which their spirituality shapes their cognitions and behaviors and can exhibit compassion for the spiritual dilemmas that parents face when selecting from competing parenting goals and methods. Yet, psychotherapists can offer parents scientifically grounded knowledge about effective ways to handle family problems and explore with parents the ways in which spirituality can inhibit or facilitate change. In a parallel way, we suggest that parents can learn to engage in spiritual dialogues with clinic-referred youths in a manner that respects parental authority while also promoting age-appropriate maturity. Ideally, the way a psychotherapist communicates with parents about spiritual matters will provide a powerful model for constructive spiritual and nonspiritual dialogues between family members. Our last case example illustrates this point.

Psychotherapists also need to communicate clearly about their stance on parents' broader cultural networks. Consistent with the APA Ethics Code, we encourage clinicians to inquire about family members' specific spiritual beliefs, practices, and values and to avoid making stereotypical assumptions based on denominational membership. We note that convergence often exists between changes that parents need to make and the values heralded by their spiritual communities. Thus, parents' allegiance to their faith community may often help motivate them to change for the better. Yet psychotherapists need to consider how they will respond if they observe a poor goodness of fit between changes the parents need to make and the values promoted by a particular faith tradition or community. Our case studies illustrate our preference to be direct with parents when we observe such discrepancies. Psychotherapists should also model good communication skills by effectively expressing their professional opinions and observations to parents while respecting parental autonomy. Again, in the context of family psychotherapy, such modeling can help teach family members who disagree about parental goals or processes how to negotiate collaboratively with each other.

Generating Parental Insight and Action

Once a psychotherapist notes that spirituality plays a significant role in shaping a parent's goals or methods, the first intervention task is to help all parties gain more insight about these issues. Of course, although we differentiate the process of assessment from that of intervention in our heuristic model, we recognize that ideal moments for a psychotherapist to increase parental insight can involve follow-up questions regarding parents' disclosures to queries at any stage of psychotherapy. An initial objective is to explore and identify with parents the distinction between their desired goals and methods of parenting. The next step is to examine how well a parent's stated destinations and pathways fit with the parents' relationship with God, reflect their views of the spiritual nature of their coparenting or parent–child relationship, and map onto messages from their spiritual community. To help parents gain insight into problematic parental ends or means, psychotherapists can provide education based on research regarding child development, parenting, and family dynamics. Taking a motivational interviewing stance (Miller & Rollnick, 2002), psychotherapists can help parents identify and articulate the short- and long-term costs and benefits of persisting in or changing their current goals or methods of parenting.

A second requirement for intervention is to clarify the ultimate goal of psychotherapy. The therapeutic process described earlier should help bring to light a clear focus for a treatment plan and engage parents as informed, active agents in the process. Our model highlights three key options for a psychotherapist to consider when negotiating the focus of treatment:

1. Accept part or all of a parent's desired goals in parenting, and focus on a parent's parenting methods as the problem that requires change;
2. accept part or all of a parent's preferred parenting methods, and focus on a parent's goals as the problem that requires change; or
3. challenge a parent to transform both desired parenting goals and methods.

We suggest that parents may be more open to change after a psychotherapist uncovers their spiritually based goals and identifies constructive means to reach their desired ends, while simultaneously addressing the developmental and psychological suitability of their selected destinations and pathways. When two or more parent figures attend psychotherapy, this dialogue can also help uncover disagreements between all primary caregivers. If irreconcilable differences emerge between the psychotherapist's and parents' opinions about appropriate treatment goals, we interpret the APA Ethics Code as encouraging the psychotherapist to refer the family to another mental health professional who may better accommodate the parents' values. Before making a referral, the psychotherapist should use clinical judgment and consultation with colleagues to decide how confrontational to be with parents about actions that violate widespread ethical norms, such as emotionally alienating a child from a coparent by portraying the coparent as being under the influence of the demonic forces. Of course, if the issues at hand involve protecting one or more family members from suspected risk of abuse or lethal harm (e.g., suicidal or homicidal threats or behavior), then the psychotherapist is also obliged to involve legal authorities.

Assuming a psychotherapist and parent mutually establish a focus for change, the psychotherapist can then work with the parent to rework the counterproductive roles played by his or her relationship with God, the sacred nature of the parent–child relationship, or the spiritual community and to identify resources within these three contexts that could be drawn on to help a parent pursue alternative goals or processes. In some cases, spirituality may not play a large role in reinforcing maladaptive parenting goals or processes, but it may still offer resources for change. However, for the purpose of this chapter, we focus on case examples in which spirituality is both part of the problem and part of the solution.

THREE CASE ILLUSTRATIONS OF INTERVENTION

We now turn to three issues that psychotherapists may encounter to illustrate our family psychotherapy guidelines more concretely. To provide a developmental dimension to our discussion, the first two topics focus on families with young children, and the next topic involves those with adolescents. Although all facets of our framework could apply to each issue, we emphasize one or two facets per topic owing to space constraints. We begin each section by presenting a case example and outlining related findings drawn from basic research.

Parental Perfectionism and Rigidity

> A 30-year-old mother, Mary, sought family psychotherapy to cope with her 6-year-old son, Matt, along with his 4-year-old brother, Sam. Two years earlier, she and her husband, John, ended their marriage of 8 years after John (age 32), a pharmacist, was sentenced to a 3-year prison term for selling prescription drugs on the black market. The couple had met at a Christian university in the Midwest and had been actively involved in a nondenominational church throughout their marriage. Mary explained that Matt had been a model toddler and preschooler and had seemed to weather the family's crisis well until recently. After entering first grade, he seemed to slip. Specifically, Mary noted that the teacher said that Matt sometimes cried when frustrated by schoolwork or when teased by peers. Mary was also alarmed by Matt's anger when Sam took Matt's toys without permission and by Matt's reluctance to do homework immediately after school, as was their custom. During the initial interview, Mary frequently reprimanded Matt for swinging his legs and failing to answer questions quickly. She would also not allow him to hold a stress ball or handle other small toys that the psychotherapist typically placed within children's reach to help them relax during sessions. According to the Child Behavior Checklist (Achenbach & Rescorla, 2001), Matt's teacher's ratings of his externalizing problems were within normal range, but Mary's ratings on these scales were elevated. On further assessment, the psychotherapist realized that Mary's threshold for child misbehavior was very low. Mary also disclosed being anxious to raise her sons so that they did not turn out to be deceptive or antisocial like their father. Thus, she had very strict rules and enforced them rigorously. She felt rejected by Matt because of his anger over her expectations.

Taken together, the results of the assessments showed that Mary exhibited excessive parental perfectionism and rigidity. We were unable to locate studies that have directly examined ties between parental perfectionism and spirituality. Yet findings that adolescents who are more religious and who have more religiously active parents tend to get better grades, be more prosocial, and engage less often in sexually risky or antisocial behavior (Smith, 2005) have suggested that more religious parents tend to have higher expectations of children from birth onward. Moreover, the more parents from a broad array of Christian denominations hold orthodox Christian beliefs about the Bible, God's role in their lives, and the authority of their religious community, the more they value child obedience (Starks & Robinson, 2007). Ironically, however, higher spiritually based standards for children's conduct may cause some parents to lose perspective on their expectations.

On the basis of initial screening questions, Mary's spiritual life and community had been a source of support to her, and she had relied heavily on her prayer life to cope with the family's crises. Thus, the psychotherapist first worked to increase Mary's insight about the role that spirituality played in her parenting goals and methods. When asked what God expected of her as a parent, she replied, "I need to make sure they know how to behave and do not turn out like John!" She viewed her children's compliance with a high moral code as her major goal as a mother. When asked about ways in which she relied on God to achieve this goal, Mary replied that God expected her to curb any sign that Matt was developing an irresponsible streak, and she prayed for help to follow through on strict disciplinary tactics and tolerate Matt's sulking when he was given consequences. When asked what parenting weaknesses God wanted to help her overcome, Mary anxiously replied that she had often caved in to pressure from her ex-husband to relax her moral standards to win his approval. She was now determined to resist caving in to Matt to win his affection. On the basis of further questions about God's views on her marriage, Mary explained that she felt she had disappointed God by having premarital sex with John and that she had reconciled herself to this decision by marrying him. John's ability to cut loose had especially attracted Mary to him, and he had helped her be more playful, but she now felt as though she and her children were paying a high price for the couple's pleasure. In short, Mary had two core problematic spiritual beliefs about her parenting: (a) God's desired goal for her was to produce perfect children to help rectify the past, and (b) God supported counterproductive parenting tactics to elicit child compliance.

To arrive at a clear treatment goal, the psychotherapist reviewed her understanding of Mary's parenting goals and methods. Specifically, she validated Mary's goal to help her children internalize a high moral code but also raised questions about whether Mary's standards were unrealistic and whether her goal to rectify the past was possible or necessary according to her faith. The psychotherapist also provided education that although Mary's parenting strategies to elicit Matt's compliance worked in the short term, she ran a higher risk of Matt's failing to internalize her values over the long term. The psychotherapist asked Mary about her comfort with making the parenting goal of maintaining a close emotional bond with Matt equal to the goal of eliciting compliance. The psychotherapist explained how balance between warmth and control (i.e., authoritative parenting) could be beneficial. Mary responded positively to this suggestion, explaining that she also felt God wanted her to be close to her children.

The psychotherapist helped Mary reconsider her understanding of God's desires about her parenting goals and methods. A major focus of psychotherapy involved working through Mary's goal to rectify the mistakes Mary felt she and John had made in the past by both her and her sons being perfect in the present. The psychotherapist explored whether Mary believed God expected her to undo the past. Mary responded tearfully that her desire to fix the past was probably more her own issue than God's. Mary was eventually able to turn to God for self-forgiveness and to be less anxious and more accepting of her own and her children's typical human faults. With more education about child development and family system issues, Mary became more understanding about Matt's resistance to her rigidity. She came to view being more flexible with Matt as a way of modeling God's acceptance of her. She was also able to recognize key differences between caving in versus being responsive to Matt's needs when his noncompliance was triggered by feeling tired, stressed, sad, or overwhelmed. With input from the psychotherapist, Mary was able to develop skills and invest more energy into playful, silly activities with both sons as a means to reach the goal of more closeness to them, which also motivated her children to please her and internalize her values. Paradoxically, Mary was ultimately able to reach both major parenting goals of more child compliance and emotional closeness with Matt by relying on God to become more relaxed and flexible in her parenting methods.

Religion-Related Child Abuse: Child Physical Maltreatment

> Jack, age 55, and Eileen, age 53, were mandated by child protective services to obtain family psychotherapy after Jack was reported for being physically abusive to their 8-year-old grandson. A neighbor had called authorities after witnessing the grandson being tied to a tree in the couple's backyard in the hot Texas sun as a punishment. On investigation by authorities, the grandfather acknowledged striking both the grandson and his 7-year-old sister with kitchen spatulas on numerous occasions. Three years earlier, the couple's youngest daughter (now age 26) had signed her parental rights to her children over to the couple and moved to a different state with one of a series of cohabiting partners. Jack and Eileen had converted to a fundamentalist form of Christianity in their 40s, after prior scant involvement in organized religion. The couple insisted that their spiritual obligation was to raise their grandchildren so that they would not end up using drugs and acting out sexually as their mother had. Jack had told the grandchildren that their mother's soul was lost, and God would punish both children similarly if they engaged in wrongdoing. Both grandparents believed heavy reliance on harsh physical discipline was necessary to restrain the grandchildren's evil natures.

However well intentioned their actions were, Jack and Eileen illustrate a phenomenon called *religion-related child abuse*, coined and documented by Bottoms, Nielsen, Murray, and Filipas (2003). Specifically, Bottoms et al. gathered retrospective reports from college students in a large, urban university in the Midwest about their experience of severe child physical aggression as a minor, such as being injured by an act of aggression or being punished with a belt, cord, or hard object. Of the 126 respondents, 21% reported religion-related physical maltreatment, with another 36% reporting nonreligious maltreatment. The incidents of religion-related abuse involved the following characteristics: occurred in a religious setting (35%); the perpetrator had religious authority or a leadership position (31%); the victim was told that God would punish disclosure (20%); the perpetrator justified aggression with religious texts (31%); the perpetrator said the victim was possessed by devils or evil spirits (8%); and the perpetrator thought God, another spiritual figure, or a religious text required the action for reasons other than discipline or possession (12%). In another, older study, 27% of school-age children from a Midwestern region of the United States reported that at least one of their parents told them God would punish them if they were bad (Nelsen & Kroliczak, 1984). These studies have suggested that parents can rely on scripture or spiritual authority figures to justify the use of physical aggression or verbal threats of divine punishment. A psychotherapist's job involves uncovering and addressing such practices.

Yet psychotherapists also need to avoid falling into stereotypical assumptions about parents who belong to conservative religious groups. For example, the assumption that devout, conservative Christian parents are more likely than other parents to justify child physical abuse on religious grounds has not been directly researched. The closest study we know of found that the odds that college students would be abusive to hypothetical children on the basis of their responses to the Child Abuse Potential Inventory were not influenced by their religious tradition, attendance, or orthodoxy or by the centrality of religion to their daily life (Dyslin & Thomsen, 2005). Only those who used religion for extrinsic or self-centered purposes were at greater risk of being abusive. Moreover, frequent religious attendance across traditions by parents has been found to substantially decrease, rather than increase, their risk of being physically abusive to their children over time (Mahoney, 2010). Thus, despite the fact that U.S. parents who belong to conservative Protestant groups or have literalistic views of the Bible are more likely than other parents to spank children (Mahoney, 2010; Mahoney et al., 2001), adults who take their faith seriously appear to be less likely to be physically abusive to their future children than adults who do not.

In the preceding case, the psychotherapist began by obtaining more information about Jack and Eileen's goals for their grandchildren to become well-adjusted, productive adults (e.g., employed and not caught up in drug use) and their sense of failure in meeting this goal with their daughter. In assessing the role of spirituality in parenting, the grandparents conveyed a sense of guilt in the sight of God for their daughter's fate. Jack said that his conversion experience made him very aware of his own sinful past (e.g., alcohol abuse, explosive anger, chronic unemployment). Also, Eileen was less afraid of Jack after his conversion because he developed better control over his hostile impulses and was better able to hold down a job. Jack felt obligated by his understanding of the Bible to rely heavily on physical discipline so that his grandchildren stayed on "the straight and narrow path." The psychotherapist also assessed the methods that the grandparents had used to raise their daughter. Jack and Eileen reported some sense of confusion that she had not turned out right because Jack had relied just as heavily on physical punishment when raising her. The main difference was that Jack was generally more engaged in parenting the grandchildren because of pressure from Eileen.

To clarify treatment goals, the psychotherapist differentiated the grandparents' goals and methods of parenting. She identified the couple's desire for their grandchildren to grow up to be sober and vocationally well adjusted, and she summarized how these goals reflected the grandparents' spiritual values. After she voiced the spiritual significance of the grandparents' parenting goals, both of them became less defensive. The psychotherapist then challenged the couple by pointing out that they were relying on the same method to reach their parenting goal as they had used with their daughter. She questioned why they were committed to a pathway that had not worked for them previously, explained why physical discipline can backfire, and explored whether they would be willing to use alternative strategies to fulfill their hopes. In the process, Eileen disclosed that she had pushed for the couple to take responsibility for the grandchildren out of a sense of obligation to God and that Jack had mixed feelings about their decision. Thus, she often felt a need to protect the children from Jack's anger. Jack admitted ambivalence about being responsible for the children, seeing the task partly as a form of spiritual repentance. But he also resented Eileen, who had during an argument given him the ultimatum of either taking on the role of raising the grandchildren or divorcing, the latter of which was entirely unacceptable given that Jack viewed the marriage as a sacred vow that could not be broken for risk of eternal damnation. Over several months, it became apparent that Jack was overwhelmed by the prospect of being a full-time parent until he retired, and his underlying resentment fueled his hostility toward his wife and grandchildren. With the psychotherapist's help, the couple realized that they were re-creating the same family dynamics that contributed to their daughter's poor adjustment. Nevertheless, Jack remained ambivalent and was unable to make major shifts in parenting practices, and Eileen did not press forward on her threats of divorce.

In terms of solutions, the couple eventually worked with the child protective system to transfer their grandchildren to another family in their church who were foster parents and open to adopting the children, while maintaining visitation rights. This transition was aided by the grandparents learning that the foster parents felt spiritually called to provide a stable, nurturing home to the children. Yet the foster couple also rejected the notion that God mandates physically abusive parenting, which helped the grandparents revise their understanding of biblically based parenting. In a similar fashion, parents who engage in religion-related abuse can be referred to clergy for education about a given tradition's religious teachings and to draw on their spiritual community to facilitate change in abusive attitudes or practices. Notably, major world religions in Western society do not condone physically abusive parenting (Onedera, 2008).

Adolescent Identity Individuation: Focus on Adolescent Sexuality

> Bob, age 57, and Joan, age 52, sought psychotherapy for their 16-year-old daughter, Sophia, after discovering that she had a prescription for oral contraceptives. Sophia was furious that her mother had searched through her purse after overhearing her phone conversation with her 18-year-old boyfriend of 3 months, Dan. Sophia had admitted she was contemplating having sex with Dan but told her parents she was still a virgin. Sophia attended a private Roman Catholic high school, where she was a straight-A student and debate star, and she did not want to risk pregnancy, which would complicate her long-term plans to become an obstetrician–gynecologist. Bob and Joan were devout Catholics who had devoted themselves to their only daughter after having struggled for a decade with infertility. As part of the initial intake process, the psychotherapist met with the parents and Sophia separately. Unbeknownst to her parents, one of Sophia's childhood girlfriends had disclosed to her the prior summer that she was a lesbian. To reconcile this news with her own strong sense of spirituality, Sophia began doing Internet searches about religion, same-sex marriage, and sexuality. In the process, Sophia became acquainted with liberal Christian writings on same-sex sexual relations outside of marriage, realizing she could justify nonmarital sexuality. Yet in an individual session, Sophia disclosed feeling guilty and spiritually conflicted about having impulsively engaged in consensual sex with a senior boy when intoxicated at a party the prior summer, who then spread rumors about her. She had managed to keep the incident a secret from her parents but tended to overreact emotionally to any questions by her parents about sexuality.
>
> Bob and Joan privately reported that they both had regrets about their sexual conduct in their late teens and early 20s. Joan felt she had traded sex for affection with three partners who then rejected her. Bob reported his first girlfriend became pregnant but miscarried. A key factor that

bound the couple together was their joint conviction that renewing and deepening their Catholic identities after college helped them to resolve their guilt related to sexuality. Yet they both wondered if their struggles with infertility had been a logical consequence from God for their earlier sexual explorations. As a result, throughout Sophia's upbringing, they had emphasized virginity as a virtue, never revealing their own premarital sexual histories because they feared such disclosures would send her the wrong message. After having had no major parenting issues, the couple was taken off guard by Sophia's anger toward them. In particular, they were at a loss as to how to handle Sophia's accusations of hypocrisy when she pointed out that they wanted her to follow Catholic teaching prohibiting premarital sex, but she knew they had gone against Catholic teachings to use fertility drugs to help them achieve pregnancy.

This case illustrates the treacherous waters that families face when adolescents begin to grapple with complex spiritual and moral decisions about sexuality. To put Sophia's sexuality into perspective, psychotherapists need to know that the majority of even the most religiously active American teens engage in sexual behaviors that may contradict their parents' wishes. For example, in 1995, 53% and 68% of 13- to 17-year-olds who attended church weekly or monthly, respectively, reported having had sexual intercourse (Regnerus, 2007, p. 121). Similarly, 56% and 73% of teens who said religion was "very important" or "fairly important," respectively, had sex by the time they could vote (the overall base rate is 66%). With regard to Sophia's lesbian friend, 6.3% and 10.4% of adolescent girls who said that religion was "very important" and "somewhat important," respectively, had engaged in consensual sexual relations with a female peer. For boys, the parallel figures for same-sex relations were 3.1% and 4.2% (Regnerus, 2007, p. 77). The following percentages pertained to the number of teenage girls and boys, respectively, from different religious groups who reported having had same-sex relations: 10.6% and 0.8% of evangelical Protestants; 6.5% and 0.7% of mainline Protestants; 12.1% and 4.2% of Black Protestants; 5% and 5% of Catholics; 10.8% and 11.6% of other religions; and 24% and 4.7% of no religion (Regnerus, 2007, p. 77). Thus, although greater religious involvement decreases the likelihood of adolescent sexual behavior, many teens engage in nonmarital sexual relations, heterosexual and same sex, that their parents may disapprove of on spiritual grounds. Yet Regnerus (2007) persuasively argued that few religious teens have internalized the sexual ethic taught by their denominations, with "don't do it until you're married" being the only message that is getting through. Moreover, young adults may often see nonmarital sex in a very different spiritual light from their elders. For example, Midwestern college students at a state university commonly viewed sexual intercourse in their current loving relationship as possessing sacred qualities (e.g., holy, sacred, blessed; Murray-Swank, Pargament, & Mahoney, 2005). Moreover, the more strongly these students held this view, the more frequently they had previously had sex and with more partners. Overall, parents and youths in contemporary societies face challenges to reconcile the traditional theological stance of "just say no" to nonmarital sex given the fact that about 90% of men and 85% of women engage in sex before marriage (Chandra, Martinez, Mosher, Abma, & Jones, 2005). Although many religious families appear to take a pragmatic "don't ask, don't tell" approach to nonmarital sexuality (Regnerus, 2007), this strategy undermines open parent–child communication, leaving adolescents on their own to integrate their spiritual and sexual identities.

Returning to our case study and conceptual model, the psychotherapist first worked to gain an understanding of how parental spirituality was part of both the problem and the solution. In this case, Bob and Joan were struggling to reconcile their parenting goals. They wanted to help their daughter uphold the sanctity of sexuality within marriage and to avoid engaging in sexual behavior that would create dissonance in her ties to God and her religious community. Yet they also wanted to maintain a close relationship with their daughter, another sacred endeavor for them. In terms of methods to achieve their goals, the parents tended to engage in highly intellectualized debates with Sophia about religion and sexuality. Although their intention in these discussions was to treat Sophia as though she was an adult, these disputes merely exacerbated the conflict and distance between them and their daughter and failed to facilitate understanding about the underlying thoughts or feelings on either side of the generational fence.

This case illustrates the dilemmas that parents may encounter when discrepancies emerge between the spiritual values promoted by their religious tradition around sexuality and the choices that teens may view as legitimate in contemporary society. The psychotherapist explained that she did not see her role as adjudicating whose position (parents' or adolescent's) was morally valid, although she could provide descriptive information about general rates of nonmarital sexuality. Moreover, she noted that parental pressure and supervision could not stop Sophia from making her own decisions about her sexual behavior. Rather, the psychotherapist articulated that she viewed her job as helping the parties communicate with each other in a manner that would protect the goals of sustaining the quality of their relationships with each other, God, and their spiritual community. She explained that from her perspective, the family members needed alternative methods to discuss sexuality so that the spiritual struggles each person faced were addressed using communication methods that matched the family's spiritual values of being loving and patient. After the parents considered and accepted this treatment agenda, the psychotherapist modeled and taught better communication skills between the family members. She facilitated dialogues between the parents and Sophia about their ultimate goals.

The parents became more open about why they felt an obligation to protect Sophia's spiritual, psychological, and physical well-being. Using "I" statements, they revealed more about their feelings in a way that helped Sophia understand their views. In turn, Sophia was able to articulate her desire to be treated as an autonomous, responsible agent, but she was better able to talk honestly about her past sexual behavior and her dissatisfaction with Roman Catholic teachings about sexuality. In the process, the parents were more influential than they might otherwise have been, helping Sophia to consider whether her boyfriend deserved the emotional risks that she would take by engaging in sex and how to be intentional about safe sexual practices.

This case illustrates that psychotherapists can facilitate candid dialogue between teens and parents about sexuality, helping to uncover complex feelings of all parties. A psychotherapist can also alert families to the fact that diverse theological perspectives exist on human sexuality. Some parents and teens may find comfort and strength in adhering to well-articulated conservative theological arguments that reserve sexuality to bind partners together within a committed marital relationship that is ready to handle a pregnancy (e.g., Zink, 2008). Other families may find that progressive theological thinking provides a spiritual platform to discuss the notion that sexual intercourse should be reserved for loving relationships marked by mutual love, respect, nonexploitation and justice, and intentional efforts to prevent sexually transmitted infections or undesired pregnancies (e.g., Cook, 2008). In either case, a psychotherapist can facilitate dialogues that engage parents and youths in difficult discussions that might otherwise be avoided, and thereby help an adolescent be more informed and equipped to make thoughtful decisions about sexuality.

More broadly, this case illustrates how our model could help psychotherapists address spirituality in a wide range of cases in which parent–adolescent conflict emerges because the youth begins to explore or develop an identity that is at odds with the spiritual goals of his or her family of origin. Parents from religious groups with highly conservative social values, for example, may become uncomfortable when their teens move toward more permissive attitudes or actions regarding media, alcohol use, or socializing with more socially liberal groups. Conversely, parents committed to religious groups with liberal social values as well as parents who eschew organized religion entirely may become uncomfortable if their teen seeks out close ties with conservative religious groups, fearing the teen will become excessively intolerant or exclusionary. Parents who try to exert control laden with conservative or liberal religious ideology that opposes the direction in which the youth is headed may end up pushing the teen to differentiate his or her identity in ways that are even more out of line with the parents' (and the teen's) faith. A psychotherapist can facilitate dialogue between parents and youths that deescalates the polarization process, helps both sides articulate their respective goals, and encourages them to discriminate between conflicts about destinations versus pathways. The psychotherapist can identify preserving open communication in parent–teen dyads as a goal that is distinct from conflicting goals the parents and adolescent may have about what kind of identity the youth eventually adopts. The psychotherapist can discuss with the parents and teen the pros and cons of being locked in patterns of arguing or avoiding versus engaging in open dialogue. The psychotherapist can help family members consider whether counterproductive communication dynamics over disagreements may do more damage in the long run to parent–teen relationships than the disagreements themselves. The psychotherapist can also explore whether the parents think that maintaining a bond will make their teenager more likely to allow the parents to participate in the teen's process of differentiation. In addition, psychotherapists can explore with parents the spiritual resources they could rely on to meet their goals. Religiously conservative parents, for instance, can turn to their connection with God to help them engage in constructive dialogues and hope that the teen may return to his or her original faith training more readily if the parent models the virtues of patience, respect, and love while the teen explores his or her identity. Similarly, religiously progressive parents can strive to rely on their spirituality to live out principles of tolerance and open-minded engagement with their teens.

CLOSING COMMENTS

Although ample medical literature exists regarding the refusal of medical interventions by extremely fundamentalist and highly conservative branches of some religious groups, we were unable to find controlled studies on whether parents' spirituality discourages reliance on mental health resources to address family or child difficulties. For example, research is needed on spiritual beliefs that may perpetuate fears of seeking family psychotherapy and medication for childhood disorders. On the basis of our clinical experiences and other clinicians' anecdotal accounts (e.g., Walsh, 1999), we suspect that parents may sometimes attribute a child's mental health disorder to some "sin" in the child's life and thus resist secular interventions to alter parenting goals or practices because such approaches seem to free the child from spiritual accountability for his or her wrongdoings. Moreover, accepting a mental health diagnosis may represent a threat to a parent's assumptions that a sacred family is a unit headed by parents who have emotionally and behaviorally well-adjusted children. We would suggest that psychotherapists who are willing to explore parents' spiritual concerns about secular mental health interventions will be in a better position to provide parent education about research on causes of children's mental health and developmental disabilities and better able to explore with parents the pros and cons of accepting a psychotherapist's help to alter their parenting. We look forward to more empirical research in upcoming decades on the benefits and challenges of addressing parental spirituality in the context of family psychotherapy.

In the meantime, in this chapter we have offered a heuristic model for family psychotherapists to use to address ways in which spirituality can be part of the problem and part of the solution when dysfunctional parenting occurs. We have focused on parents' relationships with God, family members, and faith communities as three relational contexts within which spirituality may reinforce maladaptive goals or methods of parenting. We have suggested that therapists can help clients uncover and reevaluate these linkages and potentially draw on faith to help parents transform their parental goals or methods. Finally, we have emphasized that addressing the underlying spiritual dimensions of parental goals or methods may decrease resistance and paradoxically help parents to make changes.

REFERENCES

Abu-Raiya, H., Pargament, K. I., Mahoney, A., & Trevino, K. (2011). On the links between perceptions of desecration and prejudice toward religious and social groups: A review of an emerging line of inquiry. *Implicit Religion, 14*, 455–482.

Achenbach, T. M., & Rescorla, L. A. (2001). *Manual for the ASEBA School-Age Forms & Profiles*. Burlington: University of Vermont, Research Center for Children, Youth, & Families.

American Psychological Association. (2010). *Ethical principles of psychologists and code of conduct (2002, Amended June 1, 2010)*. Retrieved from http://www.apa.org/ethics/code/index.aspx

Bartkowski, J. P., Xu, X. H., & Levin, M. L. (2008). Religion and child development: Evidence from the early childhood longitudinal study. *Social Science Research, 37*, 18–36. doi:10.1016/j.ssresearch.2007.02.001

Baumrind, D. (1967). Child care practices anteceding three patterns of preschool behavior. *Genetic Psychology Monographs, 75*, 43–88.

Bottoms, B. L., Nielsen, M., Murray, R., & Filipas, H. (2003). Religion-related child physical abuse: Characteristics and psychological outcomes. *Journal of Aggression, Maltreatment & Trauma, 8*, 87–114. doi:10.1300/J146v08n01_04

Carothers, S. S., Borkowski, J. G., Lefever, J. B., & Whitman, T. L. (2005). Religiosity and the socioemotional adjustment of adolescent mothers and their children. *Journal of Family Psychology, 19*, 263–275. doi:10.1037/0893-3200.19.2.263

Chandra, A., Martinez, G. M., Mosher, W. D., Abma, J. C., & Jones, J. (2005). Fertility, family planning, and reproductive health of U.S. women: Data from the 2002 National Survey of Family Growth. *Vital and Health Statistics, 23*(25).

Cook, C. J. (2008). The practice of marriage and family counseling and liberal Protestant Christianity. In J. Duba (Ed.), *The role of religion in marriage and family counseling* (pp. 73–87). New York, NY: Routledge.

Cotton, S., Yi, M. S., & Weekes, J. (in press). The interface among spirituality, religion, and illness in families of children with special health care needs. In K. I. Pargament (Ed.), *APA handbook of psychology, religion, and spirituality: Vol. 2. An applied psychology of religion and spirituality* (pp. 405–420). Washington, DC: American Psychological Association.

Demo, D. H., & Cox, M. J. (2000). Families with young children: A review of research in the 1990s. *Journal of Marriage and the Family, 62*, 876–895. doi:10.1111/j.1741-3737.2000.00876.x

Dyslin, C. W., & Thomsen, C. J. (2005). Religiosity and risk of perpetrating child physical abuse: An empirical investigation. *Journal of Psychology and Theology, 33*, 291–298.

Hodge, D. R. (in press). Assessing spirituality and religion in the context of counseling and psychotherapy. In K. I. Pargament (Ed.), *APA handbook of psychology, religion, and spirituality: Vol. 2. An applied psychology of religion and spirituality* (pp. 93–124). Washington, DC: American Psychological Association.

Howard, C. S., Westefeld, J. S., Olds, V. S., Ansley, T., Laird, N., & Olds, G. R. (2007). Spiritually based parenting workshop: An outcome study. *Mental Health, Religion & Culture, 10*, 417–434. doi:10.1080/13674670600913857

Maccoby, E. E., & Martin, J. A. (1983). Socialization in the context of the family: Parent–child interaction. In P. Mussen & E. M. Hetherington (Eds.), *Handbook of child psychology: Volume 4. Socialization, personality, and social development* (4th ed., pp. 1–101). New York, NY: Wiley.

Mahoney, A. (2005). Religion and conflict in family relationships. *Journal of Social Issues, 61*, 689–706. doi:10.1111/j.1540-4560.2005.00427.x

Mahoney, A. (2010). Religion in families 1999-2009: A relational spirituality framework. *Journal of Marriage and the Family, 72*, 805–827. doi:10.1111/j.1741-3737.2010.00732.x

Mahoney, A., & Krumrei, E. J. (in press). Questions left unaddressed by religious familism: Is spirituality relevant to non-traditional families? In L. Miller (Ed.), *The Oxford handbook of psychology of spirituality and consciousness*. New York, NY: Oxford University Press.

Mahoney, A., Pargament, K. I., & Hernandez, K. M. (in press). Heaven on Earth: Beneficial effects of sanctification for individual and interpersonal well-being. In J. Henry (Ed.), *Oxford book of happiness*. Oxford, England: Oxford University Press.

Mahoney, A., Pargament, K. I., Swank, A., & Tarakeshwar, N. (2001). Religion in the home in the 1980s and 1990s: A meta-analytic review and conceptual analysis of religion, marriage, and parenting. *Journal of Family Psychology, 15*, 559–596. doi:10.1037/0893-3200.15.4.559

Miller, W. R., & Rollnick, S. R. (2002). *Motivational interviewing: Preparing people for change* (2nd ed.). New York, NY: Guilford Press.

Murray-Swank, N. A., Pargament, K. I., & Mahoney, A. (2005). At the crossroads of sexuality and spirituality: The sanctification of sex by college students. *International Journal for the Psychology of Religion, 15,* 199–219. doi:10.1207/s15327582ijpr1503_2

Nelsen, H. M., & Kroliczak, A. (1984). Parental use of the threat "God will punish": Replication and extension. *Journal for the Scientific Study of Religion, 23,* 267–277. doi:10.2307/1386041

Onedera, J. D. (2008). *The role of religion in marriage and family counseling.* New York, NY: Routledge.

Pargament, K. I. (1997). *The psychology of religion and coping: Theory, research, practice.* New York, NY: Guilford Press.

Pargament, K. I. (2007). *Spiritually integrated psychotherapy: Understanding and addressing the sacred.* New York, NY: Guilford Press.

Pargament, K. I., & Mahoney, A. (2009). Spirituality: The search for the sacred. In S. J. Lopez & C. R. Snyder (Eds.), *Oxford handbook of positive psychology* (2nd ed., pp. 611–620). New York: Oxford University Press.

Patterson, J., Hayworth, M., Turner, C., & Raskin, M. (2000). Spiritual issues in family therapy: A graduate-level course. *Journal of Marital and Family Therapy, 26,* 199–210. doi:10.1111/j.1752-0606.2000.tb00289.x

Regnerus, M. (2007). *Forbidden fruit: Sex and religion in the lives of American teenagers.* New York, NY: Oxford University Press.

Richards, P. S., & Bergin, A. E. (2005). *A spiritual strategy for counseling and psychotherapy* (2nd ed.). Washington, DC: American Psychological Association. doi:10.1037/11214-000

Smith, C. (with Denton, M. I.). (2005). *Soul searching: The religious and spiritual lives of American teenagers.* New York, NY: Oxford University Press.

Starks, B., & Robinson, R. V. (2007). Moral cosmology, religion, and adult values for children. *Journal for the Scientific Study of Religion, 46,* 17–35. doi:10.1111/j.1468-5906.2007.00338.x

Stokes, C. E., & Regnerus, M. (2009). When faith divides family: Religious discord and adolescent reports of parent-child relations. *Social Science Research, 38,* 155–167. doi:10.1016/j.ssresearch.2008.05.002

Walsh, F. (1999). *Spiritual resources in family therapy.* New York, NY: Guilford Press.

Weaver, A. J., Revilla, L. A., & Koenig, H. G. (2002). *Counseling families across the stages of life: A handbook for pastors and other helping professionals.* Nashville, TN: Abingdon Press.

Zink, D. W. (2008). The practice of marriage and family counseling and conservative Christianity. In J. Duba (Ed.), *The role of religion in marriage and family counseling* (pp. 55–71). New York, NY: Routledge.

4

SPIRITUALLY ORIENTED INTERVENTIONS IN DEVELOPMENTAL CONTEXT

HEATHER LEWIS QUAGLIANA, PAMELA EBSTYNE KING, DAVID PETER QUAGLIANA, AND LINDA MANS WAGENER

Imagine the following case.

Five-year-old Joseph was referred for psychotherapy because of severe separation anxiety from his mother. He was terrified to go to his kindergarten class and was extremely worried about separating from his mother. Joseph's Korean American family identified as having a Christian faith. Joseph said that he loved God and knew God was watching him and his mother from heaven. Prayer, scripture reading, and religious discussion were common daily practices in the family. However, Joseph's religious beliefs were also tied into his separation anxiety. For instance, although he believed that God was watching over him, he also believed that if he disobeyed his mother, God might punish him by taking his mother away.

Given the importance of Joseph's faith and its relevance to his presenting problem, his psychotherapist determined that the use of spiritually oriented interventions would be appropriate and make sense to Joseph

DOI: 10.1037/13947-005
Spiritual Interventions in Child and Adolescent Psychotherapy, D. F. Walker and W. L. Hathaway (Editors)

and his family. In attempting to assess and then work with Joseph's God image (see Chapter 9, this volume), his psychotherapist encouraged Joseph to talk more about God. She emphasized that God was always there for him. After this intervention, Joseph's fears increased. After consulting with a supervisor, she learned that, consistent with his level of cognitive and moral development, Joseph believed that the ever-present, all-knowing God was primarily monitoring his behavior to punish his bad thoughts and deeds. Understandably, Joseph's anxiety increased because he felt God was always watching him, waiting for him to disobey and respond by taking his mother away from him. Joseph's conception of God was limited. Although his psychotherapist had initially tried to comfort Joseph by explaining that God was always present, this was a scary concept rather than a comforting thought. Because Joseph was 5 years old and he could not physically see God with him, he was frightened as to where God might be hiding and wondering whether God would sneak up on him.

With her supervisor's help, Joseph's psychotherapist corrected her error and intervened with Joseph in a developmentally sensitive way by encouraging his family to help correct Joseph's image of God by praying, reading scripture, and telling stories from their own life that depicted God as loving and forgiving. They began to read the Narnia series of children's books, which were consistent with their Christian tradition. In sessions, the psychotherapist used a technique of coconstructed story telling with Joseph in which God was a loving and comforting presence for children.

CHAPTER OVERVIEW

Developmental theory offers a context for understanding children's and adolescents' functioning across several domains or areas, including, but not limited to, the psychosocial, cognitive, and spiritual. In this chapter, we suggest that an understanding of developmental theory should guide treatment in a psychotherapeutic context, including those interventions that are spiritually oriented. We also argue that effective clinical work requires an understanding of the client's developmental competencies.

Thus, in this chapter, we provide an overview of developmental theory as relevant to spiritually oriented interventions in psychotherapy. Our aim is to provide a broad overview of what children's spiritual development may look like in early and middle childhood and adolescence to better equip clinicians to address the spiritual concerns of the young people in their care. After presenting a conceptual model for considering spiritual development, we also offer a series of case studies across developmental domains demonstrating a developmentally sensitive approach to the use of spiritually oriented interventions with children and teens. The case studies that are presented are amalgamated and have identifying information removed to protect client confidentiality.

Youths, of course, have as many spiritual concerns as any other clients. These concerns may be seen in what they hold sacred, beliefs about ultimate reality, understanding of good and evil, core values, quest for meaning and purpose, and religious faith and practices. Although these issues may be expressed differently by a 4-year-old than by a 14-year-old, they are frequently relevant to the clinical setting and can be an aid to those clinicians who are open and willing. As just one example, imagine a 4-year-old, born with a very fragile skeleton that has resulted in dozens of broken bones and stunted growth, asking, "Why did God make me this way?" Although a psychotherapist may not have an answer for the child, he or she may perceive and explore the underlying spiritual concerns that accompany such a question. On a basic level, such a child is asking, "Why am I different? Did I do something to deserve this? Is God angry with me? Am I loved?"

To help psychotherapists understand a process for helping children to answer such questions, we address an understanding of spirituality and offer a framework of spiritual development based on developmental systems theory to understand spiritual interventions. First, we begin by defining *relational spirituality*.

DEFINING *RELATIONAL SPIRITUALITY*

Of particular importance to us in this chapter are several related questions that may influence how psychotherapists choose to implement spiritual interventions in psychotherapy. For example, how do young children seek or experience the sacred? How do they incorporate religious beliefs? What do religious or spiritual rituals mean to a young child? What do they mean to an adolescent? Throughout this chapter, we consider questions related to spiritual development from a developmental systems approach. Over the past several decades, developmental theory has evolved from an emphasis on describing universal stages to a broader contextual approach. Although there may be commonalities among youth at various broadly defined stages in the life span, development is influenced by the various contexts and systems in which a young person interacts (Bronfenbrenner, 1979). Development is also relational and does not occur in isolation. Neither contexts nor relationships are one-directional means of influence on a developing child or adolescent. Rather, they are reciprocal (Lerner, 2002). That is, the child has an impact on the contexts in which he or she is embedded, and the contexts have an impact on the child. Considering the importance of reciprocity in relationships, we argue in this chapter for an overarching approach to understanding children's spiritual development, referred to as *relational spirituality* (King, Ramos, & Clardy, in press).

Consistent with the movement toward a broader contextual approach within developmental psychology over the past several decades, King et al.'s (in press) relational spirituality model suggests that spiritual development takes place through the interactions of a young person and the many systems in which he or she lives. It is through these interactions, or relationships, that young people experience something of significance beyond them and gain a growing sense of transcendence. This connection can be to a divine other (i.e., God); it can involve a sense of all of humanity; or it may pertain to a specific religious community, to peers, or perhaps even to nature. Such experiences are spiritual when they are imbued with meaning that goes beyond provincialism or materialism and express authentic concerns about the world (Reich, 1998). As such, spiritual transcendence provides meaning for young people and serves to motivate their contribution to the well-being of the world of individuals beyond themselves. From this perspective, seminal to spiritual development is the interaction between the self and some generalized or specific other that informs one's beliefs and commitments and propels the young person to live in a manner mindful of his or her part in a broader web of meaning and connection.

King et al.'s (in press) relational spirituality model of spiritual development also emphasizes the significance of relations that lead to transcendence. A young person's experience with God, a higher power, absolute truth, nature, connection to humanity, or belief in an ideology may all be sources of transcendence. Furthermore, Lerner, Roeser, and Phelps (2008) suggested that when a young person transcends a cognitive and emotional focus on the self, he or she gains an awareness of *other* and is provided with meaning and noble purpose that motivate a way of living that is responsible to both self and other. Another way to think about this is from a narrative perspective (McAdams, 2006). Young people derive meaning from their overarching understanding of existence, human nature, creation story, and ultimate reality. They derive their purpose from their understanding of how their personal story fits within the larger narrative. Both meaning and purpose are constructed within their particular network of relationships and contexts, including personal experience, family, peers, neighborhoods, schools, churches, societies, and cultures.

One of the big questions that remain for psychotherapists is how this process is different for children and adolescents at different ages and developmental periods. Additional questions include inquiring about the "nutrients," or spiritual assets, that children have been immersed in—their family's beliefs and practices, their peers' beliefs and practices, and whether they have received religious education or been exposed to religious ritual. King et al.'s (in press) relational spirituality model aids in theoretically conceptualizing development in the psychotherapy room.

Another consideration in applying spiritual interventions in psychotherapy is to remember to emphasize children's strengths and abilities rather than to simply focus on limitations at different developmental periods. An emphasis on competency ought to be as common in clinical practice with youth as the search for psychopathology. This approach, aligned with concepts of positive youth development (PYD), advocates cognitive and social competencies as foundational across all developmental periods for children (Catalano, Berglund, Ryan, Lonczak, & Hawkins, 2002). Furthermore, PYD acknowledges the importance of moral competencies (Catalano et al., 2002) valued across diverse spiritualities such as service to others, participation in a religious community, honesty, and social justice (Benson, 2003). It is true that there are, at times, limitations to a child's cognitive understanding of certain concepts, abilities to regulate emotions and impulses, and relational sophistication. However, even the youngest of clients are engaged in addressing ultimate concerns. Although clinicians must be prepared to be developmentally appropriate in their interventions, they should not avoid spiritual issues out of a fear that such issues are too complicated for a young person.

Highlighted in this chapter are the following spiritually oriented interventions: acceptance, spiritual awareness, reference to sacred texts, prayer, God images, and forgiveness. We believe that these practices can help guide clinicians in what might be developmentally appropriate for children and adolescents. Although we do not review all of these practices in depth, we provide an overarching developmental framework for psychotherapists that can be applied to any of these spiritual interventions. Effective clinical work will be informed by understanding the developmental competencies and limitations of the client as well as attention to the client's relationships and cultural and religious contexts.

SPIRITUALLY ORIENTED INTERVENTIONS ACROSS DEVELOPMENTAL PERIODS

Although we emphasize a systems or contextual perspective of development, age differences in how children may interact with their developmental systems are important to note. Cognitive, social, and spiritual competencies can thus be understood as contextualized by both a child's age and his or her external environment. For the latter, this approach would suggest that psychotherapists will benefit from taking an inventory of the environmental resources in a child's life that contribute to or compete with PYD assets to best understand the role that the psychotherapeutic relationship will play in the environmental context to facilitate competency development. Regarding the former, traditional stage theories can be helpful in providing general guidelines as long as one keeps in mind that particular expressions of developmental differences may vary depending on context.

At each developmental period, different competencies are achieved across multiple areas of development. To illustrate, we consider the primary domains or areas of cognitive, psychosocial, and spiritual functioning. Each of these domains has considerable theory and research that have contributed to understanding the developing child or adolescent. We discuss developmental competencies in light of their implication for spiritually oriented interventions. For example, how do developmental periods and competencies affect the work of psychotherapy and, more specifically, spiritually oriented interventions such as prayer, God images, use of sacred texts, and forgiveness? We believe that taking a relational spirituality (King et al., in press) perspective allows for an overarching theoretical view of development that integrates the child's and adolescent's contextual, cognitive, psychosocial, and spiritual experiences. A summary of developmental tasks across various developmental periods is provided in Table 4.1. Models of relational spirituality (King et al., in press) and PYD (Benson, 2003; Catalano et al., 2002) do not appear in Table 4.1 because they provide overarching perspectives through which to understand development. We should note that the domains or various areas of development are overlapping and not mutually exclusive. This is particularly evident in early childhood because in this developmental period so much of development in one domain (e.g., cognitive) depends on development in another domain (e.g., psychosocial).

DEVELOPMENTAL CONSIDERATIONS IN EARLY CHILDHOOD

It is important for the clinician to consider how development in the cognitive, psychosocial, and spiritual domains may affect psychotherapy during early childhood. More specifically, the use of spiritually oriented interventions should be developmentally appropriate for young children given both their competencies and limitations during this period.

Cognitive Development

Children in early childhood are achieving a great many competencies across multiple domains. Children's understanding of things related to spiritual-

TABLE 4.1
Developmental Overview of Childhood and Adolescence

Developmental tasks	Age: Preschool (ages 4–6)	Middle childhood (ages 7–12)	Adolescence (ages 13–18)
Social milestones	Social and sex roles; social values and beliefs	Social group formation; peer and group identity	Identity formation; dating
Competencies	Socialization; role learning; emotional regulation; imagination	Self-esteem; sense of productivity; group membership	Personal myth; complex problem solving; self-reflection
Play: psychosocial stages (Erikson, 1968)	Imaginative: initiative vs. guilt	Games: industry vs. inferiority	"Hanging out": identity vs. role confusion
Cognitive stages (Piaget, 1929/1967)	Intuitive	Concrete operations	Formal operations
Faith stages (Fowler, 1981): spiritually related psychopathology	Intuitive–projective: fears, separation, anxiety	Mythic–literal: perfectionism; abiding sense of "badness"	Synthetic: conventional nihilistic despair; loss of autonomy
Appropriate inputs	Play therapy: emotional awareness	Narratives: story gives meaning to coherence	Synthesis of faith with personal values and identity

ity such as prayer and meditation and God image is affected by their development in the cognitive domain (Gorsuch & Walker, 2006). For example, in a particular case a clinician may believe that it is beneficial for a religious preschool client who has experienced abuse to understand that "bad things happen to good people, and God is not punishing them." Yet the client may believe that the abuse is a punishment from God for his or her behavior. In fact, the client may be told this by the abuser. According to Kohlberg and Hersh (1977), children in this punishment and obedience orientation believe that physical consequences of actions determine their perceived goodness or badness, regardless of other meaning or value that might otherwise be attributed to outcomes.

In such an instance, a clinician's job is not simply to convince the child that bad things can happen to good people. A more productive intervention would be to discuss the child's understanding of punishments and rewards related to his or her behavior (Kohlberg & Hersh, 1977). Afterward, the psychotherapist could work within the child's paradigm, using the child's language (i.e., acknowledging that sometimes children feel punished even when they have not done anything wrong or do not deserve it).

Understanding children's spiritual beliefs adds another layer to this example. Children's understanding of God is most often tied to their experience of their relationship with their parents and caretakers (Dickie et al., 1997; Hertel & Donahue, 1995). However, children's schemas for authority relationships (their social cognition) are fairly limited and dominated by their experience of their parents. This process incorporates not only cognition but also emotion. As children's experiences of relationship with authority figures broaden, their schema for relationships becomes more differentiated. With a richer relational context that includes not only parents but grandparents, teachers, coaches, pastors, rabbis, and so forth, their schema for God can also become richer and less closely tied to their experience of their parents. A psychotherapist using interventions involving God images and concepts must be aware of a child's understanding of his or her relationships with parents and caregivers because this will provide insight into how a child may be experiencing God or a higher power.

Consider another example of a spiritually oriented intervention, prayer. A psychotherapist can effectively use prayer with a preschool-age client by understanding a child's cognitive competencies at this age. For example, children in early childhood are better able to use symbols in their play and thought than are infants and toddlers (Piaget, 1929/1967). However, children in early childhood are still developing the skill of perspective taking (Piaget, 1929/1967; Piaget & Inhelder, 1967). Competencies and limitations will be evident in children's prayers. Psychotherapists should not try to alter the content of children's prayers but should rather understand the newly developing skills that are evident in such an intervention. For example, children may find praying for loved ones in their lives comforting and empowering, yet the content of the prayer will most likely be from their perspective (for an example, see the case study at the end of this section). Prayer is an example of a spiritually oriented intervention that must also be considered in a developmental context.

Bamford and Lagattuta (2010) contrasted developmental differences in what motivates prayer. They found that young children (ages 4 and 6 in their sample) believe people should pray when they are feeling positive emotions; this was in contrast to 8-year-olds and adults, who noted negative emotions as the primary motivator. Furthermore, Bamford and Lagattuta noted that children's prayers become more goal directed and have more overt purpose as they transition from early to middle childhood. Applying this information to the use of spiritually oriented interventions in psychotherapy, it is important to note that the content of young children's prayers is most likely positive, and most likely an intervention should be linked to children's positive emotions and experiences during their preschool years. Therefore, encouraging a young child to pray about negative thoughts and emotions may be an ineffective intervention.

Psychosocial and Spiritual Development

Preschool-age children are in a psychosocial stage of development that Erikson (1950) referred to as *initiative versus guilt*. In the initiative-versus-guilt stage, children are taking more responsibility for themselves and wanting to do more tasks on their own. Responses from their social environment either reinforce this initiative or cause a sense of guilt to occur. This is in line with other social competencies achieved during this developmental period, such as learning and practicing social roles. An understanding of the psychosocial domain in early childhood is vital for psychotherapists to understand in tailoring spiritually oriented interventions for their clients for several reasons. First, a psychotherapist is shaping a psychotherapeutic context in which children should feel safe enough to take initiative. This initiative is also evident in spiritually related content that the child brings to a session. Children are learning to take more initiative on their own in spiritual practices such as prayer and understanding of sacred texts. Within the psychotherapeutic context, PYD internal assets are developed as a child's initiative is not only accepted but also demonstrated to have value and influence (Benson, 2003).

Second, the psychotherapeutic context is a relational, social context that allows for activation of beliefs, values, and connectedness outside oneself, including a young child's experience of transcendence (King et al., in press). King et al.'s (in press) relational spirituality approach to development provides the theoretical underpinnings of understanding the importance of spiritually oriented interventions. God images, sacred texts, prayer, and forgiveness are all interventions that activate a young child's sense of transcendence and connectedness to something outside him- or herself. The psychotherapist not only explores in session ways in which the child can activate transcendence but also explores the spiritual beliefs, values, and ideologies from familial and social influences that have helped shape the young child's developmental context. This can be achieved in very nonthreatening ways with young children, such as play and art.

Children's spirituality is evident in play themes. This is true for children who use their spirituality as a resource and those who may be working through a spiritually related issue. Clinicians need to be attuned to the role that spirituality plays in their young clients' lives. For example, if spirituality is a coping resource for a child, a clinician may invite the child to draw themes from his or her spirituality or faith system that comforts the child such as a prayer or verse from a sacred text. Conversely, a clinician may be aware that a young child's spirituality is a source of discomfort or anxiety for the child. As mentioned earlier in the chapter, a child may have a fearful attitude toward God, based on a relationship with an angry, unforgiving parent. Clinicians can use either structured or unstructured interventions within the expressive realm. As an example, asking a child to draw God or a picture of "goodness" can give the clinician relevant material to best understand how a child is processing the spiritual realm.

Case Study: A Developmentally Sensitive Approach to Spiritually Oriented Interventions in Early Childhood

John, a Caucasian boy, was brought for psychotherapy because of symptoms of depression and anxiety stemming from the loss of his mother when he was 3 years old. At the time of his initial intake, John was 5 years old and was just starting to have memories of his mother and express sadness over her absence. John's father became particularly concerned because John expressed sadness over not having a mother to his schoolteachers, classmates, and other parents. John would become tearful when other mothers would pick up their children from school and openly express, "I do not have a mother, she died, she's in heaven." Yet, John did not quite understand the permanency of death or the abstract religious concept of heaven.

In the initial intake and assessment with John's father, it was discovered that John and his family identified as Christians, specifically a Pentecostal Protestant tradition. They attended Sunday school and church weekly and relied heavily on their faith as a coping resource. In fact, John and his father described their yearly ritual around the mother's death that involved sending a balloon to heaven as mommy watching over them, as well as visiting the grave to connect with the deceased. This experience of transcendence helps to illustrate how King et al.'s (in press) model of relational spirituality plays out in a psychotherapeutic context. John and his father were connected to the spiritual realm outside of themselves. Their beliefs and ideologies about heaven and the afterlife actively shaped their coping.

Multiple strategies and techniques were used in psychotherapy, but most techniques with John focused on play and art psychotherapy interventions, given John's developmental period. John's father was also provided with psychoeducation regarding children's responses to death and the lack of permanency children may experience with such a loss. Specifically, John's father shared that over the past 2 years, he would say prayers with John that involved asking God to "take care of mommy in heaven." John's father was particularly interested in the content of John's prayers. John would pray that his mom would come back. The psychotherapist explained to John's father that this was developmentally appropriate as John wrestled through death and its permanency.

Because John and his father believed that his mother was in heaven, John was asked to draw a picture of himself before and after his mother's death, as well as a picture of his mother to process changes in identity that occur as a result of such significant loss. John's picture of himself was very typical of a grieving child. He drew himself with a happy face before his mother died and a sad face afterward. John's drawing of his mother before she died involved a specific event the two shared, and the picture after his mother's passing involved her being in heaven. The idea of heaven was comforting to John, but also frustrating because he was unable to comprehend the permanency of death and the abstractness of an afterlife.

A pivotal point occurred when John was invited to make a worry doll. This art technique is used with children who may experience feelings of anxiety to help provide a tangible reminder of coping skills learned in psychotherapy. Over the course of several sessions, the worry doll became a worry angel. For several weeks, John decorated and clothed the doll with care. Near the completion of the doll, John said, "Can this angel be mommy?" When John was able to tangibly represent his mother clothed as an angel in heaven, his mother "got her wings," flew up to heaven, and watched over John and his family. John's art signified his process to accept the death of his mother. Cognitively, John still grappled with the finality of death but sought comfort in spiritual imagery of heaven. Socially, John felt the absence of his mother, and such a loss made him different from his peers, but he still felt some sense of spiritual connection with his mother as she looked down from heaven. John also found sense of connection with other children at school who had experienced the loss of a parent, reiterating the importance of relational spirituality (King et al., in press) and connectedness outside oneself and one's own experience in the psychotherapeutic process.

DEVELOPMENTAL CONSIDERATIONS IN MIDDLE CHILDHOOD

Middle childhood is a developmental period with unique achievements across the cognitive, psychosocial, and spiritual domains. Clinicians ought to consider how development in these various domains affects the use of spiritually oriented interventions in psychotherapy with school-age children.

Cognitive Development

Children in middle childhood are beginning to develop more logical thought. Thought patterns are still concrete in nature, but that does not mean that children are incapable of more sophisticated thought and mental representation (Piaget, 1929/1967). A child's development in the cognitive domain is going to affect a psychotherapist's use of spiritually oriented interventions with him or her. Consider again the example of working with children's God images in psychotherapy. Children in early and middle childhood have some striking similarities in that their experiences of parents and caregivers inform their understanding of God. However, Dickie et al. (1997) noted a difference between early and middle childhood in that older children are more likely to attribute maternal characteristics to their understanding of God, whereas younger children are more likely to attribute paternal characteristics to their understanding of God. Thus, there appears to be a developmental progression in the way in which children understand and attribute parental characteristics to their understanding of God (Dickie et al., 1997). Applying this developmental competency to spiritually oriented interventions means exploring a child's concepts of both maternal and paternal figures and assisting a child in beginning to understand how parental qualities inform the relationship to God. For example, a psychotherapist may find it beneficial to discuss the spectrum of characteristics that their client in middle childhood associates with maternal figures, particularly in how both positive and negative qualities have helped shape the client's understanding of God or a higher power.

Of particular importance in the social context during middle childhood is the growing influence of peers. Before middle childhood, parents and caregivers tend to be the primary influences. Ecologically speaking, Bronfenbrenner (1979) suggested that children in middle childhood experience a broadening of their systems and the resulting influence of peers. For example, Benson's (2003) developmental assets model of PYD advocates for the importance not only of the family environment but also of a caring school climate with clear boundaries, rules, and consequences, thus indicating the value of encouraging relationships with teachers and peers in creating an environment for positive development. A clinical implication of this tendency is that the content of sessions, and thus the content of spiritually oriented interventions, with a child in middle childhood may be more likely to contain material related to peers and school concerns because of the increasing influence of others in these domains. Consider again the example of prayer as applied to middle childhood. Children in middle childhood have a more sophisticated understanding of prayer than preschool-age children. For example, they identify negative emotions as a primary motivator for praying. They are also attuned to how prayer applies relationally to God or a higher power (Bamford & Lagattuta, 2010). This is perhaps because of their increased focus on the social aspect of things.

Psychosocial Development

According to Erikson (1950), middle childhood encompasses a psychosocial stage involving conflicts around industry versus inferiority. A child is now comparing himself or herself with others. As a result, children's school context becomes central to their development, and a sense of emerging industry and productivity compared with same-aged peers occurs. Again, feedback from children's social environment can either reinforce a sense of industry or cause a sense of inferiority. This sense of industry is also evident in children's play preferences, such as competitive games, and focus on building self-esteem, and these will most likely be topics of focus in psychotherapy.

Spiritual Development

With such a focus on social competencies, themes related to relational spirituality are evident. There are a variety of opportunities for transcendence because children are eager to connect to others. An excellent example of a specific spiritually oriented intervention combined with relational spirituality is forgiveness. Several authors (Enright & Fitzgibbons, 2000; Worthington, Jennings, & DiBlasio, 2010) have given increased attention to the developmental progression of forgiveness and suggested that reasoning abilities affect children's and teens' understanding of forgiveness. With increasing focus on the social domain, children may be afforded more opportunities to engage in or discuss forgiveness.

Consider an angry 9-year-old child who has been wronged by a friend. This opportunity may afford the psychotherapist the opportunity to discuss the variety of responses the child may have. Enright and Fitzgibbons (2000) acknowledged two methods commonly used by children in dealing with anger: denying it or expressing it. Enright and Fitzgibbons further asserted that few children understand that forgiveness is a third option that is available to them. The relational context of psychotherapy may serve as a sounding board for consideration of responses congruent with one's faith system, as well as provide opportunities for deeper social and relational connection.

Children in middle childhood are still excellent candidates for expressive therapies; however, they are more capable of verbalizing or participating in talk therapy because they have increased language development compared with children in early childhood. Therefore, clinicians may more readily integrate both verbal and nonverbal methods because children in middle childhood benefit from telling their story and engaging in a more narrative perspective. For example, a psychotherapist may still use play and art in psychotherapy while inviting verbal discussions of the content of such interventions. This enables children to tell their story in a variety of methods.

Case Study: A Developmentally Sensitive Approach to Spiritually Oriented Interventions in Middle Childhood

Lionel, at age 10, was a highly anxious African American fifth grader who had multiple competencies. His highly educated family had no religious tradition but could be considered secular humanists. He was socially well integrated with several good friends, a decent athlete, and an excellent student. Yet he had a persistent and preoccupying fear that his mother was going to die. Traditional cognitive–behavioral interventions had led to some relief in his general level of anxiety as he diligently worked on trying to change his cognitions and practiced deep breathing, yet he was not able to fully let go of his specific fear regarding his mother's death and his more general questions about what happened after death. In some ways, his fear was rational; he was intensely aware that death is inescapable for all who live.

Despite Lionel's intelligence, he was limited cognitively and emotionally in his ability to live with ambiguity. The paradox of death as the endpoint of life was one example. The fact that he both loved his mother and was angry with her for favoring his younger brother was another. His cognitive capacity was advanced enough to allow him to ask existential questions about life but not enough to be comfortable with the lack of answers.

The psychotherapist, recognizing that Lionel was unable to use abstract thought to resolve the existential questions that plagued him, kept their conversations to the observable, the concrete, and the pragmatic. As one example, he consistently observed that people feel multiple emotions. Love and anger can and do coexist. Together, they worked on increasing Lionel's skills in identifying and expressing his conflicting emotions. The psychotherapist coached the parents and children as a family to begin to practice forgiveness. They increased their comfort with communication around anger. First in role plays during the therapeutic sessions and later at home, they practiced both giving and receiving forgiveness when they had experienced a wrong. This practice gave Lionel something concrete to do when he was angry and greatly reduced Lionel's chronic anger with his mother and brother. This in itself relieved the tension generated by his mixed emotional state.

As another example, they worked on the concept of mystery—the common experience of not knowing answers. Lionel loved to read mysteries. The therapist could point out that much of the fun of a good mystery was not knowing the answers and having to wait for the "reveal." Finally, they also researched the various ways in which humans have dealt with the question of what happens after death. Lionel read books of mythology and developmentally sensitive versions of scriptures from several major world religions from his school library. As a result, he was able to use his good academic skills to write a report on the various cultural answers to this ultimate concern. Although Lionel continued to be sensitive to anxiety, he developed a set of tools to recognize and deal with complex questions and emotional states.

DEVELOPMENTAL CONSIDERATIONS IN ADOLESCENCE

Lerner et al. (2008) argued that because of the marked changes in body, mind, and social relationships that adolescents face, many youths seek earnestly to find their place in the world by defining who they are and how they matter. The synthesis of cognitive, psychosocial, and spiritual changes in adolescents causes them to work toward a more complex and adultlike understanding of contextualized self. Although adolescence has typically been bounded by the onset of puberty and age 18, the tasks undertaken in adolescence are increasingly recognized to extend further in both directions—undertaken within social contexts before puberty and continued into college-age development and beyond in today's culture (Lerner & Steinberg, 2009).

Cognitive Development

Cognitive development in adolescence involves the dawn of hypothetical reasoning, abstract thought, and more complex problem solving. The richness of these added perceptual abilities allows the psychotherapist to replace representative play and concrete psychoeducation about emotions with more adult-typical verbal processing and reflection in the psychotherapy process. These must be approached with caution, however, because the complex reasoning skills are newly emerging ones. Therefore, in use of sacred texts, a psychotherapist might assist an adolescent in realizing that individuals might interpret texts differently, encouraging the adolescent to consider multiple interpretations of a particular passage and ways to discern his or her own understanding of it. Adding similar complexity to the use of forgiveness in session might mean helping an adolescent to realize that forgiveness is a complex construct related to relationship rather than merely a behavioral act of stating acceptance of an apology or resolution of anger and hurt.

Psychosocial Development

There is an inherent connection between this added complexity of thought and the degree to which an adolescent is aware of and self-reflective regarding his or her disposition in multiple spheres of social influence. Thus, psychosocial development in adolescence involves heightened awareness of both self-perceived identity and the way in which social interaction defines identity. Adolescence brings a reduction in the role of family in a person's identity, as physical changes bring attention to the self as an individual and social and emotional changes increase the priority of social acceptance. These two factors come together to bring about a social-referencing process of individual identity formation. Marcia (1966) referred to the challenging of the beliefs gained through family tradition, positing that the accomplishment of identity achievement requires a reflection on alternatives to parentally instilled values and a conscious choice of values and identity. In this process, adolescents seek an identity (e.g., Erikson, 1959, 1968; Harter, 2006) that gives them a stable self-concept and a sense of belonging and enables them to matter to peers, family, and society.

Increasingly, U.S. culture has influenced adolescents to conceive of identity in terms of how they "seem" or represent themselves to others—hence the increased focus on body image, clothing and accessories, and piercings and other markings (Sweetman, 2000). This approach to identity stands in stark contrast to basing this construct on "being" an identity laden with certain personal skills, beliefs, and other personality characteristics (Becker, 2004). Similarly, the dominance of technologically assisted interaction, such as social networking websites (e.g., Facebook, Twitter), has accentuated the degree to which identity is seen by adolescents as an image constructed for the observation of others rather than as a genuine representation of self-perceived internal traits and overall personality. As a psychotherapist, one would be wise to acknowledge the way in which this "seeming" aspect of identity appeals to the growing importance of peer identification and acceptance. The concept of empowerment in the formation of an identity can be valuable as adolescents realize sources of identity beyond their parents. Psychotherapists can overtly discuss ways in which adolescents have the power and responsibility to determine aspects of their identity rather than passively rely entirely on peer pressure or parentally transmitted sources of self. In this process, it is possible to help adolescents learn to observe the underlying values (spiritual or otherwise) and competencies being explored in this process of identity formation through social comparison. A positive iteration of the social referencing in adolescence is that this search can impel young people to transcend a cognitive and emotional focus on the self, becoming aware of and motivated by ways to seek to contribute in important and potentially noble ways to their world (Lerner, Warren, & Phelps, 2011). Through these experiences of transcendence, young people are infused with a sense of meaning, which informs their beliefs, values, and worldviews. Such rich and meaningful transactions help shape one's identity and result in a sense of fidelity to an abstract worldview.

Spiritual Development

As adolescents reflect on their newly realized transcendent possibilities, aspects of spirituality previously beyond their comprehension come into view. Moving beyond the "what" of religious practices and moral behavioral norms, adolescents are more adept at asking why one's values and behaviors matter in the complex world beyond their immediate sphere of interaction. Psychotherapists can assist adolescents to integrate hypothetical reasoning, abstract thought, and more complex problem solving with transcendent social awareness to consider the potential impact of their spiritual identity on the world. A psychotherapist can use an adolescent's growing experience with transcendence to illustrate how forgiveness can be seen as more than a young person's reconciliation with a peer. For example, forgiveness played a foundational role in the racial, legal, and political landscape of postapartheid South Africa (Tutu, 1999). Psychotherapists have an opportunity to model the use of transcendent reflection and meaning making in identity formation to help adolescents negotiate an identity with fidelity to familial, spiritual, and general cultural relationship navigation.

In harmony with ecological or systems models, the psychotherapist has opportunities to have an impact not only on an adolescent but also on his or her system. Often, a psychotherapist not only works with an adolescent client but also interacts directly with parents, siblings, and educators in the adolescent's life.

Interactions with parents often reveal that they have difficulty welcoming the social influences playing increasingly influential roles in their children's lives. The phenomenon of "helicopter parenting" as a cultural norm, in which parents provide high levels of structure and assistance with interactions to ensure successful outcomes, has decreased the degree to which children have learned independent skills for navigating their relationships and experiences from birth to adolescence and beyond (Arnett, 2004). This, in turn, has created increased dependence on parents and others in the process of identity formation. Additionally, in more conservative religious cultures, parents frequently respond with stronger explicit statements about expectations that their children adopt their parents' values, beliefs, and other aspects of identity. These messages are often accompanied by explicit expression of fears of the dangers anticipated by parents in the process of exploring nonparental sources of value and identity for their children. By assisting parents in accepting young people's normative development of socially referenced identity formation, the psychotherapist can facilitate a parent–child relationship conducive to Marcia's (1966) identity achievement through development of critical evaluation of sources for identity formation.

Also helpful to parents and psychotherapists in thinking about spiritually oriented interventions is a PYD perspective, which emphasizes a vision of a child's maturation into adulthood to extend beyond avoidance of teen pregnancy, violence, drugs, and other deficit-focused outcomes. Instead, PYD models provide helpful constructs related to the characterological development sought by parents such as prosocial involvement, fostering spirituality, promotion of moral competency, and positive values (e.g., integrity, social justice, and responsibility; Benson, 2003; Bundick, Yeager, King, & Damon, 2010; Catalano et al., 2002). Furthermore, fundamental to PYD is the notion that young people will thrive when they transcend themselves, developing community-conscious personal assets (e.g., social justice, cultural competence, sense of purpose) and connecting with a source of ultimacy so that it transforms their identity and fuels a life of purpose and contribution.

In direct interaction with teenage clients, the psychotherapist has an opportunity to model, perhaps for the first time and likely in the most explicit way yet experienced, a relationship with an adult built on the foundation of self-determination and empowerment. This relationship models a developmentally appropriate shift from value transmission based on rules and boundaries, providing a safe space in which adolescents can self-reflect and gain insight regarding the role of nonparental influences on their perceived identity. Illumination of the opportunities and risks involved in social referencing provides an opportunity for adolescents to perceive adults as seasoned guides in the navigation of these new sources of information rather than as obstacles to their newfound priority of freedom and independence from a middle childhood perception of adult–child interaction. Such a role is crucial, given the previously discussed importance of relational and contextual conceptualizations of the child and the work he or she is doing in psychotherapy. More important, if such a client–psychotherapist relationship is achieved, it provides the opportunity for illumination of and assistance in the navigation of the identity formation process.

Specifically, when such a trusting adolescent–psychotherapist relationship is achieved, the psychotherapist can become a resource for integrating the adolescent's parentally transmitted ideas of character (including but not limited to those directly involving spirituality), newly explored alternative belief systems, and developing self-concept. As stated earlier, adolescents are increasingly defining identity as the formation of an image to present to others in pursuit of social acceptance (Becker, 2004). Psychotherapists can contextualize this oversimplified model of identity formation within a more healthy pursuit of reciprocal interaction between personal values and their implications in societal interaction, illuminating ways to act in fidelity to espoused core traits while allowing the adolescent to cocreate such identity traits with transcendence beyond self into a social context. Teens can be encouraged to see this newly prioritized social world as one in which they seek not only acceptance but also self-authorized impact on the world. Such emphasis on reciprocal interaction between self and society can empower adolescents to overcome an oversimplified emphasis on presentation of a "seeming" identity, often focused on outward appearance, and emphasize transcendence through transactions that transform identity in a purposeful and productive manner.

Such an approach can lead the adolescent client and the psychotherapist to open dialogue about, rather than resistance toward discussion of, familial spiritual beliefs. Such exploration can assist adolescents in the development of a spiritual identity that incorporates dialogue with opposing views. Ultimately, this will allow an adolescent to be resilient against existential hopelessness and identity stagnation in response to simple exposure to new or different values, philosophies, or religious ideologies. This process may involve the use of sacred texts and related commentaries, behaviors and rituals such as prayer, or discussion or engagement in other specific activities by the client, such as community service or organizational involvement. These resources have been used at previous stages of development, but the reflection on their role in character and identity development is much more explicit with adolescents than with clients at earlier stages of life.

The psychotherapist thus plays a crucial role as a seasoned and collaborative guide in the adolescent's striving for a sense of identity that is now more explicit in the client's awareness and is influenced by rising awareness of the individual's place within a system of peers, family, and other aspects of local and global cultural context. The process of achieving fidelity in such an identity incorporates spirituality both in exploration of explicit religious models and in reflection on the interaction among reciprocal social influence, spirituality, and personal beliefs and values. Adolescents seek connection and acceptance in relationships with peers and others, but they also seek meaning and identity in their lives. Such transcendent and existential reflection is a newly forming opportunity for a level of spiritual identity previously inconceivable before adolescence. Consequently—and of particular importance from a clinical perspective—the emergence of transcendent awareness and reflection allows adolescents to experience something bigger than themselves—God, a belief system, higher power, social impact, a cause—something that is beyond the mundane of life. This will enable them to gain broader perspectives and create an identity that is committed to something bigger than themselves with self-perceived and self-authorized spiritual significance.

Case Study: A Developmentally Sensitive Approach to Spiritually Oriented Interventions in Adolescence

Josie was a senior in high school who came for treatment of depression and separation anxiety regarding her decision to leave home to attend college. She was a committed atheist who disdained organized religion. Although she had little that she did believe in, she was very clear about what she did not believe in. She grew up in a Caucasian liberal household in the northeastern United States with parents who had been raised in religious traditions (Christian and Jewish) but had rejected their parents' belief systems.

Josie's depression had begun at the age of 10 when one of her schoolmates died unexpectedly from a viral infection while alone at home. In some ways, she exhibited symptom behavior more congruent with that of a young child. She had frequent nightmares and night terrors. She found the thought of living away from her mother almost intolerable. She was unable to project herself into the future in a way that provided a sense of meaning and purpose. Without that, she had little to undergird her as she faced the questions raised by entrance into adulthood. What kind of person would she be? What would she do with her life?

Josie's spiritual development was stunted by the lack of a context that addressed fundamental questions of existence. In the absence of exposure to the various ways in which people have addressed the question of what makes life good, she was bereft of resources that she needed to find comfort in separation and grief. She lacked both vocabulary and concept to struggle with pain and suffering. Her crisis came to a head when her father died. This event forced her to confront the emptiness of her belief system and begin a spiritual quest. In her search for answers, she began to read and take coursework in philosophy as well as comparative religions. During this time, she read a number of sacred writings from various spiritual traditions. These materials were a useful adjunct to the work she did in psychotherapy, where she began to construct a narrative of her own life in the larger context of her family history, middle-class North American culture, and personal giftedness, values, and morality. She remained an atheist and materialist who did not believe in either a spirit world or an afterlife, but she found that a humanistic philosophy provided her with a spiritual and moral framework that could guide her life decisions and support her adult development.

CONCLUSION

Spiritually oriented interventions must be considered in a developmental context across several areas of functioning: cognitive, psychosocial, and spiritual. Relational spirituality (King et al., in press) offers an overarching perspective on how to understand development and its relevance in the psychotherapeutic relationship and interventions. A variety of spiritually oriented interventions help to inform the importance of a psychotherapist's attunement to a child's or adolescent's developmental level. Prayer, the use of sacred texts, the God image, and forgiveness are all interventions used across developmental periods, but nuanced according to the child's or adolescent's developing competencies. Responsible use of spiritually oriented interventions with children and adolescents demands a working knowledge of developmental psychology to best meet clients at their developmental level.

REFERENCES

Arnett, J. J. (2004). *Emerging adulthood: The winding road from late teens through the twenties*. New York, NY: Oxford University Press.

Bamford, C., & Lagattuta, H. (2010). A new look at children's understanding of mind and emotion: The case of prayer. *Developmental Psychology, 46*, 78–92. doi:10.1037/a0016694

Becker, A. E. (2004). Television, disordered eating, and young women in Fiji: Negotiating body image and identity during rapid social change. *Culture, Medicine, and Psychiatry, 28*, 533–559. doi:10.1007/s11013-004-1067-5

Benson, P. L. (2003). Developmental assets and asset-building community: Conceptual and empirical foundations. In R. M. Lerner & P. L. Benson (Eds.), *Developmental assets and asset-building communities: Implications for research, policy, and practice* (pp. 19–43). New York, NY: Kluwer Academic.

Bratton, S. C., Ray, D., & Rhine, T. (2005). The efficacy of play therapy with children: A meta-analytic review of treatment outcomes. *Professional Psychology: Research and Practice, 36*, 376–390. doi:10.1037/0735-7028.36.4.376

Bronfenbrenner, U. (1979). *The ecology of human development: Experiments by nature and design*. Cambridge, MA: Harvard University Press.

Bundick, M. J., Yeager, D. S., King, P. E., & Damon, W. (2010). Thriving across the life span. In W. F. Overton (Eds.), *Handbook of life span development: Vol. 1. Methods, biology, neuroscience, and cognitive development* (3rd ed., pp. 882–923). Hoboken, NJ: Wiley.

Catalano, R. F., Berglund, L. M., Ryan, J. A. M., Lonczak, H. S, & Hawkins, D. J. (2002). Positive youth development in the United States: Research findings on evaluations of positive youth development programs. *Prevention and Treatment, 5*, Article 15.

Dickie, J. R., Eshleman, A. K., Merasco, D. M., Shepard, A. S., Vander Wilt, M., & Johnson, M. (1997). Parental child relationships and children's images of God. *Journal for the Scientific Study of Religion, 36*, 25–43. doi:10.2307/1387880

Enright, R. D., & Fitzgibbons, R. P. (2000). *Helping clients forgive: An empirical guide for resolving anger and restoring hope*. Washington, DC: American Psychological Association. doi:10.1037/10381-000

Erikson, E. H. (1950). *Childhood and society*. New York, NY: W.W. Norton.

Erikson, E. H. (1959). Identity and the life cycle: Selected papers [Monograph]. *Psychological Issues, 1*, 1–171.

Erikson, E. H. (1968). *Identity: Youth and crisis*. New York, NY: Norton.

Fowler, J. W. (1981). *Stages of faith: The psychology of human development and the quest for meaning*. New York, NY: HarperCollins.

Gorsuch, R. L., & Walker, D. F. (2006). Measurement and research design in studying spiritual development. In E. C. Roehlkepartain, P. E. King, L. Wagener, & P. L. Benson (Eds.), *The handbook of spiritual development in childhood and adolescence* (pp. 92–103). Thousand Oaks, CA: Sage.

Harter, S. (2006). The self. In W. Damon & R. M. Lerner (Series Eds.) & N. Eisenberg (Vol. Ed.), *Handbook of child psychology: Vol. 3. Social, emotional, and personality development* (6th ed., pp. 505–570). Hoboken, NJ: Wiley.

Hertel, B. R., & Donahue, M. J. (1995). Parental influences on God images among children: Testing Durkheim's metaphoric parallelism. *Journal for the Scientific Study of Religion, 34*, 186–199. doi:10.2307/1386764

King, P. E., Ramos, J. S., & Clardy, C. E. (in press). Searching for the sacred: Religion, spirituality, and adolescent development. In K. I. Pargament (Ed.), *APA handbook of psychology, religion, and spirituality: Vol. 1. Context, theory, and research* (pp. 513–528). Washington, DC: American Psychological Association.

Kohlberg, L., & Hersh, R. H. (1977). Moral development: A review of the theory. *Theory Into Practice, 16*, 53–59. doi:10.1080/00405847709542675

Lerner, R. M. (2002). *Concepts and theories of human development* (3rd ed.). Mahwah, NJ: Erlbaum.

Lerner, R. M., Roeser, R. W., & Phelps, E. (2008). Positive development, spirituality, and generosity in youth. In R. M. Lerner, R. W. Roeser, & E. Phelps (Eds.), *Positive youth development and spirituality: From theory to research* (pp. 3–22). West Conshohocken, PA: Templeton Foundation Press.

Lerner, R. M., & Steinberg, L. (Eds.). (2009). *Handbook of adolescent psychology: Vol. 1. Development, relationships and research methods* (3rd ed.). Hoboken, NJ: Wiley.

Lerner, R. M., Warren, A., & Phelps, E. (Eds.). (2011). *Thriving and spirituality among youth: Research perspectives and future possibilities*. Hoboken, NJ: Wiley.

Marcia, J. E. (1966). Development and validation of ego identity status. *Journal of Personality and Social Psychology, 3*, 551–558. doi:10.1037/h0023281

McAdams, D. P. (2006). *The redemptive self: Stories Americans live by*. New York, NY: Oxford University Press.

Piaget, J. (1967). *The child's conception of the world* (J. Tomlinson & A. Tomlinson, Trans). London, England: Routledge & Kegan Paul. (Original work published 1929)

Piaget, J., & Inhelder, B. (1967). *The child's conception of space* (F. J. Langdon & J. L. Lunzer, Trans.). New York, NY: Norton.

Reich, K. H. (1998). Psychology of religion: What one needs to know. *Zygon: Journal of Religion and Science, 33*, 113–120. doi:10.1111/0591-2385.1301998130

Sweetman, P. (2000). Anchoring the (postmodern) self? Body modification, fashion, and identity. In M. Featherstone (Ed.), *Body modification* (pp. 51–76). London, England: Sage.

Tutu, D. M. (1999). *No future without forgiveness*. New York, NY: Doubleday.

Worthington, E. L., Jennings, D. J., & DiBlasio, F. A. (2010). Interventions to promote forgiveness in couple and family context: Conceptualization, review, and analysis. *Journal of Psychology and Theology, 38*, 231–245.

II

INTERVENTIONS

5

ACCEPTANCE

STEVEN A. ROGERS, LEANNE STEEN, AND KERRY McGREGOR

Love your neighbor as yourself.

—Luke 10:27 (NIV)

In most schools of psychotherapy, the concept and application of acceptance do not assume any particular spiritual training or affiliation. Although most spiritual and religious systems contain either implicit or explicit assumptions about the role of acceptance, it is also true that some spiritual or religious orientations discourage acceptance, either of oneself in favor of striving for approximate perfection or of others by championing exclusivity in their faith's access to the hereafter.

However, acceptance is central to interpersonal relationships and is considered a core element of some therapeutic approaches. In this chapter, we describe *acceptance* as a spiritual approach to psychotherapy built on a belief in the innate ability of children to strive toward personal and spiritual growth and a deep and abiding belief in the child's ability to be. Ways in which acceptance functions therapeutically are discussed across different theoretical orientations. In addition, we also review personal attributes on the

DOI: 10.1037/13947-006
Spiritual Interventions in Child and Adolescent Psychotherapy, D. F. Walker and W. L. Hathaway (Editors)

part of the psychotherapist that foster acceptance in therapy. We begin by discussing the therapeutic function of acceptance in object relations therapy, then we discuss acceptance in child-centered therapy. Across each approach, we provide one or more case studies involving actual clients whose personal information has been deidentified to illustrate the use of acceptance within each approach.

ACCEPTANCE WITHIN OBJECT RELATIONS PSYCHOTHERAPY

Object relations psychotherapy may appropriate acceptance as a particularly important intervention for those clinicians who have a spiritual orientation. In this section, I (Steven Rogers) review object relations theory and describe the function of acceptance as a therapeutic intervention within object relations therapy. I then present two case studies demonstrating the therapeutic application of acceptance before concluding by describing acceptance as an explicit spiritual intervention within object relations theory.

The actual concept of acceptance may be placed in an important dialectic in spiritual and psychoanalytic circles. In the former, acceptance is often pitted against a striving for betterment, perhaps with the serenity prayer at one end of the spectrum and an active dissatisfaction with oneself as a prerequisite for successive levels of spiritual growth or enlightenment at the other. In the case of many psychoanalytic schools, this dialectic may take a different form, with acceptance as a therapeutic goal placed in opposition to a necessary disruption or perturbation of one's defenses and relational patterns. Among the misleading connotations of this dialectic is that acceptance as a therapeutic intervention is either antithetical to change or cannot be its own form of frustration, something many of those struggling with anxiety might dispute. One of the branches of the psychoanalytic approach in which these tensions may disappear, however, is in object relations therapy, in which acceptance is not only a necessary part of the path toward clients' growth and change but can also subserve as a distinctly spiritual intervention. Both the theory and interventions in object relations therapy allocate acceptance a premium position that is friendly to those with spiritual orientations. What follows is an attempt to understand how acceptance within an object relations approach to therapy can itself represent a powerful spiritual intervention.

Object Relations Theory and Therapy

To better understand the place of acceptance and its spiritual role in object relations therapy, it may help to start with a quick overview of the theoretical principles of the theory, its understanding of psychopathology, and its approach to psychotherapy. Among the central contributors to this theory and therapy were Melanie Klein, Ronald Fairbairn, and Donald Winnicott. Each of these individuals created his or her own particular brand of object relations, but common among them is dissatisfaction with the mechanistic and heavily instinctual focus on classic Freudian theory. Without discounting the importance of neurobiology, they emphasized the impact of early relationships on human development and psychological well-being. They assumed that relatedness and mutuality are the primary motivators for human behavior, so that health and psychological constitutions are a function of the quality and type of relations with past and current objects, namely, significant others (McDargh, 1983; Wenar & Kerig, 2000).

These object representations of oneself and others appear to arise through a series of distinct developmental stages. Mahler, Pine, and Bergman (1975) described these stages as symbiosis, differentiation, and individuation–rapprochement, which loosely map onto Fairbairn's (1946) stages of infantile dependence, transition, and matured dependence. According to both theories, the developmental process begins at birth with the child engaging in a symbiotic relationship with the caregiver, assuming complete dependence on the caregiver as an object for satisfying the child's basic needs. In the mind of the infant, there is no separation or boundary between the infant and the caregiver; the infant's actions directly elicit the effects of the parent, making it the autistic center of a one-sided universe in which it can reign in blind omnipotence. Because virtually all of the infant's basic needs are met, the enmeshed parent becomes perceived as inherently good and incapable of harm (McDargh, 1983).

Beginning around 6 months of age, however, the infant becomes increasingly aware of the reality of the caregiver's separateness and limitations. This is the stage of differentiation, which inevitably emerges because the caregiver fails to fully satisfy the child's complete needs. Other family members demand attention, food is delayed, and frustration emerges because the caregiver is separate. According to object relations theorists, this frustration and betrayal are not only inescapable, but also necessary because the child is forced to accept both the good and the bad polarities of the independent parent. Among the child's possible responses to this newly conscious awareness are perceived alienation and abandonment, giving rise to anger toward the caregiver and ambivalence about one's desire to maintain enmeshment and yet assert independence. This response naturally causes a separation, a discarding of the outdated object representation of the parent as symbiotic and flawless, to be replaced by the adoption of a new parent relationship characterized by a more accurate internal representation that accepts and integrates the separateness and polarity of the caregiver.

To the extent that this differentiation is accomplished, the self has individuated and reached the rapprochement stage, declaring itself free from defining the parent according to its own needs and able to finally accept the parent's unique dimensionality and identity (Mahler et al., 1975). With this maturation, the representations of oneself and others have become capable of accepting and integrating both good and bad traits. This frees the subject and object to have mature, healthy relationships, in which there is not complete identification but rather mutuality in experiencing and accepting both the strengths and the limitations of the other.

Psychological problems arise from the unsuccessful accomplishment of these stages of separation and differentiation. Ideally, the child is able to accept and internalize mental representations of the parent and the self that are realistic and healthy, such as accepting both the positive and the negative aspects of oneself and one's parents. This happens if a parent is just good enough to create a holding environment that is safe, secure, and nurturing, supporting the separation–individuation process. This environment or zone of safety is what Winnicott (1988) called the *third space*, in which the child learns the difference between subject and object, caregiver and self. If children experience poor relationships with primary caregivers, however, these relationships get perpetuated in inner reality through the formation of unhealthy representations of others and inaccurate representations of themselves (Fairbairn, 1958). In the case of abusive parents, children may develop templates of others as angry and themselves as powerless and worthless. Those children whose parents are unable to withdraw and separate often develop view of others as overprotective and themselves as unable to be mature and tolerate frustration (Burns-Smith, 1999). Consequently, life is spent replaying this dysfunctional relational drama, using the same unhealthy script and simply casting different individuals to play the same character roles.

Acceptance as an Intervention in Object Relations Therapy

The disruption of this drama is the aspiration of object relations therapy, with acceptance serving as both a critical attitude and a primary technique. Granted, acceptance is not exclusive to object relations therapy; quite the contrary, almost all therapeutic traditions likely champion some form of acceptance, either as a posture of the therapist or as a goal for the client. However, each therapy tradition differs in the meaning and definition given to acceptance. Within object relations, acceptance is a therapeutic tool and attitude aimed at helping clients achieve two forms of their own acceptance, namely acceptance of the reality of others and acceptance of the reality of themselves. Specifically, the goal of the therapist is to help clients learn to differentiate their views of themselves and others from early relational templates so that they can see themselves and others in a realistic and integrated way that is only minimally influenced by early representations. According to object relations therapy, this most potently occurs in the relationship between the therapist and the client. Object relations therapists attempt to provide corrective emotional and relational experiences in which clients do not replay old reconstituted roles and they foster a healthy and more accurate understanding of the client and his or her interpersonal environment.

Central to accomplishing this is the acceptance of all aspects of the client, including all feelings, thoughts, actions, and sensations. This is deliberately aimed at counteracting a failed acceptance that likely occurred in early relationships. Most children experience their caregivers as generally positive and fulfilling, but caregivers invariably and necessarily disappoint and fail, so their children need a way to resolve this conflict. For many children, this resolution is achieved by internally dividing the caregiver into good and bad components, psychically splitting off one from the other. As a result, both the internal and the external worlds become bifurcated into frustrating and destructive objects and gratifying and loving objects (Cashdan, 1988). One of the unfortunate by-products of this splitting is a division of the self into good and bad elements. Those aspects that are perceived as positive remain conscious and expressed, but those perceived as negative are often subject to any number of mechanisms aimed at concealing their acknowledgment or ownership, such as projection, sublimation, repression, and projective identification. When a child first experiences a caregiver's failure and frustration, for example, the prior feelings of love and affection toward the caregiver might become accompanied by anger and fear. Uncertain of how the caregiver may respond to these difficult emotions, and afraid of rejection and abandonment, the child may cast off or repress these unacceptable emotions, perhaps as a way to protect against exploitation, hurt, and annihilation of the self (Burns-Smith, 1999).

Ideally, all of these disparate or mixed feelings can be tolerated and accepted by the caregiver. For many clients, however, conditions have been placed on their feelings and impulses, so only certain aspects of their selves were accepted and acknowledged by their caregivers. For clients with somatic complaints, often physical dependency has been accepted and independence rejected. For clients consumed by the desire for power, neediness may have been rejected. For still other clients, ingratiation may have been accepted, with demonization of a healthy demandingness. Object relations therapists strive to redress this goodness–badness balance of the self by accepting all those parts that have been fragmented or split off from consciousness or acceptable expression. For the client whose parents accepted only a part, be it the somatic, the athletic, or the academic, the therapist tries to accept all parts, both strengths and vulnerabilities. For the person who tries to present as intelligent and culturally refined, the therapist will likely need to accept the client's mundanity and naïveté. For the person who is overzealous in his or her attempt to appear gregarious and morally certain, it may be necessary to accept his or her deep existential angst and doubt. Ideally, any and all aspects of the client are worthy of acceptance. This means accepting the negative and hateful feelings of the client, his or her sinister affects and destructive motivations, and his or her grandiosity, idealistic strivings, and yearning for inviolability (Skolnick, 2006).

The value of the therapist's acceptance is not simply in validating previously invalidated parts of the client's self but also in facilitating the client's self- and other acceptance. When clients are enveloped by the therapist's acceptance of previously unintegrated experiences, they are offered space for an expanded sense of self where they can integrate the reality of those feelings and sensations that were either previously discouraged or cast out of conscious awareness. For clients who struggle to contain overwhelming, intolerable negative affect, the therapist's ability to accept and contain the negative affect helps clients to share in the acceptance and mutually discover new ways of stumbling, repairing, tolerating, and modulating the affect. Because of the therapist's acceptance, there is an integration of disconnected feelings and realities that enables the client to experience greater peace with him- or herself, so energy is directed away from keeping unacceptable parts unexposed and toward wholeness and self-acceptance. In other words, as the therapist attempts to repair failures in acceptance, the client can form a new bond between or acceptance of his or her own self and self-object (Gehrie, 2011). This promotes a change in relationship to the client's self, so new bonds with undesired parts are formed, resulting in new consequences when these undesired elements are experienced.

Not only is the therapist's acceptance internalized in a way that minimizes self-fragmentation, but it also helps clients completely accept others in their lives. According to object relations theory, a child's ability to accept the conflicting emotions toward his or her caregiver, especially after the symbiotic phase is shattered by a parent's failure and disillusionment, allows for an internal representation of others not as symbiotic and flawless but rather as realistic, with strengths and liabilities. In the same way, if a client achieves self-acceptance of difficult emotions and thoughts, which is facilitated by the therapist's acceptance of those disconnected parts, then the client is better able to develop more accurate internal representation of others. This then frees the client to see and accept the reality of others, without self-serving blindness to others' flaws or enviable virtues. Clients are able to more clearly accept others' sordid optimism, paranoia, or dependency so that new and mature ways of being with others are cultivated. In a sense, they can come to accept others as neither flawless nor hopelessly flawed (Skolnick, 2006), with imperfection and virtue, frustration and love, danger and gratification, because their representations of themselves and others can realistically accept both the good and the bad. Such a profound change in one's relationships with others and oneself follows from what might seem simplistic and trite, namely, the therapist's acceptance.

There are myriad ways in which therapists from an object relations orientation foster acceptance. Certainly warmth and accurate empathy allow for the emergence and acceptance of split-off parts of the client. Collaboratively imagining the possibility of difficult emotions or sensations, such as naming the possibility of hate or lust or helplessness, can cultivate an environment in which clients' deepest fears and pain can be accepted and explored. Looking for the positive in clients and not being stingy with supportive, albeit genuine statements can be particularly helpful for those who see themselves as all bad. Observations or interpretations that link the client's current views of him- or herself and others with his or her past relationships or that unveil the process between the client and therapist, can be ways of accepting and fostering the return of banished parts of the self. Each of these communicates that the therapist can accept and tolerate whatever clients bring into the therapy relationship, that the space between therapist and client is not only a place in which clients can address and develop those parts of themselves they are reticent for others to see, but also a place in which the totality of the client can safely and effectively meet the totality of the therapist.

More often, though, acceptance in object relations therapy does not happen through codifiable techniques, but rather through specific verbal and nonverbal exchanges in the therapeutic relationship. This makes sense considering that most psychological struggles are problems of object relationships, so acceptance likely serves as the strongest agent of change in the context of the therapeutic relationship. One example relates to the way in which therapists respond to their own failure. In ironic fashion, the disillusionment of one's client is an inevitable part of object relations therapy. This does not mean that object relations therapists purposefully fail or disappoint clients; quite the contrary, they attempt to show warmth and empathy in meeting the unmet relational needs of their clients, and they attempt to avoid therapeutic mistakes. However, in the same way that caregivers' invariable disappointment of their children potentiates their children's acceptance of their complete selves and others, object relations therapists do not avoid the disillusionment of clients. They do not strive for an illusion of perfection and can accept clients' potentially difficult feelings about their therapeutic failures and betrayals. To wholeheartedly avoid clients' rage, perceived rejection, and guilt in response to one's therapeutic imperfections might risk keeping clients in a symbiotic phase of omnipotence or perpetuate a fragmented internal world in which certain aspects of the client are disowned. In short, this would be antithetical to acceptance because avoiding one's own reality fails the client in accepting his or her own internal reality and the reality of the external world (Parker, 2008).

In contrast, when clients' responses to the failure of therapist are met with acceptance and nondefensiveness, clients can better bridge the gap between their good and shameful parts, as well as better determine how to meet their internal needs in an imperfect world. Seeing the same therapist who at one time attends to a client's needs and at another time forgets an important event in the client's life allows the client to accept him- or herself as the same individual who gets excited or disappointed or feels strong or helpless. Therefore, the way in which object relations therapists respond to clients' disillusionment becomes a vehicle for clients' acceptance of their disconnected feelings and the development of a more realistic view of others. This is, however, predicated on the therapist's willingness to not avoid clients' disillusionment.

Case Study: Responding With Acceptance to Client Disillusionment

As an example, several years ago a college-age adolescent client of mine (Rogers) took the courageous step of disclosing about a history of sexual assault she had endured in a psychiatric treatment facility. Early in therapy, she had alluded to a traumatic event that facilitated her posttraumatic stress disorder, but she had been understandably reluctant to share about the nature of the trauma, particularly with another professional serving in the same field as the one that caused the trauma. When she finally risked sharing about the sexual assault, I sat with her tears in silence for a while and empathized with her pain, but I then made a marked clinical mistake. In my eagerness to help and normalize her reaction to the trauma, I tried to fill the silence by gently wondering about the details of what happened and even suggested a couple of possibilities about these details. Immediately after I posed this wonderment, I knew it had been a mistake. Although my intentions were to cultivate a safe environment for her to share, to know that any detail would be accepted, the question re-created a sense of violation in her, restripping her of power over the event. She left the session in silent anger and pain, despite my desperate apologies and feeble attempt to share the truth of my intentions.

After the session, I was afraid I would not see her again, but to my surprise, she returned the following week, saying, "The only reason I am back here is because I have no one else to talk to. If I had any shred of dignity and self-respect, I wouldn't be here. That's how pathetic I am." Then, getting visibly angry, she said,

> What were you thinking? At best, you are a social moron, and at worst, you are a sick bastard who enjoys hearing the details of sexual abuse. I even hate that you are probably thinking of some way of defending yourself, and even more, I hate that I gave you my feelings about what you did, because that gives you power, that gives you want you want.

Deciding to accept her anger rather than defend myself, I replied,

> Maybe there is no defense for what I did. Not only was it an inappropriate question, which does reflect social ignorance, but it was probably for my own needs, my own desire to help, that I asked it, which again re-created trauma and violation in you, without considering what you need and how you hurt. I am truly, truly sorry.

We were able to end the session with some repair of the relationship, and I offered her a second session that week, which she gratefully accepted. To be sure, her rapid response to my mistake might reflect damage from early object relationships that primed her for assault when it was not intended, but rather than offer such an intellectualized interpretation, it seemed better to accept her loss and anger as a way to facilitate (a) her own connection with her hurt and emptiness and (b) a realistic relationship that she might recall when others invariably fail her.

Acceptance in the Reception of Clients' Love

Another example of the way in which acceptance can be used in the therapeutic relationship is the reception of clients' love. Although recently highlighted by Skolnick (2006), this is one of the less commonly discussed aspects of acceptance in object relations therapy. In an attempt to reverse the classical psychoanalytic view of love as a sublimated expression of the drive for sex, Fairbairn (1952) instead argued that the need to establish and maintain loving connections is fundamental to human nature. Not only does the development of a healthy internal self-image and external relationships require the reception of love from others, but it also presumes the ability to express love, even if it is to ensure connection with others and one's own capacity for love. Developmentally, this implies that parents facilitate their children's maturation by loving them in accepting ways and unconditionally accepting their children's love. An example might be a young son who, getting ready for dinner, carefully looks through all his options of plates with animal designs on them and selects one for him and another for his mother. He is grateful that his mother provides him food for dinner, which is necessary for an internalized sense that he is worthy of love and that others can meet his needs, but if his mother elects not to use the plate that her son selected, even if it is under the guise that she wants to selflessly keep them for his later use, then she might inadvertently be rejecting his loving side. If this deficit in the embrace of a child's love reoccurs on several occasions, it can lead to a weakened sense of self-efficacy, a devaluation of ambitions and dreams, feelings of worthlessness, and difficulty believing in the loving intent of others (Skolnick, 2006).

For similar reasons, it seems equally important for therapists to accept their clients' expressions of love and care. This concept might be difficult for many clinicians who feel more comfortable in the role of giving than receiving, perhaps because of parentification, of needs for meaning that are fulfilled in service, or simply as the result of a paradigm of therapy in which any form of gift, including love, is discouraged on theoretical grounds. Yet many therapists have heard comments from clients such as, "I feel like you give so much to me, but I don't feel like I have given you anything." Other therapists have had a client bring them a cup of coffee, pay them a compliment, or express concern at a misfortune or joy in the therapist's research or writing outside of the office. In these moments, a significant danger might be overinterpreting or rejecting these offers, which could essentially collude with a tendency to split off the positive, loving, productive, and caring side of clients, thereby perpetuating fragmentation. To instead accept a client's love reinforces the message that all emotions and expressions are acceptable in the therapeutic space, allowing the client to also become more whole in his or her own ability to give and receive love from him- or herself and others. As Skolnick (2006) so aptly stated, therapists need to "climb into the heavens with our patients' positive feelings, just as we dove into the mud of their negative feelings" (p. 17).

Acceptance of Client Projective Identification

A final example of how object relations therapists engender and communicate acceptance is in the way they handle projective identification. As with the concept of repression in Freud's classic psychoanalytic tradition, projective identification keeps unacceptable thoughts, feelings, and impulses expunged from the self. It seems to particularly unfold in a three-stage process. First, unacceptable impulses are split off and projected onto another. Then the projecting individual pressures the recipient to feel the disowned impulses and behave consistently with the projected fantasy. Finally, the recipient responds to the feelings and responses that have been induced, reacting to the projecting person as though the recipient owns the projection. Put more simply, it involves another person becoming the repository for the feelings and inner representations of the individual doing the projection (Cashdan, 1988), so the receiving individual feels pressured to think, act, and feel consistent with the projected self- and other representations.

A projective identification of sexuality might serve as a good example. Driven by the need to establish and sustain relationships through sexual venues, some clients attempt to induce an erotic response in others, perhaps out of fear that the relationship would dissipate in the absence of sexuality. To illustrate, a highly attractive college-age adolescent female client of mine (Rogers) had a tendency to become quickly sexual with most men she met. She was unusually flirtatious, dressed suggestively, and often went home with men she had met that same evening. In itself, this sexual expression is not unusual or necessarily troubling, except for the compulsive regularity with which it occurred. Even in our first session, she asked the question, "Do you trust yourself to stay on that side of the room?" Independent of comments such as these, I was highly attracted to her, but she was evoking sexuality and then responding to it in a quicker way than most individuals, as if ensuring that I remained attracted and connected to her.

In situations such as this, object relations therapists strive to accept these projections and gradually help clients reown the dissociated aspects. Often this means reframing the aim of the projective identification as having a positive rather than a negative purpose, linking it to past object relationships, and clarifying the legitimate reason why the client had to disown and project the dissociated element, such as protecting others, preserving self-esteem, or responding to family rules (Slipp, 1991). Presupposed within this process, however, is that the object relations therapist allows him- or herself to accept the project and emotionally respond to it. This does not equate to responding as though the projection is accurate. To yield to the projective identification without helping the client reintegrate it only confirms a client's fantasy and fears (Cashdan, 1988).

An analogous concept might be object usage, in which the client does not relate to the therapist as a projection of his or her internal fantasies but rather recognizes the therapist as an object other than the client's own projections, with his or her own right to desires and needs, but who can still help the client (Parker, 2008). Just as a caregiver's survival of a child's projections launches the child into a more realistic and objective relationship with the caregiver, so too can a client experience a new relationship with her- or himself and the therapist after seeing the therapist tolerate and withstand the disowned elements. According to Parker (2008), this new relationship is one of being able to use others in a healthy fashion for mutual satisfaction of needs, which essentially means recognizing them as more than projections.

Case Study: Acceptance of Client Projection of Sexuality

In the case of the previously mentioned client, this process took shape through the acceptance of her projection of sexuality, namely, feeling and affirming the intended sexual arousal, then exploring the role of sexuality in her early object relationships, and finally wondering how men's sexual interest served an important purpose for her. Through this process, she came to recognize how her attractiveness and worth to men were centrally located in her ability to create sexual interest. Her father's unfiltered and age-inappropriate discussions about his own sexual fantasies contributed to her assumption that inciting his sexual arousal and interest was the primary way to attain his love and attention. Fortunately, as she progressed in therapy, the appearance of a new relationship with men quietly emerged, perhaps most cogently captured in one therapeutic exchange.

During this particular session, she mentioned that she had gone to a bar the previous evening, but then went home with a man with whom she became more physical than she was comfortable. Sexual intercourse was a boundary she refused to let men cross, so they did not have sex, but she felt as though he distinctly objectified her. Disregarding her objections, he asked her to take off her clothes and stand in front of him naked and then stimulate him to orgasm. After relaying this, she looked down and asked, "Are you upset at me?" This type of question was distinctly new. In much earlier sessions, she might have relayed a similar story with intent to incite my sexual arousal or even jealousy, but she never asked about feelings other than sexual interest in her. I genuinely responded, perhaps with some incredulity, "How could I be upset with *you?*" "Well, I feel like you could be disappointed in me for doing this." Surprised, I countered, "No, I'm actually angry at this guy and sad for you." She responded,

> Really? That's a completely different reaction than I anticipated. This surprises me because very few men in my life care about what I feel, about those things that hurt me. Your anger toward him and sadness for me is new. My dad never wanted to protect me from boys who stopped by the house. He never even asked me to keep my bedroom door open when I had boyfriends over. I guess I never knew if he cared about protecting me from them.

Granted, she was likely still viewing me in a paternal role, but I hope my response was a corrective paternal exchange that yearned to protect and help her recover her sexuality. Had she felt uncomfortable initially projecting her sexuality, and had I been unwilling to accept it for months and then gradually explore its meaning, she might not have been able to internalize her own sexuality and see others as more than her own projections. Because someone accepted her experiences and emotions in a way that early caregivers could not, she could experience a more integrated self and a more balanced view of men as not just sexual but self-controlled, loving, and valuing her boundaries.

Acceptance as an Explicit Spiritual Intervention in Object Relations Therapy

Not unlike prayer, meditation, or the use of holy writings, acceptance may serve as a powerful and potent spiritual intervention in object relations therapy. This becomes most clear when considering how clients' spirituality is not immune to the processes involved in the formation of internalized self- and other representations. As Hall (2007) so cogently described, "Clients' spirituality is a manifestation of their deep structure of internalized relationships with emotionally significant others," so their subjective experiences of spiritual entities, such as God, Allah, or Buddha, "provide a mirror of their gut level experiences of early relationships" (p. 5). Put differently, one's early relationships are not only internalized in the form of schemas of oneself and others, but also as representations of God, the spiritual, or the divine. According to Ana-Maria Rizzuto (1979), a South American psychiatrist and psychoanalyst, people's concept and views of God and spirituality are constructed directly out of the mold of their early experiences with primary objects (i.e., principal caregivers). This suggests that clients unconsciously organize their relations with the sacred or spiritual in a way that corresponds with how they unconsciously organize their construction of others.

There is considerable empirical support for this idea that the quality of one's object relations determines the quality and nature of one's representations of the sacred (Hall, Brokaw, Edwards, & Pike, 1998). Adults with a history of secure attachments are likely to envision God as loving and accessible, whereas those with histories of avoidant attachments are most likely to describe themselves as agnostics and atheists (Kirkpatrick, 1999; Kirkpatrick & Shaver, 1992). Similarly, those who see God as offering providence but not closeness have parents who provided limitless material provision but little emotional connection (Gattis, Sorensen, & Lawrence, 2001). These God representations are not only formed out of one's internalized representations from childhood but are also continually transformed and reshaped as new experiences are incorporated into one's internal representations. The level of a client's object relations development therefore informs his or her spiritual representations.

If object relations theory is correct and clients' spirituality is formed in the crucible of their early relationships, then spirituality may also be a way to facilitate the development of more realistic, accurate, and healthy representations of self and others. According to Winnicott (1971), the third space of therapy may be a sacred space, an illusory space between the subjective and objective inner and outer realities out of which spirituality and religion emerge. It is not unlike the transitional space that exists between a child and caregiver, in which the child differentiates her- or himself from the caregiver, the *me* from the *not me*. In this role, therapy serves as a good-enough holding environment and place for experimentation and play in which the child or client can experience mixed emotions, relationships, and sensations, ideally coming to accept each of these with their good and bad qualities.

It is in this space that the therapist's acceptance of the client can facilitate both the spiritual's acceptance of the client and the client's ability to form a more mature relationship with the divine. In many cases, the experience of having disowned and undesirable parts accepted by a spiritual entity can exceed the weight of the therapist's acceptance. Moreover, the therapist's acceptance and the acceptance of a spiritual entity also engender a new relationship with the divine, in which new and previously unseen dimensions of the holy or spiritual, be they grace or disappointment or hurt, are appreciated. This often happens through a process of disillusionment with the spiritual, similar to the failures created by the caregiver and the therapist. In the same way in which therapists do not retreat from the disillusionment of their clients, most spiritual systems assume some inevitable frustration of believers' needs, even if it is the by-product of living between the now and the not yet. Many new converts to spiritual systems experience a symbiotic closeness with their spirituality or divine entity, but much as the necessary disillusionment that occurs in children, almost all believers will experience distance and dissatisfaction with their spirituality (Parker, 2008). In many spiritual systems, this distance and disappointment are necessary so that God, Allah, or Buddha is experienced as real. Disillusionment is an agonist for believers to distinguish reality from fantasy, the latter being the unceasing fulfillment of their needs by a spiritual entity (Parker, 2008). As clients experience God or their spirituality's acceptance of their resulting disappointment, anger, and fear, they not only come to accept these elements in themselves and thereby become more real themselves, but they also allow their spirituality to become more whole and real, rather than a fantasy. In Buddhist terms, when Buddha accepts and survives clients' fantasies and projections (good and bad), the Buddha is allowed to be who the Buddha truly is, and the reality of the clients is able to relate to the wholeness and reality of the Buddha (Parker, 2008).

This stronger relationship with oneself and the spiritual is predicated, though, on the therapist's acceptance of the client. This initial acceptance, which likely represents a repair of an initial failure of acceptance, helps the client own difficult elements and encounter the reality of the therapist. In turn, this allows the client to experience acceptance by the spiritual, rather than the feared destruction, which grants the spiritual a freedom to be independent and exactly what it is. In the process, a new internal landscape is also carved out in the client, in which the client can experience him- or herself more fully, without fantasy. The acceptance of the therapist, therefore, creates a transitional psychic space, not only in which older representations of the self and others are replaced with more accurate and whole representations, but also in which the sacred is encountered in a way that enables clients to more fully relate with themselves and their spirituality (Burns-Smith, 1999).

For those object relations therapists who are spirituality minded, one of the direct implications of this is that their acceptance should also extend to clients' spiritual doubts and uncertainties. Acceptance of clients' spiritual skepticisms or misgivings might not seem like a particularly spiritual intervention, especially if it results in the abandonment of the spiritual system. According to object relations theory, however, the need for immutable truths is part of the symbiotic fiction, based on the idea that complexity, ambivalence, and doubt threaten survival (Skolnick, 2006). Certainty and truths that demand absolute adherence are not only the anathema of acceptance, but the obliteration of doubt comes dangerously close to being the plaything of primitive defense mechanisms, such as splitting or projection. Therapists whose acceptance is not inclusive of these doubts and reservations risk perpetuating clients' disownership of difficult impulses and musings. They also risk hampering clients' ability to more fully relate to others and the divine. God and other spiritual entities only become real when they are not fantasies, yet unquestioning faith locks these entities in the realm of fantasy and splits off important aspects of oneself, so that individuals end up relating not to their reality but to their fantasized selves.

ACCEPTANCE WITHIN CHILD-CENTERED PSYCHOTHERAPY

In child-centered play therapy, as in object relations psychotherapy, the relationship is the agent for change. In understanding the relationship, acceptance is the core. What is acceptance? According to Landreth (2002), acceptance is unconditionally prizing the child, despite difficulties with behaviors or coping, as a unique growing human. The therapist has an unshakeable belief in the child's capability to find his or her own way. Axline (1969) posited that only in the environment of true acceptance is the child free to come out of the shadows and into the sun to direct behavior and ultimately experience selfhood. Landreth (2002) outlined acceptance as creating an atmosphere of all-encompassing trust with the child. The child will trust the therapist to the point at which he or she feels safe enough to reveal any part of the self without fear of criticism.

An important part of accepting a child is seeing the child as a person, not a person in waiting. There is no age of maturity at which a person is suddenly eligible for respect. The child-centered play therapist views the child as an individual who has inherently earned respect simply by being a fellow human. One way to respect a child is to meet the child where he or she is. This is why the playroom is so important. Play is a language that children use naturally to communicate and process their experiences (Landreth, 2002). The therapist does not expect a child, developmentally in a different place in life, to be capable of engaging in the same therapeutic procedures often used with adults. The play therapist meets the child in the child's world, using the child's language, and uses a playroom to facilitate the child's comfort and mutual respect. In the special playroom, the child is afforded the complete attention of the therapist, who notices the child's feelings, capabilities, needs, attributes, and even weaknesses, such as giving up.

Because the play therapist is accepting and attentive to the child's communications through play, the child is able to understand that the therapist is there to help. According to Landreth and Bratton (2006), in the therapist's being fully present with a child and communicating his or her understanding of the child's needs, wants, experiences, feelings, and so forth, the child becomes more open to healing through what Landreth called "the healing messages":

1. "I am here"—I am fully present. I will feel no need to evaluate once I really become part of the child's world—evaluation comes from objectivity, not empathy.
2. "I hear you"—I must allow you to be separate and different from me.
3. "I understand"—This message is communicated verbally and nonverbally through attending, reflection of feeling and content, and limit setting.
4. "I care"—if I communicate the first three, the fourth is automatic.

In my (LeAnne Steen's) experience, *acceptance* is the effect of accepting my own imperfections and allowing the child to share his or hers with me. The faith the therapist must convey in self, in child, and in human potential is strong and invaluable to the experience. The child who has given up on self, whose parents and teachers have resigned, defeated at the idea that this child is just different, experiences an almost constant sense of exasperation in relationships. A child-centered play therapist will recognize the strengths, self-control, ability, and even functionality of this child's way of being and trust the child to find his or her own way to the truth and a new way of being. Lessons are not learned, they are experienced. The play therapist offers the child the opportunity to experience, therefore offering the child the opportunity to grow.

Children are more emotional than they are cognitive. Their emotional memory will override how they feel about childhood (Campbell, 1977). A child who evokes exasperation in others will remember feeling confused, hurt, angry, and unimportant. He or she will not remember the details of the events or how others became exasperated by the child's behavior. This is an important feature of unconditional acceptance and positive regard. Until the child feels this from the therapist, the child will not be able to reflect and find another way of being. The stress of feeling hurt, angry, unimportant, and confused locks the child into a pattern of recycling the same behaviors, yearning for the acceptance of another in that cycle.

Acceptance as a Spiritual Intervention in Child-Centered Play Therapy

The child-centered play therapist is unique in that he or she must trust in self, in the universe, and in humanity that the child is the best determiner of his or her own personal reality (Landreth, 2002). Landreth (2002) also suggested that psychotherapists must have an unshakeable belief in the child's ability to find his or her own way. This is easy when the child is exhibiting mild adjustment issues and possibly acting out. This trust in and complete acceptance of a child who is having major adjustment problems, exhibiting oppositional defiant disorder typology, and possibly even prone to violence is much more difficult.

Axline (1947/1989) outlined eight guiding principles to help the play therapist develop an atmosphere of unconditional positive regard and a facilitative relationship:

1. Establish rapport.
2. Accept the child completely.
3. Establish a feeling of permissiveness.
4. Recognition and reflection of feelings
5. Value of limits
6. Therapy cannot be hurried (Cannot be FORCED to bloom!).
7. The child leads the way.
8. Maintain respect for the child. (pp. 73–74)

Landreth (2002) discussed Rogers's (1951) 19 propositions and condensed them to provide a framework for conceptualizing play therapy, guiding the therapist to find acceptance and unconditional positive regard. According to Landreth, the play therapist views the child as

1. being the best determiner of personal reality,
2. behaving as an organized whole,
3. desiring to enhance the self,
4. goal directed in satisfying needs,
5. best able to perceive the self,
6. being able to be aware of the self,
7. valuing experiences,
8. interested in maintaining self-concept,
9. behaving in ways consistent with self-concept,
10. not owning behaviors inconsistent with self-concept,
11. experiencing psychological tension by admitting or not admitting certain experiences of self (Dissonance),
12. responding to threat by being behaviorally rigid,
13. willing to admit into awareness experiences inconsistent with self-concept if the self is free from threat,

14. being understood by others if a well-integrated self-concept exists, and
15. moving from self-defeating to self-sustaining values. (pp. 64–65)

In understanding how the therapist views the child and the tenets of child-centered play therapy theory, the meaning and value of acceptance are clear. For the therapist, releasing the belief that one has to help this child and allowing the child the space to find his or her own way is difficult, confusing, and sometimes painful. The acceptance of the therapist-self as good enough and the relationship as sufficient is imperative. It is a spiritual connection that allows one to do what one does—to trust the process.

Psychotherapy Implications of Acceptance

One of the most important implications of acceptance rests in the psychotherapist's ability to have faith in the child's inner healing process. The client-centered model of psychotherapy is strongly rooted in the belief that the client can achieve self-directed healing. Consequently, it is the psychotherapist's job to be the facilitator of this healing. When the client is a child, the therapist needs to be even more aware of his or her role as a facilitator, because only a child can truly be an expert at childhood (Landreth, 2002). Therefore, accepting the child in this model is not about accepting the child's limits, but instead accepting the fact that children have no limits. It is not therapists' job to go into the therapy room feeling as though they understand; instead, therapists need to humble themselves to recognize that they can never know all there is about childhood.

In a play therapy context, the psychotherapist seeks to create an environment of acceptance wherein the child is given the time he or she needs to discover and explore his or her own personality. As the child is able to achieve his or her own healing, the therapist never suggests that the child play other games or talk about more important topics. In fact, the psychotherapist takes every care to ensure that he or she does not discount the feelings and thoughts of the child. In this way, it is especially important that the therapist meet the child where the child is at and refrain from talking down to the child (Landreth, 2002). The psychotherapist's role is to help enable the child's journey without ever trying to guide or lead the child. To succeed in creating the therapeutic conditions for growth, two main aspects need to be considered: nonpossessive warmth and empathy. These two things work together to create an accepting environment in which a child can flourish.

Nonpossessive warmth is a large contributor to creating a healthy, successful relationship with the child. To do this, one must first show interest in getting to know the child as well as recognize that this feat can certainly not be done immediately. Throughout the therapist's relationship with a child, he or she is likely to be introduced to many different sides of the child's personality, and some of those personality traits might even be hard to deal with. However, nonpossessive warmth is a continual tool in that it is used despite the mood state the child might be in. Therefore, one accepts the child to the same degree when he or she is being moody and defiant as when he or she is being loving and well behaved (Landreth, 2002). If this show of warmth is continual, then the child gets the sense that he or she is accepted as a whole, not just in selected pieces.

Empathy is equally important, most especially in developing a trusting bond with the child. When the child feels his or her therapist's empathy, he or she recognizes and understands that the psychotherapist is meeting the child at his or her level. This allows the child the ultimate feeling of safety and acceptance. The empathy displayed by the psychotherapist needs to be all encompassing, especially in situations that deal with painful experiences and emotions. If the child does not feel empathy and acceptance in these painful moments, then the child begins to feel that it is not acceptable to have these emotions (Landreth, 2002). Therefore, empathy should be used when walking in the child's shoes and teaching the child that whatever he or she feels is legitimate.

Role of Limit Setting in Communicating Acceptance of a Child

Acceptance is of the person of the child, not always the behavior of the child. In child-centered play therapy, the psychotherapist is always aware of conveying acceptance of the child's feelings, regardless of behavior. Without this communication, the child will internalize from others that his or her feelings are wrong, which is again confusing. The few limits that do exist in the playroom are mostly around safety. Limits are not punitive, and limit setting is, in fact, therapeutic. In my (Steen's) opinion, there is no place in child-centered play therapy and theory in which acceptance is more important than in limit setting.

Limits are a reminder of the rule with an option for getting the child's needs met in a more appropriate form. For example, I tell children, "I am not for hitting in the playroom," even when a child is angry with me, but that they can hit the bop bag. Most children will follow a therapeutic limit when it is set appropriately. The accepting psychotherapist acknowledges the feeling, wish, want, or need, then expresses the limit and offers an alternate option. Because the child-centered play therapist is so focused on conveying acceptance of the feeling, wish, want, or need, the child is more capable of finding his or her own self-control and redirecting his or her own behavior. According to Landreth (2002), psychotherapists need to provide children with experiences, not answers. This experience of self-control by children is an opportunity afforded in the playroom, not easily found in many of their other experiences.

In the playroom, the child is free to choose how to use the time, and limits are minimal. The psychotherapist facilitates a feeling of permissiveness and freedom. The therapist must let go of his or her own preconceived ideas, allowing the psychotherapy to unfold. I had a child create what looked like a spider's web out of scotch tape one time. He was delighted that he could use all of the tape and create what he wanted with it. Many times, children are not allowed that much freedom in their play. It would be wasteful and must not be done. In the special playroom, the child can use all the supplies. This is done so that the therapist does not have to set unnecessary limits.

Personal Therapist Attributes That Facilitate Children's Acceptance of Themselves

Engaging in play therapy is like going on an adventure with the child. One does not guide the child through the obstacles, but instead becomes the child's companion. A psychotherapist is committed to journeying with the child wherever the path goes, whether it leads to joyful, sunny places or dark, scary destinations. A therapist will be present in all moments of this journey. Although there are many important attributes to develop if one wants to become a play therapist, there is perhaps none so important as a personal delight in the experiential world of children and the children themselves. Acceptance is not merely a therapeutic tool, but a way of life. If the love of children is not present, then the acceptance can never truly be genuine. This is especially important considering that play therapists, Landreth (2002) in particular, have felt that the most important thing that therapists have to offer in the therapeutic process is themselves. A psychotherapist can be trained to use skills and techniques, but, really, the fact that a therapist is a person who wants to engage his or her heart and be present with another person is the greatest gift one can give.

Before one can extend acceptance to others, one must first accept oneself. Therefore, among the most important attributes that one can have as a play therapist are self-awareness and self-understanding. Children are excellent models of this because they accept others unconditionally, never considering that others should earn this acceptance. Thus, the first step to achieving this self-awareness is recognizing that it can never be just a therapeutic technique, but an ideology that must infiltrate one's entire life. One must first accept that the psychotherapist is a human being with thoughts and feelings of his or her own. Therefore, therapists need to be cognizant that these emotions and thoughts can affect their relationship with the child in both positive and negative ways. It is the psychotherapist's job to understand the motives behind their feelings and to be willing to express them when appropriate. This is especially important when the therapist is dealing with negative emotions or his or her own weaknesses. There is no room for pride in the therapy room, and the psychotherapist must continually humble him- or herself to ensure that these negative feelings do not affect the play therapy in harmful ways. However, there should not be an intense dwelling on the negative. The psychotherapist should always seek to recognize his or her own continuous development and accept personal imperfections (Landreth, 2002). In that sense, a strong sense of forgiveness is necessary. It is never expected that any human, therapist or not, should be perfect.

Another invaluable trait for the play therapist to have is the ability to be truly present in the moment. The play therapist never assumes that his or her mere physical presence is enough for the child. Instead, the therapist seeks to be fully present with the child in all areas, paying attention to their thoughts, feelings, and actions without distraction. There is some flexibility inherent in this process, because the therapist has to accept and adapt with an attitude of willingness. There is never an attempt by the psychotherapist to impose conforming behavior on the child. Acceptance is a continual, in-the-moment process, and the therapist must always be openminded to where the child wants to lead. This openmindedness comes when one lets go of one's own views of reality and enters the child's reality. This process must be accompanied by a high tolerance of ambiguity because the child needs to be the guide (Landreth, 2002).

Case Study: Acceptance in Child-Centered Play Therapy

In this section, I present a child-centered play therapy case involving a 7-year-old boy named Franco, adopted at age 6 months from Central America by White parents. This case has been deidentified to protect the client's confidentiality. Franco's parents were concerned that he might have attachment issues, and they knew very little about his biological parents. He was in an orphanage when they adopted him, and according to his pediatrician, he had been malnourished in infancy before his parents gave him to the orphanage for better care. He appeared in my playroom to be a happy boy, easy to engage and talkative. I felt a deep connection with him immediately, as though I knew his soul, and I could sense that he was highly intuitive. At the time, I was recovering from the loss of my own infant, who had died shortly after birth 1 year earlier (my daughter was a twin, and her twin survived the birth). His fantasy play was very intense, and he lost no time getting right into it. So there we were, in our first session together, and he was being my doctor. He was sitting very close to me, in front of me, and he was checking my eyes, ears, and throat. Suddenly he said, "Did your baby die?" I was stunned, and immediately felt my hands go cold. I found a whisper and said, "Do you want me to say yes, or no?" "Yes," he said. So I said, "Yes, doctor, my baby died." "That's OK, you can still see her." I felt my own emotions begin to rise, and I felt a spiritual connection to this child, even deeper than that I had felt before. I wondered whether God was sending me a message, and I struggled to maintain a connection to this child that was not around my own pain. I realized, even in that moment, that something very special, something spiritual, had just happened in this new relationship. Somehow, this child connected to the one thing I was trying to push away.

As we continued our time together, I began to work with his father more. His father had problems with acceptance. What I mean by this is that he had problems with patience that the child experienced as a lack of acceptance. This child, being intuitive, was particularly capable of pushing a few buttons with his parents. His father often engaged in minor power struggles and felt disrespected. Acceptance and trust in the individual's ability to find his or her own way is the keystone of a child-centered play therapist's work. I began teaching the father how to have play sessions at home with his child and how to use the play times to practice acceptance and unconditional positive regard. In the sessions, the child asked whether we could invite his father into the play sessions, so we did. I was happy because the father and I could take turns responding to Franco, and I could coach and model the unconditional responses in the live sessions.

Franco began to play out the power struggles he had experienced in his family. He asked me to be a tornado (I waved my arms around in the air and made wind sounds), and he would come close to the tornado and get caught inside. Then he would call for his father, who would come and try to pull him from the tornado. I would pull back, and a power struggle would ensue before the tornado would give in and Franco would be returned safely to his father. This play was repeated within sessions and between sessions for months. I believe that Franco was communicating his need to be accepted by his father and also communicating the chaos he felt inside when he perceived his father to be incapable of acceptance. Luckily, his father was able to receive the communication that was coming through. Their relationship grew tremendously. When they terminated therapy, in the final session we had all together, the child set up the tornado theme again. This time, he was not trying to communicate something to his father; rather, he wanted to revisit something that he had done months earlier. The feel of the tornado and the power struggle was completely different. The child was playful and giddy, joking and laughing with his father. He also chose to get out of the tornado one time without the help of his father. It was clear that he was on the right path in his journey to healing and that acceptance from me, from his father, and ultimately of himself had brought him to a new place.

CONCLUSION

In this chapter, we have described acceptance of the client as an intervention that is both therapeutic and inherently spiritual. Throughout our discussion, we have demonstrated that acceptance functions in slightly different ways depending on the theoretical orientation of the psychotherapist. Inveterate questions about acceptance still remain, such as where acceptance stands on the continuum from resignation and tolerance to experiencing private events free of entanglement and regulation (Block-Lerner, Wulfert, & Moses, 2009). Most likely, pursuit of either extreme is problematic. Acceptance of difficult parts of oneself does not eclipse the value of trying to improve oneself, nor does acceptance of the reality of others obviate the hope or yearning for a stronger relationship with others. Neither is there an assumption that complete and unconditional acceptance is entirely possible. Such types of questions about the most suitable form or expression of acceptance, including whether it should also be followed by forgiveness, are highly important, but they risk overshadowing the simple value of acceptance in therapy. The power and potency of acceptance as a spiritual intervention should not be dismissed or overlooked, however simplistic and self-evident it seems.

REFERENCES

Axline, V. (1989). *Play therapy*. London, England: Ballantine. (Original work published 1947)

Block-Lerner, J., Wulfert, E., & Moses, E. (2009). ACT in context: An exploration of experiential acceptance. *Cognitive and Behavioral Practice, 16*, 443–456. doi:10.1016/j.cbpra.2009.04.005

Burns-Smith, C. (1999). Theology and Winnicott's object relations theory: A conversation. *Journal of Psychology and Theology, 27*, 3–19.

Campbell, R. (1977). *How to really love your child*. New York, NY: Penguin.

Cashdan, S. (1988). *Object relations therapy: Using the relationship*. New York, NY: Norton.

Fairbairn, W. R. D. (1952). *Psychoanalytical studies of the personality*. London, England: Routledge & Kegan Paul.

Fairbairn, W. R. D. (1954). Object-relationships and dynamic structure. In *An object-relations theory of the personality* (pp. 137–161). New York: Basic Books. (Original work published 1946)

Fairbairn, W. R. D. (1958). On the nature and aims of psycho-analytical treatment. *International Journal of Psycho-Analysis, 39*, 374–385.

Gattis, J., Sorensen, R. L., & Lawrence, R. (2001, August). *A free, web-based scoring program for the Lawrence God Image Inventory*. Presented at the 109th Annual Convention of the American Psychological Association, San Francisco, CA.

Gehrie, M. J. (2011). From archaic narcissism to empathy for the self: The evolution of new capacities in psychoanalysis. *Journal of the American Psychoanalytic Association, 59*, 313–334. doi:10.1177/0003065111406270

Hall, T. W. (2007). Psychoanalysis, attachment, and spirituality, Part 1: The emergence of two relational traditions. *Journal of Psychology and Theology, 35*, 14–28.

Hall, T. W., Brokaw, B. F., Edwards, K. J., & Pike, P. L. (1998). An empirical exploration of psychoanalysis and religion: Spiritual maturity and object relations development. *Journal for the Scientific Study of Religion, 37*, 303–313. doi:10.2307/1387529

Kirkpatrick, L. A. (1999). Attachment and religious representations and behavior. In J. Cassidy & P. Shaver (Eds.), *Handbook of attachment* (pp. 803–822). New York, NY: Guilford Press.

Kirkpatrick, L. A., & Shaver, P. R. (1992). An attachment-theoretical approach to romantic love and religious belief. *Personality and Social Psychology Bulletin, 18*, 266–275. doi:10.1177/0146167292183002

Landreth, G. (2002). *Play therapy: The art of the relationship*. New York, NY: Routledge.

Landreth, G., & Bratton, S. (2006). *Child parent relationship therapy (CPRT): A 10-session filial model*. New York, NY: Routledge.

Mahler, M. S., Pine, F., & Bergman, A. (1975). *The psychological birth of the human infant*. New York, NY: Basic Books.

McDargh, J. (1983). *Psychoanalytic object relations theory and the study of religion: On faith and the imaging of God*. Washington, DC: University Press of America.

Parker, S. (2008). Winnicott's object relations theory and the work of the Holy Spirit. *Journal of Psychology and Theology, 36*, 285–293.

Rizzuto, A. (1979). *The birth of a living God*. Chicago, IL: University of Chicago Press.

Rogers, C. R. (1951). *Client-centered therapy: Its current practice, implications, and theory*. Boston, MA: Houghton Mifflin.

Skolnick, N. J. (2006). What's a good object to do? *Psychoanalytic Dialogues, 16*, 1–27.

Slipp, S. (1991). *The technique and practice of object relations family therapy*. Northvale, NJ: Jason Aronson.

Wenar, C., & Kerig, P. (2000). *Developmental psychopathology: From infancy through adolescence* (4th ed.). New York, NY: McGraw-Hill.

Winnicott, D. W. (1971). *Playing and reality*. New York, NY: Basic Books.

Winnicott, D. W. (1988). *Human nature*. New York, NY: Schocken Books.

6

SPIRITUAL AWARENESS PSYCHOTHERAPY WITH CHILDREN AND ADOLESCENTS

LISA MILLER

Spiritual awareness psychotherapy (SAP; American Psychological Association, 2005) holds that the human journey is to evolve by finding harmony with the universe. Human purpose, health, and wholeness are derived by drawing into alignment with the universe, the great teleological force of life that is true, teaching, and healing. SAP with a child and family relies on the greater awareness youths have of the universe, such that listening to the child guides the family toward alignment. Adolescents, who are often in a phase of spiritual awakening as part of a deep individuation, can be supported in treatment to find harmony by relying on the direct wisdom that they receive.

In this chapter, I describe the use of SAP with children and adolescents. First, I provide a theoretical overview of this type of psychotherapy. Next, I discuss a developmentally sensitive application of the therapy. Each section includes two clinical case studies illustrating the use of this approach with both a child and a teenager. I conclude the chapter with some thoughts on the future of SAP with children and adolescents.

DOI: 10.1037/13947-007
Spiritual Interventions in Child and Adolescent Psychotherapy, D. F. Walker and W. L. Hathaway (Editors)

The primary assumption of SAP is the spiritual dialectic: We are in dialogue with a living universe, of which we are emanations. This assumption is a radical departure from the normative stance of 20th-century mainstream psychotherapy, marked in its formulation by ontological silence and generally taught and practiced from an assumptive stance of secular materialism. For instance, cognitive–behavioral therapy (CBT) is silent on ontological assumptions surrounding healing and mental illness or wellness. Although the point may rarely gain reflection by cognitive–behavioral psychotherapists, CBT can be and actually has been conducted from a broad range of ontologies, including a secular–materialist or spiritual perspective. CBT as practiced generally mirrors the personal ontology of the psychotherapist. This means, in a field of much secular materialism, marked by individualism, that treatment often buttresses the ego dimensions of self as being "better," more worthy, more appealing than the client's depressive self-cognition. This psychotherapeutic tact misses an opportunity for personal evolution. The notion of the self as given to a sacred calling or as designed to find the spiritual path as part of a great purposeful universe does not enter into the view of suffering, awareness, or healing.

These mainstream psychotherapies hold that we make meaning from an inert universe—lessons come from our construction, post hoc, of random or untoward events. In the past decade, however, we have entered an era of postmaterialism (Miller, 2010) in which spiritual reality is increasingly viewed as ontologically real (Sperry, 2011). Sperry (2011) elegantly offered conceptualization of and treatment formulations for understanding Axis II mental illness as occluding and distorting our spiritual awareness. At the very least, over this past decade psychotherapists have once again become accountable for understanding their ontological assumptions, and clients can gain this clarity in their work with a psychotherapist.

A strong and explicit ontological view shapes SAP in its assumptions, frame, process, and therapeutic stance. The central five principles of SAP are:

1. The universe is alive, loving, and guiding—every bit of the universe.
2. We are in dialogue with the universe, which brings us toward greater alignment with the nature of the universe, which is our nature. The dialogue helps us evolve toward living the spiritual axioms of the universe.
3. We hear the guiding universe through inner and outer experience: outer experiences such as synchronicities, messengers, and relationships and inner experiences of dreams and an imagina-

tion that detects, as well as constructs, and is divinely inspired. The continuousness of inner and outer experiences, such as that of a premonition, visitation, or awareness of an external event in answer to an internal question, reveals the oneness of the universe beyond the boundaries of atomistic human being.

4. We are made out of the same sacred stuff as the great universe that is in us, through us, and around us.
5. The spiritual clock always runs, but it is most apparent at the edges of birth, life chapter transformation, and death.

SAP as a postmaterialist psychotherapy is heavily informed by the principles of Carl Jung (see Jung & Hall, 1981, for a review of Jung's work). SAP, as with Jungian analysis, views our dialogue with the universe as transformative, guiding, and individually honed toward the next step in our evolution. Jung's conviction regarding archetypal changes associated with development, such as awakening in adolescence and the second half of life, also informs SAP in its emphasis on spiritual chapters in the human life. That the universe carries axioms with which we harmonize through spiritual growth is a linchpin of SAP consistent with Scott Richards and Allen Bergin's (2003) conceptualization of the spirit of truth, which they conceived of as a set of absolute laws in living that inherently bring forward wellness (forgiveness, commitment, family).

The need for awareness and honoring of universal spiritual principles as axiomatic to health became clear to me in working with a broad range of people in New York. The suffering we create for ourselves and others consistently struck me as emanating from our blindness to spiritual principles. Spiritual principles are readily learned, if not already known, through direct experience and can be stated within and outside of religion. Spiritual principles include allowing each person to walk his or her spiritual path, which includes maintaining commitments versus a chase for hedonism and happiness, and being committed to right action and livelihood while surpassing illusions of ego control. These values are not selfless; they very much support the self as living within an ontological reality of connectedness and oneness. In an epidemic of cultural narcissism, psychotherapy has been inured to overfeeding and overauthorizing ego unchecked by spirit. I have seen basically good people become solipsistic and insufferably self-serving through years of a misguided psychoanalysis in which their own passing feelings were viewed as objects in themselves to be honored rather than as indicators of how they were doing as spiritual and moral beings. I have seen survivors of abuse reach out to the universe and find sustenance and awareness of the sacredness and preciousness of life. How we value the spiritual laws of the universe determines how we treat ourselves and others.

The therapeutic frame of SAP hinges on an ontological spiritual reality—it holds that the universe will do the healing if we listen and let it into the room to guide the process. This process relies on a psychotherapist who is present in the living universe—whose own inner compass aligns with the spirit for direction, not one who merely views spirituality as the client's belief (Miller, 2008). The process of SAP honors the universe as our guide; we attend to the universe, listen, and honor the direction that comes. In SAP, the psychotherapist is a fellow journeyer who offers his or her own direct experience as it emerges in relation to the client's experience, as would be expected from a postmaterialist view in which therapist and client have a shared field of intention. The psychotherapist is a lookout, something of a Sherpa who knows how to climb mountains but is not a great sage. In SAP, the psychotherapist does not present him- or herself as a spiritual teacher because the teacher is within the client and everywhere without. The transparency with which the psychotherapist works, and his or her collaborative stance with the client as one of equals in awe of the universe, can resemble that of practical current-day short-term psychotherapy. In the widespread interpersonal psychotherapy or CBT, for instance, the therapeutic stance is for the psychotherapist to show everything he or she knows and to help the client become his or her own therapist. The SAP psychotherapist does not know where treatment will go and would be unlikely to make a treatment plan. Rather, the SAP psychotherapist acts much as the Native American guide Sacajawea did with Lewis and Clark as they traveled through new terrain. Psychotherapist and client are equally in awe. Connected by a shared field of love and intention, both revere, and are often surprised by, the specific gifts and guidance of the universe.

The notion of a guiding universe makes sense to many people and carries a clear theistic understanding. The language within psychotherapy hinges on that of the client. Some clients prefer to speak of the Creator, higher power, Jesus, or God, all of which I honor. All these terms show an intentional loving universe.

RELATIONSHIPS IN SPIRITUAL AWARENESS PSYCHOTHERAPY

SAP allows the universe to more fully inform our life choices and hoist us along our journey toward growth and healing. Spiritual guidance does not come directly from the therapist but through attunement with the universe, if we remind ourselves to pay attention and revere the sacredness in life. In the sacred theater, the cues are loud if we listen. Very often, the message comes through our relationships, most commonly from people close to us, such as family.

SAP may be seen as an interpersonal approach in which relationships are spiritual instantiations, replete with purpose. We each express the Creator, and our paths cross for a crucial reason in our spiritual development. Appreciation of the purposefulness and significance of relationships comes into focus through a few central notions:

1. Relationships are sacred vehicles for spiritual evolution and reveal spiritual truths. Our work in relationships allows us to evolve spiritually. We learn love, compassion, forgiveness, justice, and many spiritual truths through loving each other in relationships. Relationships are as central to our spiritual path as other forms of spiritual work, such as individual or private contemplation and retreat.
2. All relationships are divine. The sacred clock runs every instant. We come together in relationship, a gift of the Creator. The gift is given in love and is a guided process. Just as we are created by the Divine, so too are our relationships an expression of the Creator. This does not mean that it will be easy to get along: Some relationships can be extremely full of challenges. Nobody we pass on the street, share a bus ride with, marry, debate at work, or love crosses our path without transforming us, nor do they appear accidentally. The right people come at the right time. All relationships transform us, even if we realize this in memory years later.
3. Developmental windows, such as parenthood, adolescence, and childhood bring spiritual opportunity. Similarly, dyadic and communal relationships have developmental windows, to include parenthood or grandparenthood, later adulthood's generativity toward the collective, or young adulthood's path toward spiritual awakening. New sensibilities and unexplored psychospiritual territory come forward with the advent of each developmental passage.
4. Spiritual awareness heightens around the edges of and inflection points in relationships, including birth, death, illness, crisis, and points of epiphany or trauma. Clarity regarding our fundamental spiritual nature emerges, giving us access to the prominence of spiritual reality.

SAP and its conceptual underpinnings and technique have been described at length and demonstrated with an adult case documented by the American Psychological Association (2005). In this chapter, I focus on SAP as brought to the developmental phases of childhood and adolescence.

Spiritual Awareness Psychotherapy With Young or School-Age Children and Families

Many children, particularly young children through preadolescents, come to treatment at the behest of their families or school counselors. Children tend to be carriers of the family condition, often holding within them some level of family crisis. The family is the context that permeates the feelings and state of the child. In SAP, the child is viewed as particularly prescient of the family's diagnosis because the child most acutely expresses the discordance of parental attunement to the universe.

Beyond being self-evident, the inherent spiritual attunement of the child has been shown in psychological and genetic research (Boyatzis, in press; Kendler, Gardner, & Prescott, 1997). The child is closest to the source of truth emanating most directly from the wise universe. If the child is ill, entangled, or distorted, it is as truth pushes against falsehood or error.

Beyond matters of physical and emotional safety, the crisis, most fundamentally, is a spiritual opportunity for everyone in the room, including the psychotherapist. Psychotherapists can host the regenerative process by acknowledging the guiding spiritual presence that has sustained the family in the past and precipitated the crisis and note such a great presence in bringing the family in search of healing through treatment. From the initial treatment session, the psychotherapist can acknowledge that the family in crisis may find a new and better direction than previously imagined. A letting go of the family's previous expectations may host a deeper, more satisfying situation.

The healing of the child and the family can be introduced as an act of sacred creation for the family, in that a new family life can be discovered through crisis. As in any psychotherapy, narrative accounts of positive family transformation help more than cosmology. Central to supporting families in SAP are three spiritual perspectives on the relationship of parents and child:

1. The child is closest to the source of creation, such that the child is the spiritual teacher for the family. The child's behavior, words, and style of coping are revelatory of the family challenge.
2. Parents have an opportunity to develop spiritually in tandem with their children. Childbirth is a reawakening to spirit for parents. Early childhood is, for parents, an opportunity to again be present to the sacredness in us, around us, and throughout the world. Adolescence is, for parents, a revisiting of meaning and purpose, along with a confrontation of good, evil, paradox, and hypocrisy. Any suffering of the child is a spiritual challenge to an exponentiated degree for the parent.

3. The parent is the spiritual ambassador for the child; parenting is a spiritual absolute—such as mercy, charity, or wisdom—for which divine guidance is offered by the universe. As the spiritual ambassador, the parent has the responsibility to support the child's direct spiritual wisdom and cultivate the child's awareness of the Creator.

The linchpin of SAP with families and children is to identify where the child is truth bearer. A child is inherently closer to the truth and naturally seeks alignment with the universe. The child will therefore show the incongruence between the axioms of the universe and the ego-based functioning and error of the environment. The child's suffering in play, actions, or even in his or her very body holds the truth; at other times, the child's words reveal the family struggle—a challenge that may result in a spiritual lesson if we follow the child.

To convey this process, I share the case of a family challenged by the spiritual lesson surrounding fear and grasping. The case has been deidentified for the purpose of sharing the family's key clinical points. Irrespective of material stability or security, it is often easier for parents to take the leap of faith to follow their own spiritual path than to freely allow their children to find their own spiritual path. I am often reminded of the biblical story of the sacrifice of Isaac (Genesis 22:5–14) because I see fear and grasping by well-intentioned parents who truly do love their children and strive to act in their interest.

Case Study: Spiritual Awareness Therapy With a Child

Rachel (age 32) and David (age 48) had a daughter, Sophie (age 8), who was the impetus for their family consultation. From a clinical perspective, David and Rachel both had a long history of affective disorders and related social struggles. David had a history of recurrent depression with a personality style that tended toward dominance in the relationship. Rachel recalled more than two decades of being dysthymic, with a history of double depression and a personality marked by passivity and dependence. David and Rachel were well educated and read a great deal. David was a well-compensated professional; Rachel focused on motherhood and did not work outside the home.

In terms of parent history, David, despite coming from a relatively close Jewish family, had strong emotional pain associated with his treatment by an abusive older brother. David experienced his brother as a bully who could strike at whim and destroy his world.

Rachel's parents were divorced, affluent, childlike, physically and emotionally unreliable, and absent. Neither parent offered Rachel the guidance and support she desired as a child. Her mother overtly brought home a string of sexual partners, several of whom she married over the course of four marriages. As a child, Rachel felt that home and her future were unsteady, and even the composition of her family was uncertain. She recalled that she often retreated to her childhood bedroom for comfort. Both David and Rachel had been in individual treatment sporadically for decades.

David and Rachel shared the developmental past of growing up in what felt like an unsafe world, despite plenty of material resources and personal and professional mastery. In their joint, shared marital space, the couple seemed surprisingly fearful about the future. This fear existed despite their ample intellectual, professional, and material resources.

Their daughter, Sophie, was born innately free of her parents' liability of lingering fear. At age 8, she was confident, joyful, and physically and mentally healthy. Sophie was well liked by friends and thrived socially among her classmates (although she presented as being more mature than her peers). She was verbally expressive and conversant with people of all ages. The presenting problem of "concerns about Sophie" intimated to me that Sophie might have become a magnet for her parents' anxiety about lacking safety in childhood and subsequent anxiety around events in the future.

I found it surprising, for instance, to hear David express concern that he could "see that when Sophie gets older, she may be taken advantage of by boys. She wants to please older men." Of even greater pressing concern was whether Sophie, currently in third grade, would eventually be admitted to the same Ivy League college attended by her parents. Against this prescient future point of focus, Sophie's childhood of the next decade had become merely the background.

David and Rachel feared that a potential impediment to Sophie's eventual college admission was that she might have an undiagnosed learning disability because her current academic skill level was roughly in the middle of her class. David and Rachel's final pressing concern was Sophie's potential to become overweight, because she was currently slightly less lean than her peers and did not like sports.

I wondered how Sophie experienced her parents' constant anxiety and worry. Although some of the family anxiety was expressed, some might be diffuse and hard to locate for a child. Had Sophie absorbed a general feeling of being a problem or flawed?

The pressing questions of how to manage Sophie consumed the couple, so much so that the first session was filled with unpressured speech and few pauses. It was well into the session when the couple mentioned the existence of a second child, younger than Sophie, about whom they did not yet have any worries.

Fear and grasping on behalf of our children is common, and it is usually mixed with love. Yet, the sway held over the child's daily lived reality by parentally owned issues makes an intervention worthwhile. In the case of Sophie, it became clear to me that the obsessive ruminations of her parents insidiously spawned the precise objects of their fear.

Sophie was confronted by failure at her parents' hands around academic success, normal peer interactions, and body weight. Sophie had been pulled out of relatively comparable schools twice in 3 years to find one good enough to meet her needs. Although her parents had explained to her that she had learning challenges, repeated testing had not confirmed this possibility. Parental fear laid true obstacles to the child's academic and social reality.

I felt concerned about Sophie's inner feeling of worthiness. So I invited Sophie to join her parents in the next session, during which we discussed how she experienced their involvement with her at home, in friendship, and in her academic work.

Sophie sat back and took in the room with a watchful eye. She seemed to have learned better than to jump head-first into her parents' discussions. My eyes were wide open: How had Sophie developed a way to live with the fearful, ego-based reality? What was Sophie's experience of her parents' fear and grasping? I continued to watch. Sophie's measured engagement seemed not to reveal social anxiety; she had a half-smile on her face, suggesting that our entire meeting carried irony. Then the clue: As her parents launched into their practiced concerns about her, 8-year-old Sophie *rolled her eyes*.

How fabulous! Therein was our opportunity for this process. Eye rolling did not appear to be a deliberate communication, nor an act of overt defiance, but a response to manage her inner life. Sophie already knew that the anxiety belonged to her parents, and she was throwing it back. I felt I could hear her heart say, "This mumbo jumbo is nuts." The potential of this psychotherapy was that Sophie might become a teacher for her parents, teaching them to be free and have faith beyond their usual fear, anxiety, and grasping at illusions of rescue from a deeper anxiety.

Sophie sensed the illusory nature of the anchors of academic performance and body weight against the tides of her parents' deeper anxiety. Could I help her parents to truly see that ironic smile, that Sophie's sense of humor revealed the more valid reality that Sophie was aligned with the true life force?

"Sophie, what do you most enjoy—what do you not like—about school?" I asked in front of her parents. Clear as a bell, she replied, "Art and music—and I love my music teacher. I sang in a musical, and I want to sing in musicals when I grow up." What Sophie did not enjoy was "memorizing spelling words and having to do worksheets all day."

I started to wonder what type of world might open for Sophie if her parents released their grasp. Could Sophie's parents come to see her, with her bright twinkle and ironic smile, unshrouded by their own projections and fears of elusive success and body weight?

In the next session, I shared with the parents that having met Sophie, I was impressed that she seemed full of joy, quite confident and self-possessed. She seemed rooted in her own sense of reality, not caught up in their concerns. They nodded and smiled. I then hit the point harder, asking them to consider what Sophie thought of their concerns for her. However, the parents seemed not to relate to the question. Then I felt compelled to invoke the powerful call of parents as ambassadors on the sacred journey. "The calling of parenthood is not just to make highly functional products, but to raise children who can walk the spiritual path, who are in tune with a sacred universe." They seemed surprised and a bit intrigued. It was nonetheless clear that the concept was not entirely foreign. The language was mine, not theirs, and the point penetrated because it was heartfelt, said in their best interest, and authentic and reflected a deeper reality that all people access. I shared with Rachel and David my impression that Sophie had a fabulous sense of irony, showing perspective like that of a very old woman. Then I left them with a question: "Have you noticed anything deep or wise about Sophie? Has she ever said something that struck you as spiritual?"

Over the next 2 weeks, Rachel and David started noticing more about Sophie and speaking of her in a broader way. They delighted in her passion in singing and raised the possibility that perhaps Sophie would someday go to Broadway instead of a law firm. Then came a sense that the parents were learning a spiritual lesson from Sophie. "You mentioned this sense of irony; we definitely do notice her irony. It's great. It's like she already sees it all, gets it all, and is above it all." Rachel smiled. David smiled. Then Rachel extended her insight: "Particularly when we [gesturing at David] are going on and on. It's like, 'chill, Mom and Dad, everything is fine.'"

Rachel and David were barely practicing, somewhat agnostic Jews. Three weeks later, they came back with a book, *The Blessing of a Skinned Knee*, written by psychologist Wendy Mogel, who writes out of the Jewish religious tradition. They explained, "We have talked about the idea that the job of a parent is to teach your child something more." Living with an awareness of something more was new to them. They considered, although still from something of a distance, a life that was not wrapped in fear and feelings of inadequacy, in which they did not chronically grasp the steering wheel with white knuckles. A world marked by a quest to control, an ego-based life, cracked and buckled under their feet. Their daughter, however, was given more freedom to live out her own birthright not choked by extreme ego control and fear.

Adolescents and Spiritual Awareness Psychotherapy

Adolescence marks a developmental window of spiritual awakening, as viewed through religious and cultural traditions around the world, including the Native American inipe and sun dance, Jewish bar and bat mitvah, confirmation in many Christian faiths, mission for the Latter-day Saints, and the trials of the African Kaluli. Within psychology, spiritual awakening has recently been understood as central to adolescent development (Roehlkepartain, King, Wagener, & Benson, 2006). From the viewpoint of clinical science, personal spirituality becomes far more robustly protective against depression and substance abuse in puberty (Miller & Gur, 2002) and is, more robustly than any other psychosocial variable, associated with well-being among adolescents (Kelley & Miller, 2007). In late adolescence, the influence of family wanes, and instead we augment our inherent genetic makeup with personal spirituality (Koenig, McGee, Krueger, & Bouchard, 2005). SAP embraces this developmental imperative of adolescents and focuses on validating and encouraging the emergence of direct spiritual knowing.

For many years, I have worked with adolescents in poverty, pregnant girls who are thrust from home to live with drug dealers, adolescents of depressed and previously abused parents, transgender boys on the streets of New York, and most recently, late adolescents in homeless shelters. I have found that under extreme stress adolescents can have extremely strong and clear spiritual access and a personal connection to the universe that guides them through and well beyond their current immediate circumstance. Adolescents benefit if their direct relationship with the universe is supported and validated, prioritized to become their guide through the perilous jungle of their social and emotional worlds. Work with the poorest adolescents highlights, naturally, a universal process of healing for adolescents in far less extreme circumstances.

For the past year, I have been working with my clinical research team at Covenant House of New York, a shelter for homeless youths. Covenant House helps provide food, shelter, or both to 3,000 homeless youths a year, and it is the largest homeless shelter for youths in New York City and in the country, with about 300 beds—New York's largest response to the cry of its more than 10,000 homeless youths. Of the youths (younger than age 21) who show up at Covenant House, the majority (more than 60%) are escaping physical or sexual abuse, 50% have witnessed extreme violence or murder, 30% to 40% abuse substances, 35% have aged out of foster care, and 40% were asked by their families to leave. Many of the girls have walked the streets with an infant or pregnant. The boys, too, have been abused and beaten and have fought and struggled to eat and to survive. These youths are less visible to the general public than the more familiar homeless adult. They are often passed on the street with no awareness of their struggles or their homelessness. Most of these adolescents are fundamentally healthy and resilient. Covenant House successfully helps many youths to build a very good life, rather than contacting society through mental hospitals and the justice system. Our work as psychologists is to support the teens' natural resilience and find ways to help them move forward, often with a new independent, adaptive, and unfamiliar way of living.

The dedicated leadership and staff of Covenant House show the energy, enthusiasm, commitment, and vision that comes from a strong sense of spiritual mission. They listen intently to the adolescents; they honor and respect each youth.

On my first day working at Covenant House's shelter for youths, Sharleen, a long-standing worker, pulled me aside and said, "You are a psychologist? You do know that we are *not* our stories." She repeated this point until she felt heard, enough times and with sufficient emphasis for me to remember and to contemplate the wisdom revealed through her direct experience with homeless youths.

In reflecting on my experience with youths over time, I have come to believe that Sharleen is right, for all adolescents—not exclusively the poorest but the most oppressed youths—show the way toward a deeper form of healing. The only way to move past the imprisonment of nearly global degradation, betrayal, and deceit in a young life is by strengthening a direct relationship with the Creator. A retrospective rehashing of oppression and abuse, reliving the road of painful trials without an immediate vision of opportunity, can further harm an emerging young adult in crisis. Rather, the ultimately dependable guide—greater and more true and reliable than humans, or perhaps from among the living or deceased of us humans, the one who has most taken up the sacred role of ambassador—is a sure guide.

In contrast to work with young children, SAP occurs in the context of individuation into early adulthood, focusing on inner empowerment and capacity building among youths. Severely oppressed youths often particularly benefit from an early individuation that allows them to escape from the danger of living under oppressive adults. By becoming young adults, they gain the power and opportunity to step up to adulthood ahead of the normative schedule. This takes, from a spiritual perspective, a sure and fast connection with the Creator, a loving and ultimately knowing source of guidance.

Sharleen's input confirmed my sense of working past the stories. Of primacy to the possibility of a different life lived off the streets and away from abuse is an adolescent's direct relationship with a loving guide. How might I help a youth who might not like religion connect with the loving guidance of the universe, higher power, the Creator? Traditionally, I had waited, when the urgency was less, for the sacred presence to emerge. For a youth in crisis, though, with whom there may be little time to work, this work needs to be encouraged and if possible accelerated.

As I held open this question in my heart—how might I contribute to the youths at Covenant House—the universe brought the opportunity to meet Dr. Gary Weaver, a psychologist in Utah whose work for decades has been with court-referred adolescent offenders with conduct disorder. Weaver has developed a method of encouraging direct dialogue with the Creator through spiritual visualization. His method was precisely the way in which to work with the poorest and most abused youths. Court-referred adolescents who have not benefited from rounds of traditional models of secular–materialistic psychotherapy and who now perpetrate abuse are sent to Weaver for help by the state court judge.

The universe proposed an opportunity for helping the youths with whom we work. Weaver flew to Columbia University to teach my clinical research team some of his methods. In his work with the offending adolescents, he often starts with a prayer: "Help me see your child the way that you do. Remove immediately our human judgment and sense of picking and choosing who is worthy of help." Creating a space of love and care for the spirit of the youths, Weaver guides them through spiritual visualization, such as the following:

> Imagine everyone assembled at a table who truly has your self-interest at heart. Ask them if they love you. Now put your eternal self at the table. Ask you if you love you. Now, put at the table your higher power. Ask your higher power if you are loved. Now, with all the people assembled there, ask them what right now, at this moment in your life, you need to know.

I have come to refer to Weaver's guidance as the *spiritual table* visualization. He has found that from this spiritual engagement with the universe, court-referred adolescents very often find a direct relationship with the Creator. Weaver's method uses the embodiment of love and spiritual guidance through the images of people, a view consistent with SAP, which holds that here-and-now relationships are a vehicle for spiritual guidance and growth.

In conducting SAP, I now teach my students to embrace Weaver's method of spiritually propelled dialogue through the inner presence in consciousness of meaningful people. In other words, people do not need to be present in body, but present in consciousness. Spiritual psychotherapy is predicated on a postmaterialist view of reality, in which the spiritual realm is ontologically real and operative.

Case Study: Spiritual Awareness Therapy With an Adolescent

Armondo was a nervous and withdrawn adolescent with a very painful history of trauma, drug addiction, and homelessness. I have deidentified this case study because of profound elements in Armondo's personal journey. From the age of 4, he recalled being tortured, burned with matches, and beaten when his stepfather came home drunk. He remembered knowing by the turn of key whether his stepfather would be on a rageful and violent streak. At age 7, Armondo started using alcohol and drugs. By age 11, he was using crack cocaine.

Armondo seemed quite intelligent and loved to read, although he did not like school. Growing up in a borough of New York City, he had a number of friends who led him into the music scene, and he wanted someday to be a rock musician.

Armondo claimed that when he lived on the streets, he never used his knife to harm another person but kept it in his hand as he slept to protect himself. He described feeling safer on the street than in his stepfather's home. However, he was beaten twice on the street and on occasion sold his body for food or small amounts of money to buy food.

One night, an outreach worker from a homeless shelter for youths approached Armondo, who had been sleeping under the Brooklyn Bridge with a sandwich and a card showing the address of the shelter. Armondo felt fearful of being sent back to his stepfather, so he explained that he did not need help. The worker tactfully suggested that if Armondo knew someone who might benefit from the information, to please pass on the card. Two days later, Armondo walked more than 70 city blocks to the shelter, where he asked to meet with the outreach worker.

What struck me hard in meeting Armondo was that he essentially lived a postwar existence, similar to youths in refugee camps or in post–World War II Europe. However, he absorbed the entirety of his experience as a statement of his being and worth. Although his physical stature was that of a late adolescent, his facial expression was that of a 6-year-old. His bodily composure was sunken and unconfident. Although he seemed interested in connecting, he would look at me—as if throwing a survival rope to connect—and then look quickly away.

It did not seem helpful to talk through the many abuses against this trembling spirit in a boy's body. Rather, it seemed that Armondo needed a guide, someone to help him navigate the emerging independence and self-reliance that he had achieved, albeit ahead of peers who had far more emotional and material resources. We also did not have unlimited time. Armondo would most likely not have access to care for long because finding treatment and housing for a nonpsychotic youth can be difficult. For a youth who came to a private practice or a clinic setting, I might have used SAP in a more gradual time frame, waiting to highlight the synchronicities as they emerged or for the feeling of a spiritual connection to emerge over time. Weaver provided a way to accelerate, under crisis, the work of SAP.

I invited Armondo to do Weaver's round-table spiritual visualization, in which Armondo envisioned a great aunt who had in his childhood taken him in until she became ill and died. Armondo did not find the exercise to be foreign or strange; he was utterly transfixed. Deep inside his visualization, Armondo seemed part of the table, at home with this level of spiritual access to his great aunt as ambassador for the Creator. He was still for a solid 10 or 12 minutes, and then he opened his eyes. He seemed different, with a sacred look and a glimpse of love.

I did not ask Armondo what his aunt had said. I wanted to sustain the boundary so that he could privately engage with his aunt, and the sacred guidance of his ancestors, without anyone penetrating his boundary. A week later, however, I saw Armondo on the floor of the shelter. "Dr. Lisa," he said, "that table you showed me, I've been doing it, and it's powerful—I mean it's really powerful. I've been listening to my aunt, and it's like I have a home with someone to help me out again."

Despite his mature body, Armondo's face still looked like that of a boy in early childhood, but not in a dissociated way. He had managed to live here by being aware that he was loved. He was able to speak to team members and engage enough with staff that with the generosity of the universe, he found placement at a program with stable housing and educational resources in upstate New York, where I sense that he and his aunt now live.

CONCLUSION

SAP with children and adolescents, as well as parents, engages the path of spiritual development across the life span. The child has direct access to the Creator, wittingly or first hand, free of self-consciousness. The adolescent is in a phase of spiritual awakening, leading to a direct relationship with the universe of guidance and love. Parents have the opportunity to spiritually develop in tandem with their child as they face familiar challenges on a deeper level and with more seasoned experience.

Direct dialogue with the universe guides transformation and healing for people of all ages, and this dialogue can be encouraged and supported through SAP. However, whether in childhood or adolescence, heeding the wisdom within the youth is particularly crucial when ambassadors have not taken up their sacred parental call.

SAP came to me from my clients over the past 15 years, highlighted by bright relationships and the message of the guiding universe. As the needs of clients have started to appear more urgent, with precious time passing in their lives, I have become less tentative and have shifted my stance from 90% receptive to about 70% receptive. There are more and more times when it makes sense to help clients by taking up the charge, as generously shared by Weaver, and be more proactive. Also, it has become clear that SAP can be extended to embrace any technique, conceived in love and healing intention, that invites the client into dialogue with the universe, such as the gift of the spiritual-table visualization brought just in time for the Covenant House collaboration.

Spiritual awareness holds that we evolve through a dialogue with the universe, one that we experience through the teachings of relationships and messengers all around them. The lessons are most vivid, and the effects strongest, because they come from those whom we love and who are close to us, particularly the parent ambassador and child sage. As healers, we have a chance to bear witness and listen with our clients to the sacred dialogue told through the living world.

REFERENCES

American Psychological Association. (Producer). (2005). *Spiritual awareness psychotherapy* [DVD]. Available at http://www.apa.org/pubs/videos/

Boyatzis, C. (in press). Child spirituality and the family. In L. Miller (Ed.), *Oxford University Press handbook of psychology and spirituality*. New York, NY: Oxford University Press.

Jung, C. G., & Hull, R. F. C. (1981). The archetypes and the collective unconscious. In G. Adler & R. F. C. Hull (Eds. & Trans.), *Collected works of C. G. Jung* (2nd ed., Vol. 9, Part 1, pp. 3–41). Princeton, NJ: Princeton University Press.

Kelley, B. S., & Miller, L. (2007). Life satisfaction and spirituality in adolescents. *Research in the Social Scientific Study of Religion, 18*, 233–261.

Kendler, K. S., Gardner, C. O., & Prescott, C. A. (1997). Religion, psychopathology, and substance use and abuse: A multimeasure, genetic-epidemiologic study. *American Journal of Psychiatry, 154*, 322–329.

Koenig, L. B., McGee, M., Krueger, R. F., & Bouchard, T. J. (2005). Genetic and environmental influences on religiousness: Findings for retrospective and current religiousness ratings. *Journal of Personality, 73*, 471–488. doi:10.1111/j.1467-6494.2005.00316.x

Miller, L. (2008). Spiritual awareness in life and psychotherapy. In C. A. Rayburn & L. Comas-Díaz (Eds.), *Woman soul* (pp. 221–236). Westport, CT: Praeger.

Miller, L. (2010). Watching for light: Spiritual psychology beyond materialism. *Psychology of Religion and Spirituality, 2*, 35–36. doi:10.1037/a0018554

Miller, L., & Gur, M. (2002). Religiosity, depression and physical maturation in adolescent girls. *Journal of the American Academy of Child & Adolescent Psychology, 41*, 206–214.

Richards, P. S., & Bergin, A. E. (2003). *Casebook for a spiritual strategy for counseling and psychotherapy*. Washington, DC: American Psychological Association.

Roehlkepartain, E. C., King, P. E., Wagener, L., & Benson, P. (2006). *The handbook of spiritual development in childhood and adolescents*. Thousand Oaks, CA: Sage.

Sperry, L. (2011). *Spirituality in clinical practice: Theory and practice of spiritually oriented psychotherapy* (2nd ed.). New York, NY: Routledge.

7

SACRED TEXTS

DONALD F. WALKER, SAMEERA AHMED, AVIDAN MILEVSKY, HEATHER LEWIS QUAGLIANA, AND ANISAH BAGASRA

Early one morning, a foolish young rabbit lay sleeping beneath an apple tree tucked away in a corner of a forest. As the rabbit tried to sleep, he began to ask himself what would happen if the earth were to break apart. After thinking more about this, he sat up and asked out loud, "What if the earth broke up today?" While he considered this possibility, he began to look around the forest and listen for signs of danger.

Just as he began looking around, he heard the sound of a loud crash behind him. Without turning to see what had happened, the rabbit jumped up, began running, and started yelling, "The earth is breaking up!" over and over again while he ran as fast as he could. He continued running through the forest, gathering animals with him as he ran.

Before long, a pack of rabbits, bears, elephants, and snakes were bounding and slithering through the jungle, until they ran underneath a brave lion that was perched on a mountaintop that overlooked the forest. From there,

DOI: 10.1037/13947-008
Spiritual Interventions in Child and Adolescent Psychotherapy, D. F. Walker and W. L. Hathaway (Editors)

the lion could see that unless he intervened, the herd of animals would run over the edge of the cliff they were advancing on.

The brave lion decided to help them and leapt from the mountaintop to the front of the pack. He asked them why they were running and was told that the earth was breaking up. The lion replied that the earth was not breaking up, and he struck the ground with his paw to prove it. He then asked the pack who had told them this.

When the foolish little rabbit told the lion that he had heard the earth breaking up under an apple tree, the lion had an idea, and returned with the rabbit to the tree where he had been sleeping. The lion sniffed around the tree until he found the apple that he was looking for. He told the rabbit that the sound of the apple falling had been the reason for his thinking that the earth was breaking up, and they returned to the pack of animals to reassure them that it had all been a mistake.

This fairy tale, described in *Foolish Rabbit's Big Mistake* (Martin & Young, 1985), is a story recommended for use in an empirically supported treatment manual for childhood anxiety (Kendall & Hedkte, 2000). Kendall and Hedkte (2000) have used the fable to help anxious children learn to identify cognitive errors related to anxiety by following the main character in the story. Kendall begins by teaching children to identify the foolish rabbit's thinking errors. Then, Kendall asks clients to generate adaptive self-talk and actions to help the main character in the story cope effectively with anxiety-provoking thoughts. Kendall's rationale for using a fictional story to discuss cognitive errors and practice replacing them is that using a make-believe character is less threatening to a child than asking the child to directly discuss his or her own anxiety-provoking experiences, at least initially.

Children often learn about life through stories and parables. This has been the case for generations, from Aesop's fables (Aesop, Jones, & Ashliman, 2003) to Grimm's fairy tales (Grimm, Grimm, Grimm, & Dalton, 2003). For children raised in religiously committed families, stories describing character formation, rules for living, and ways to deal with adversity are often passed down in sacred texts, including the Bhagavad Gita (Hinduism), the Holy Bible (Christianity), the Qur'an (Islam), the Tipikita (Buddhism), and the Torah and Talmud (Judaism).

Indeed, every major world religion has a way of life that is communicated through a sacred text. In counseling and psychotherapy, the incorporation of sacred texts is commonly used to address client and religious issues (Garzon, 2005; Johnson, Ridley, & Nielsen, 2000; Tan, 2007). This practice has been alternately referred to as *religion-accommodative* or *spiritually oriented psychotherapy* (McCullough, 1999; Richards & Worthington, 2010). The idea of adapting standard psychotherapy approaches with children to be more culturally sensitive to diverse populations is not new (see, e.g., Cohen, Deblinger,

Mannarino, & de Arrellaneo, 2001; Huey & Polo, 2010; Lau, 2006; McCabe & Yeh, 2009). In a sense, the approaches to incorporating sacred texts into treatment that we advocate represent an extension of culturally modified practice applied specifically to children, teens, and families for whom religious and spiritual tradition is a highly important aspect of diversity.

Thus, in this chapter, we discuss the use of sacred texts from different world religions in the context of child and adolescent psychotherapy. We provide more in-depth discussion of spiritual interventions using sacred texts in the context of empirically supported psychotherapy treatment packages. As a result, our approach to using sacred texts falls squarely within the second of the three categories for considering spiritual interventions (adding religious and spiritual content to secular treatments) identified by Post and Wade (2009). We begin the chapter by providing an overview of the sacred texts from several major world religions, with a focus on Christianity, Islam, and Judaism because these are religions that we are more familiar with. Next, we present a model for addressing spiritual and religious issues in parent training in behavioral interventions for childhood disruptive behavior using sacred texts. Afterward, we consider the role of sacred texts in the context of cognitive–behavioral treatment for childhood anxiety and depression. Then we discuss the use of sacred texts in the context of treatment for childhood physical and sexual abuse. We conclude the chapter by discussing the future of study in incorporating sacred texts in treatment for children and adolescents. Across sections, we present a series of case studies demonstrating the use of sacred texts in psychotherapy with children, teens, and families.

OVERVIEW OF SACRED TEXTS FROM MAJOR WORLD RELIGIONS

Christianity

The Christian Bible is broadly divided into two sections: an Old Testament (inherited from Judaism) and a New Testament (focusing on the life of Jesus Christ and the early church in the years after his death and ascension). Within the New Testament, four books, called the synoptic Gospels (Matthew, Mark, Luke, and John) record the life and teachings of Jesus Christ. These books were probably written between 60 and 100 AD (Walsh, 2005). At least 100 separate Christian sects exist, roughly broadly divided among Roman Catholic, Eastern Orthodox, Mainline Protestant, Evangelical Protestant, and Fundamentalist Protestant denominations. Christians are unique in their belief in the existence of one God existing in three persons: God the Father, the Son (Jesus), and the Holy Spirit. Christians of varying denominations are united in their belief that all of humanity is separated from God the Father because of sin and that belief in the person of Jesus and the atoning work of his death and resurrection are necessary for salvation from sin.

Protestant Bibles contain 66 individual books (39 in the Old Testament and 27 in the New Testament). Roman Catholic and Eastern Orthodox versions of the Bible maintain an additional 10 and 13 books, respectively, as canon. Christian denominations vary widely in their approach to interpreting the Bible. Most denominations emphasize the importance of considering the cultural context in which the original works were written. However, denominations differ widely in the importance they place on scripture as a source of authority for knowing truth. Depending on the specific sect, scripture is typically balanced against the authority of religious leaders, reason, tradition, and personal experience as sources of knowledge. Protestants and Roman Catholics differ most widely on the role of church leadership in interpreting scripture. Roman Catholics consider the Pope to have been appointed by the direct successors of the apostle Peter, and consider all of the modern-day apostles to have been appointed by the direct successors of the original apostles, or 12 disciples, of Christ. As a result, Roman Catholics are more likely than Protestant Christians in particular to weigh their own personal interpretations of scripture against those of the Pope and their religious leaders. Protestant Christians emphasize a priesthood of all believers and are more likely to interpret scripture in the light of tradition, reason, and personal experience.

Islam

The word *Islam* means "peace" and implies submission to God. Islam is a monotheistic and Abrahamic faith, and its followers are referred to as *Muslims*. The Qur'an, the Muslim holy book, was revealed to the Prophet Muhammad by God and serves as the primary source of guidance for Muslims. The Sunnah, or the sayings, actions, and approval of the Prophet Muhammad, serve as the secondary source of religious guidance for Muslims. Both the Qur'an and the Sunnah are considered sacred texts by Muslims.

Clinicians working with Muslim clients should realize that there is no hierarchical religious structure in Islam, which can result in religious scholars having differences of opinion on the interpretation of varying aspects of Islam, including issues affecting mental health. For example, parents may justify family rules for their teenager using the Qur'an and Sunnah as their evidence, but their teenager may provide evidence from the sacred texts that may have an alternative perspective, which can complicate psychotherapy.

Another issue that may affect treatment is the sometimes indistinguishable intertwining of culture and religion in different Muslim cultures. Islam consists of principles and behaviors to be adapted to one's culture, resulting in Muslim cultural traditions that differ depending on the cultural context of the individual. As a result, it is often hard for parents or their children to identify and separate which beliefs are in fact cultural and which are religious. Parents may present ethnic cultural values as Islam, which their children may have difficulty accepting because they identify more with American culture than with their parental ethnic culture. Therefore, clinicians working with Muslim families are recommended to use a religious and cultural consultant to navigate through religious and cultural issues that may affect treatment.

Judaism

The two primary Jewish sacred texts are the Bible and the Talmud. The Bible, known as the Tanach, consists of 24 books divided among three sections. The Torah ("Teaching") is the first section and contains five books (the Pentateuch) focusing on the creation of the world, the early history of the founding of the Jewish people, and the basic commandments for living. The Nevi'im ("Prophets") is the second section, concerned mainly with the Jewish prophet era following the Jewish people's entry into the land of Israel. The Nevi'im also describes the Hebrew monarchy and its division into two kingdoms and details the prophecies warning of the impending destruction of the temple in Jerusalem. The final section, the Ketuvim ("Writings" or "Scriptures"), is a collection of prophesies, reflections on living, and stories of Jewish leaders leading up to and during the Babylonian exile (McDonald, 2007).

The Talmud is a vast collection of rabbinic discussions occurring during the era of the Second Temple and the years after its destruction (100 BCE—475 CE) pertaining to the practical interpretation of the Bible. It covers the application of biblical law in daily Jewish life, including the laws of prayer, keeping the Sabbath, holidays, interpersonal matters, marital issues, and dietary restrictions (Steinsaltz, 2010). In addition to being the primary resource for understanding Jewish law, the Talmud also contains numerous discussions about living in general, including insights into the meaning of life, emotions, dreams, internal conflicts, well-being, and character growth.

Clinicians working with Jewish populations are encouraged to understand the substantial differences that exist between members of various denominations of Jews (Langman, 1995, 1999). The need for such understanding is further highlighted when considering the appropriate use of sacred texts with Jews, given the diverging approaches toward the Bible and the Talmud taken by the various denominations. The three primary denominations of Jews are Orthodox, Conservative, and Reform.

Orthodox Jews "accept that G-d gave the Torah, the Hebrew Bible, to the People of Israel at Mount Sinai, along with a divinely ordained interpretation of its commands" (Schnall, 2006, p. 277). Orthodox Jews apply the teachings of the Bible and the Talmud to all aspects of life, including daily routines, personal interactions, family life, and business matters. Because the Talmud is seen as equally authoritative as the Bible, the use of both passages from both texts would be appropriate with and accepted by an Orthodox Jewish client.

Conservative and Reform Jews practice a more egalitarian Judaism and emphasize the need to view Jewish law in the context of modernism. Conservative Jews may be more likely than Reform Jews to ascribe divinity to the Bible. However, both denominations view the Talmud as discussions with historical value but little legislative authority (De Lange, 2000). As such, the use of the Bible in therapeutic interventions may be more appropriate with Conservative and Reform Jews than the use of the Talmud.

INCORPORATING SACRED TEXTS INTO PARENT TRAINING

Two out of three psychotherapy referrals for children and teens are for behavior problems that are frequently addressed through parent training in behavioral interventions (Barkley, 2006). Highly religious parents often imbue their parenting role with sacred significance—a process some have referred to as *sanctification of parenting* (Mahoney, Pargament, Murray-Swank, & Murray-Swank, 2003). Elsewhere, we have argued that because religiously committed parents frequently view their parenting role as a sacred calling, it can be important for psychotherapists to help them understand parent training in light of that importance (Walker, Reese, Hughes, & Troskie, 2010). Three of the more prominent, empirically supported parent training treatment packages available are Barkley's (1997) Defiant Children parent training program, Webster-Stratton's (2005) Incredible Years parent training program, and Eyberg's parent–child interaction therapy (PCIT; Zisser & Eyberg, 2010). These treatments have been demonstrated to reduce disruptive behavior among children and to increase parental self-efficacy related to parenting practices (Barkley, 2006; Hood & Eyberg, 2003; Webster-Stratton, 2005).

Summary of the Three Programs

Barkley's (1997) Defiant Children parent training program is designed to provide approximately 12 sessions of parent training and can be adapted to family therapy or collateral treatment for parents or administered in a parent group format. Barkley (1997) developed the Defiant Children parent training program for parents of children with a cognitive or developmental level of at least 2 years of age but suggested in the manual that children as young as 18 months of age may benefit from treatment. Barkley also recommended a parallel version of the program for teenagers (Barkley, Edwards, & Robin, 1999).

Webster-Stratton's (2005) Incredible Years is a multidimensional treatment program for parents, teachers, and children designed to increase compliance with parent and teacher requests and to eliminate disruptive behavior at home and in school settings. The Incredible Years consists of two parent training programs, the BASIC and ADVANCE parenting programs for parents of children ages 2 to 12. Both the BASIC and ADVANCE parenting programs contain 14 sessions that have video vignettes for parents to discuss in a group context. The program begins by building parenting skills; it then addresses parental interpersonal issues, such as problem-solving skills, anger management, and social support.

Eyberg's (2005) PCIT is usually conducted in 16 sessions or fewer. It was originally developed for use with preschoolers ages 3 to 6 but has been adapted for older children. PCIT has traditionally been conducted in an individual therapy format in which the therapist first demonstrates and explains a technique to the parent and then provides live coaching for the parent with the child. Eyberg uses the acronym PRIDE to teach parents to *praise* their child for good behavior, *reflect* on what their child says, *imitate* and *describe* the ways in which their child plays, and be *enthusiastic* in building their relationship with their child.

Pretreatment Considerations for Parent Training With Religious Parents

In parent training with religious parents, we encourage psychotherapists to explore and consider ways in which a parent's religious text prescribes specific parenting practices that may or may not be compatible with empirically supported parenting interventions. This is important for several reasons. First, when psychotherapeutic practices are compatible with religious directives related to parenting, religious parents will more readily receive and apply them. Second, when psychotherapists perceive areas of conflict between religious instructions related to parenting and their treatment protocols, we believe that they should demonstrate respect for parental religiousness by openly discussing areas of potential disagreement and, if necessary, respecting the parent's right to not incorporate all aspects of the program. Finally, when religiously committed parents sense conflicts between their religious tenets and psychotherapy practices, they may passively avoid implementing them or outright refuse. Openly discussing areas of difference makes it more likely that they will choose to participate, ultimately benefiting the child client being treated. In the following discussion, we consider four common treatment modules across empirically supported parenting programs: (a) psychoeducation, (b) teaching attending skills, (c) using psychotherapeutic time out, and (d) using a token economy.

Integration of Sacred Texts With Parenting Modules

In this section, we describe the use of sacred writings in parent training modules from different empirically supported parent training programs. Our intention is to describe the use of sacred writings in such a way that practitioners can incorporate our clinical recommendations across empirically supported parent training manuals such as Barkley's (1997) Defiant Teen manual, Eyberg's (2005) PCIT manual, or Webster-Stratton's (2005) Incredible Years manual. As a result, we focus on modules that are common across these and other parent training programs.

Psychoeducation

When providing psychoeducation to parents about the causes of childhood misbehavior, psychotherapists may find it helpful to discuss parents' beliefs about religious and spiritual explanations (e.g., the role of sin) for their child's misbehavior. This is important for two reasons. First, some parents who are highly religiously committed might blame their child's misbehavior on sin or another spiritual cause on the part of the child. For example, some Muslim parents may blame mental health symptoms or child misbehavior on possession by supernatural beings referred to as *jinns*. The notion of supernatural beings does exist in Islam; however, there is a difference of opinion among scholars regarding their role in mental health symptoms. Supernatural causes are more typically attributed to symptoms and diagnoses that are difficult for the family to understand, such as psychosis, mania, or schizophrenia. Therefore, a religious consultant should be contacted in such cases. Our clinical experience has been that religious parents' spiritual attributions about child misbehavior vary to some degree depending on the religion of the parent. Some conservative Judeo–Christian parents more frequently attribute child misbehavior as being related to sin in cases in which the child has been diagnosed with a neurodevelopmental disability (e.g., attention-deficit/hyperactivity disorder) or an autism spectrum disorder and the parent or parents are unaware of the extent to which the condition results in difficulty in behavioral regulation.

Conversely, other religiously committed parents might believe that their child's spirituality naturally prevents them from having a diagnosable condition that needs treatment. One of us (Avidan Milevsky) once treated an Orthodox Jewish teenager referred by his pediatrician because of concerns over the teen's symptoms of anxiety. During the initial stages of treatment, the teen's mother said that he was a "big masmid" (i.e., someone who is extremely engaged in the study of the Bible), and as a result of this presumed spiritual maturity, she found it difficult to believe that her son needed psychotherapy.

Teaching Attending Skills

The attending skills module is a foundation for later teaching the process of giving parental commands to increase compliance in most parenting programs. In this module, parents provide positive and negative reinforcement for desired behavior, which involves selectively attending to desired behavior and ignoring mild forms of undesired behavior. When parents selectively attend to desired child behaviors, they are encouraged to provide specific, labeled verbal praise (e.g., "I love it when you play quietly like you are now"). In our parenting work, we commonly encourage parents to "catch their child being good."

In our clinical experience, some highly religiously committed parents (particularly those who self-identify as conservative or fundamentalist) object to the notion of providing positive reinforcement for desirable behaviors. Occasionally, these objections are grounded in religious instruction. For example, Jewish parents may view evil as an inclination within their children that needs to be subdued. This belief is based in part on Genesis 5:6: "The thoughts of people are evil all day." As a result, Jewish parents may believe in punishment (as opposed to positive reinforcement) as a religiously congruent parenting practice.

Other parents object to the use of positive reinforcement on the grounds that their child should behave without having to be rewarded. Furthermore, some religious parents have been taught that corporal punishment is a specifically mandated practice in their religious tradition. In response, we suggest that psychotherapists explore scriptural passages from various religious traditions that involve corporal punishment or that could alternatively be used to support selective attention and positive reinforcement as parenting practices. For example, when working with Christian parents, we encourage open discussion of a commonly cited passage that instructs parents that "sparing the rod spoils the child" (Proverbs 13:24).

Walker and Quagliana (2007) proposed an alternative interpretation of this passage that notes that in biblical times, shepherds also guided sheep with the crook of the rod rather than striking them with it. Considered in the context of child rearing, this verse could encourage parents to guide their children rather than (or in addition to) striking them with an object such as a switch or paddle. When reconceptualized this way, Christians receiving parent training could view the rod in Proverbs 13:24 as a tool that is symbolically represented by the use of selective attention.

A similar dynamic may exist in Muslim families, for whom corporal punishment may be a culturally accepted practice but one that is religiously rejected. For example, one hadith (or saying of the Prophet Muhammed) specifically states, "Do not abuse anyone." Prohibitions against abuse extend to verbally abusive behavior such as belittling children. For such parents, a reminder from the Qur'an may help reframe their behavior in religious terms: "O you who believe! Let not a group scoff at another group, it may be that the latter are better than the former" (Qur'an 49:11).

It is imperative to be aware that parental openness to considering alternative views of particular scriptural passages varies widely. In general, parents from mainline denominations (across religious faith traditions) are probably more open to considering new ways of thinking about specific passages. Parents from conservative traditions are more likely to accept a reframing of a particular scripture when it is done by a psychotherapist from their own faith tradition. In religiously mixed psychotherapy dyads, many religiously committed parents are more willing to consider an alternative reconceptualization of a particular passage if their psychotherapist has demonstrated respect for and a desire to work within their particular faith tradition.

However, some conservative or fundamentalist religious parents simply will not consider an alternative interpretation of their sacred writings, even if their psychotherapist is from the same faith tradition. One of us (Milevsky), having completed rabbinical ordination, was working in a psychotherapy setting and with Orthodox Jewish clients. Despite his ordination, he found that the parents he was working with would not consider challenges to their religious beliefs about parenting. Although he was a Jewish rabbi, he found himself having to obtain a release of information and collaborate with his clients' rabbis in order to work with them on parent training. This anecdote illustrates the danger that psychotherapists may face when challenging parental religious beliefs. We encourage psychotherapists to tread lightly when walking on sacred ground related to parenting and to collaborate as necessary with clergy members from their clients' religious traditions.

Psychotherapeutic Use of Time Out

Parents bring a wide range of experiences with time out when they present for parent training. Some parents have previously attempted time out with their children unsuccessfully and are therefore opposed to future attempts to use this intervention. Others prefer corporal punishment (often on the religious grounds that we have cited) and are opposed to a noncorporal form of intervention. Either way, time out is a crucial component of most parenting programs because it is typically the only punishment suggested for misbehavior.

We encourage psychotherapists to ask parents whether time out is an intervention that is compatible or incompatible with their religious traditions for parenting. For example, among Christian parents, time out could be considered as congruent with the idea that "people reap what they sow" found in Galatians 6:7–8. Psychotherapists might encourage parents to focus on a religious reference to the consequences of misbehavior among children and allow their children to experience natural consequences associated with their behavior (Walker & Quagliana, 2007). In a similar manner, Muslim parents may be encouraged to use the following verses from the Qur'an to assist parents and their children to understand that behaviors have consequences: "Whoever chooses to follow the right path, follows it but for his own good; and whoever goes astray, goes but astray to his own hurt; and no bearer of burdens shall be made to bear another's burden" (Qur'an 17:15).

Creating a Token Economy

This treatment component is a prescribed part of the Defiant Children manual developed by Barkley (1997) and an optional part of treatment within PCIT. In implementing a token economy, parents must link individual rewards to specific desired behaviors. In addition, behaviors must be reinforced immediately, through verbal praise, the use of a small token, or both. Finally, rewards are stratified so that these tokens are then exchanged for daily privileges or larger rewards that the child can earn over time. Within Barkley's (1997) system, in particular, a key feature of the module is that particular rewards are tailored to the child's unique interests.

We encourage psychotherapists to highlight ways in which token economies are compatible with religious prescriptions for parenting. For example, among both Jewish and Christian parents, an often-cited scripture about parenting declares, "Train a child according to his way; even when he is old he will not depart from it" (Proverbs 22:6). This verse can be used to emphasize to Judeo–Christian parents the importance of flexibility in parenting and the need to tailor parenting (including rewards) to the individual needs of a child. Use of this verse can be integrated when working with parents on challenging some of their faulty cognitions about the musts of parenting. For Jewish parents specifically, the Talmud (Tractate Sabbath, 156a) expands on this concept by stating, "If an individual is born with a violent disposition he may become a murderer or a medical practitioner or a circumciser." Similarly, in the Sunnah of the Prophet Muhammed, it is recorded that he said, "Don't take upon yourselves, except the deeds which are within your ability" (Bukhari). These statements reinforce the importance of assessing an individual's disposition and steering the individual toward adaptive outcomes on the basis of his or her unique temperament. Thus, authoritarian parents who insist on specific behaviors that their children must abide by can be draw into a therapeutic discussion using scripture about the need to treat each individual child according to the child's unique temperament and personality.

Case Study: Parent Training Using Sacred Texts

One of us (Sameera Ahmed) saw a 7-year old girl named Fatima because of her repeated angry outbursts, irritability, defiance, and acting-out behavior. During her initial intake, her parents indicated that these behaviors only took place at home and that her teachers at school reported that she was a model student.

Exploring family dynamics revealed that the mother was the disciplinarian of the family and was overwhelmed by demands at work and loneliness because of a lack of her family and a social network. Fatima's father was supportive of his wife but unable to assist her because of long work hours and feeling unsure of how to parent Fatima. Her parents reported difficulties with setting limits with their daughter and giving mixed or unclear messages about their expectations of her, and they were inconsistent in following through with discipline. Exploring Fatima's daily schedule, Ahmed observed that Fatima was often sleep deprived, lacked relaxation time because of a stressful family schedule, and ate junk food to substitute for main meals. The lack of developmentally appropriate needs being met, coupled with a stressful home life and the need to enhance parenting skills, appeared to be contributing to the negative parent–child interaction. While assessing for sources of social support, the family indicated that Islam served as a source of spiritual direction for how they lived their life. In addition, they reported obtaining great support from their religious community.

The initial session began with helping Fatima's parents reframe the presenting problem. Ahmed reminded them of a Qur'anic verse, "But it may happen that you hate a thing which is good for you, and it may happen that you love a thing which is bad for you. Allah knows, what you know not" (Qur'an 2:216), to reframe their child's behavior as an opportunity to adjust the present family lifestyle and dynamics. She provided psychoeducation about normative developmental needs for sleep, nutrition, and relaxation to promote Fatima's development. The next few sessions involved parent training that focused on building the following parenting skills: identifying Fatima's behavior patterns, increasing opportunities for positive parent–child interaction, and communicating effectively.

During the early stages of psychotherapy, Fatima's parents expressed concern about increasing opportunities for positive parent–child interactions as a parenting goal. Both parents felt that Fatima had been very disrespectful and should be expected to comply with parental requests even in the absence of a nurturing interaction from them. To challenge this belief, Ahmed reminded Fatima's parents that the Prophet Muhammad was known to have taken time out to play with children and encouraged others as well to strengthen the attachment between children and caregivers. She quoted the following hadith, in which the Prophet Muhammed said, "Those who have a child should act like a child with him."

During the early phases of psychotherapy, Fatima's father also admitted that he was uncomfortable providing emotional and physical displays of affection to her. In response, Ahmed processed his discomfort in giving Fatima affection. She also quoted a hadith showing how the Prophet Muhammad encouraged the display of affection with children:

> A man passed by as the Prophet Muhammed was kissing his grandson and said, "I have ten children, yet I have never kissed anyone of them." The Prophet replied, "We have nothing to do with those harsh hearted people. A person who shows no mercy to others, God will show no mercy to him."

In subsequent sessions, Ahmed then helped family members identify physical sensations associated with anger and taught relaxation exercises and activities to be practiced by Fatima and her parents at home. In identifying activities to calm one's anger, Ahmed reminded the family of the varying hadiths of the Prophet in which he advised that a person in a state of anger should either change his or her position or make ablution (a ritual wash with water) to decrease his or her state of anger.

The sessions that followed helped Fatima and her parents to do a situational analysis and identify negative self-statements that were contributing to their anger during negative parent–child interactions. The family then used the following Qur'anic verse as a springboard toward developing more positive communication:

> O you who believe, let not a group scoff at another group, it may be that the latter are better than the former. . . . Nor defame one another, nor insult one another by nicknames. How bad is it to insult one's brother after having good faith. And whosoever does not repent, then such are indeed wrongdoers. (Qur'an 49:11)

Through this process, Fatima and her parents were able to establish more positive communication and develop a positive parent–child relationship. The final sessions focused on effective problem solving within the family to help equip the family for future challenges.

COGNITIVE–BEHAVIORAL THERAPY FOR CHILDHOOD AND TEENAGE ANXIETY AND DEPRESSION

In this section, we consider the use of sacred texts in the context of cognitive–behavioral therapy (CBT) for childhood anxiety and depression. We begin by reviewing secular protocols for each of these disorders. Next, we discuss ways to incorporate sacred writings into treatment components of protocols for each disorder. We conclude by presenting a case study using amalgamated client data demonstrating the incorporation of sacred texts into the treatment of childhood anxiety and depression.

Cognitive–Behavioral Therapy for Childhood Anxiety

Kendall and Hedtke's (2006) Coping Cat manual is a widely used, empirically supported treatment for childhood anxiety (Kendall, Hudson, Choudhury, Webb, & Pimentel, 2005). The manual was developed for children ages 7 to 13 and is designed to complete treatment in 17 sessions, although Kendall has encouraged psychotherapists to apply the manual flexibly. *Coping Cat* refers to a drawing of a cat that is used in the child's companion workbook to the psychotherapist manual. Throughout treatment, the Coping Cat is present to illustrate treatment concepts and to allow the child to practice them in workbook exercises. As part of the treatment, children are taught a four-step procedure, summarized by the FEAR acronym: (a) *feeling* frightened? (b) *expecting* bad things to happen? (c) *attitudes* and actions that will help? and (d) *results* and rewards. Treatment using the Coping Cat manual begins with rapport building with an anxious child client. Next, a psychotherapist using the Coping Cat manual will help the child to identify anxious feelings and somatic responses to anxiety. Afterward, relaxation training is introduced, in which the child is taught diaphragmatic breathing and muscle relaxation. Once the child has practiced relaxation training, several sessions are typically spent teaching the child about self-talk and assisting the child in modifying his or her self-talk in anxiety-provoking situations. As part of this process, the child is encouraged to evaluate the likelihood that something negative will happen, notice his or her own self-talk, then modify this self-talk and corresponding actions to more effectively deal with whatever stressor is causing the child anxiety. Finally, the child client is taught to evaluate the results of his or her efforts to cope and to reward him- or herself with praise or tangible rewards for successfully coping in anxiety-provoking situations. A separate, parallel manual exists for adolescents called the *C.A.T. Project* manual (Kendall, Choudhury, Hudson, & Webb, 2002).

Parental involvement in the program is also encouraged for several reasons. First, some parents may themselves have anxiety that could be contributing to their child's anxiety. In addition, nonanxious parents are also encouraged to participate to reinforce the coping lessons that their children are learning. A number of outcome studies have demonstrated that the Coping Cat manual is more effective than placebo, no treatment, or an alternative form of treatment across different clinical trials (Kendall, Furr, & Podell, 2010).

Cognitive–Behavioral Therapy for Childhood Depression

In addition to treatments for anxiety, several evidence-based treatments have also been developed for childhood and adolescent depression (see Stark, Streusand, Krumholz, & Patel, 2010; and Weersing & Brent, 2010, for reviews). The ACTION program developed by Stark et al. (2010) is a group psychotherapy and assumes that there are multiple pathways to childhood depression, including difficulties stemming from neurochemical, behavioral, family, and cognitive causes. Stark et al. further suggested that disturbances in these areas are reciprocal, such that psychotherapeutic changes in any one area will subsequently improve functioning in other areas contributing to childhood depression. Similar to Kendall and Hedtke's (2006) Coping Cat manual, Stark et al.'s ACTION program is currently geared toward children (specifically 9- to 13-year-olds), and they have focused recent research on the application of the model in treating depression among girls, but the manual itself can be used with boys as well.

Writing for school-age children, Stark et al. (2010) summarized the main goals and psychotherapeutic steps in the program in the following manner:

1. If you feel bad and don't know why, use coping skills.
2. If you feel bad and you can change the situation, use problem-solving skills.
3. If you feel bad and it is due to negative thoughts, change the thoughts. (p. 94)

According to Stark et al. (2010), the group is intended to last to last for 20 sessions, with two individual meetings for participants (although additional meetings can be scheduled). During the group meetings, participants are taught the interrelationship among thoughts, feelings, and behaviors; coping skills for depression; and then problem solving and cognitive restructuring.

Weersing and Brent (2010) have used cognitive–behavioral interventions in individual psychotherapy with adolescents. The focus of their treatment model involves identifying and changing cognitive distortions, encouraging adolescents to engage in activities that promote a positive mood, and teaching problem-solving skills to cope with their negative emotions.

Using Sacred Texts in Empirically Supported Treatments for Anxiety and Depression

Tan and Johnson (2005) contended that sacred writings are compatible with CBT in several ways. For instance, both emphasize beliefs as the foundation for understanding psychopathology and healing. They also focus on learning, which parallels a teacher–disciple dynamic found in many world religions. Finally, they give prominence to modifying one's thoughts and behavior, which parallels exhortations to change one's heart and behavior in many people's spiritual traditions. Furthermore, CBT treatment packages that use sacred texts from major world religions have been developed for Christian, Jewish, and Muslim clients (see Tan & Johnson, 2005). The bulk of outcome studies using these spiritually oriented forms of CBT have been done with adult and adolescent participants. Spiritually oriented CBT typically uses scripture in several ways. These include (a) cognitive disputation using passages from sacred texts to challenge clients' irrational beliefs, (b) use of religious imagery to alleviate anxiety, and (c) readings from sacred texts in or outside of session as an adjunct to homework assignments for psychotherapy (Tan & Johnson, 2005).

Challenging Irrational Beliefs and Replacing Self-Talk Using Sacred Writings

Our clinical experience has been that elements from the evidence-based practices for childhood anxiety and depression are particularly effective with religiously committed child or adolescent clients when sacred texts are incorporated into treatment. Sacred texts are used in several ways. First, telling the child (regardless of age) that the treatment that he or she is engaging in is consistent with tenets from the child's religious and spiritual tradition makes it more likely that the child will engage in it. It also makes it more likely that the parent will participate and that the parent will believe in its effectiveness, if the parent bringing the child in for treatment is of the same faith tradition as the child.

Second, we have found that using scriptural passages is particularly helpful when helping clients to challenge irrational beliefs and replace damaging self-talk related to their irrational beliefs. As Tan and Johnson (2005) pointed out, disputation using sacred writings can occur at several levels. At an indirect level, a psychotherapist can indirectly refer to truth from a client's scripture without citing specific chapters or verses. For example, in developing a cognitive–behavioral treatment for anxiety, Rosmarin, Pargament, and Mahoney (2009) disputed irrational beliefs related to anxiety among Jewish clients by asking them to consider whether God and anxiety can coexist. This disputation is consistent with what Jewish people know about God from the Bible, without guiding a client to a specific chapter or verse.

Cognitive disputations using sacred texts can also occur when using more specific references to scriptural passages at varying levels of direct reference. For instance, a clinician might refer to specific teachings or examples from a client's sacred text without including a chapter and verse where it might be found. For example, a Christian teenage client with depression who reports feeling all alone might be reminded that Jesus said that he would never leave us or forsake us without attempting to identify a specific passage in which Jesus said this. More directly, disputation using sacred writings can occur when a psychotherapist uses scriptural passages from a client's faith and references chapter and verse in the disputation. For example, a Muslim teenage client who reports feeling depressed and focuses on negative details in his or her life might be challenged to focus on positive events in his or her life using the following verse: "And He gives you all that you ask for. But if you count the favors of Allah, never will you be able to number them. Verily, man is given up to injustice and ingratitude" (Qur'an 14:34).

A third way in which sacred writings can be used in CBT with children and teens is by drawing on sacred texts for religious imagery in situations in which guided imagery is called for. For example, a Christian child who is struggling with anxiety might be asked to imagine Jesus holding him or her while engaging in guided imagery for relaxation training.

CBT also often involves completing homework assignments outside of the psychotherapy office. Passages of scripture can be assigned for homework and then discussed in session. We present the application of this practice in the next section, in which we offer a case study demonstrating the use of sacred texts in CBT for a teenager experiencing anxiety and depression. Although the case is an amalgamation from several clients, the interventions were used in each of the cases that were drawn on for this case presentation.

Case Study: Use of Sacred Texts in the Treatment of Teenage Anxiety

One of us (Milevsky) provided psychotherapy for Sarah, a 17-year-old ultra-Orthodox Jewish girl, at the recommendation of one of her teachers at an all-girls religious high school. Her teacher referred Sarah for psychotherapy after Sarah confided in her about her pervasive fears and anxieties related to her own health and safety. Sarah presented with pervasive fears about getting sick and acute anxieties pertaining to personal injury and safety concerns. During her initial intake, she reported that every time she felt a minor headache or pain, she feared that she had cancer. In addition, Sarah indicated that she was anxious being alone at night for fear of experiencing a home invasion. Milevsky, an ultra-Orthodox Jew himself, engaged Sarah in CBT and helped her challenge some of the irrational aspects of her fears. As part of the cognitive restructuring, he integrated discussions about trust in God and how Sarah's beliefs about God's daily interventions, referred to as *Hash'gacha Pratis* (personal supervision), were antithetical to experiencing anxiety. Milevsky encouraged Sarah to read the classic Jewish text dealing with trust in God, *Duties of the Heart* (Ibn Pekuda, 1996), specifically the chapter titled "The Gates of Trust." This chapter highlights the various aspects of belief in God, including the idea that God has knowledge of, and power over, the workings of all aspects of the world and that God in his mercy is compassionate to all. These ideas helped counter the client's anxious feelings by challenging her low tolerance for uncertainty with the realization that although she may be uncertain about her health and safety, God has knowledge of her situation, is in control of it, and is concerned for her welfare.

After several weeks of spiritually oriented CBT using sacred texts, Sarah experienced a minimization of her fears and anxieties.

TRAUMA-FOCUSED COGNITIVE–BEHAVIORAL THERAPY FOR CHILDHOOD PHYSICAL AND SEXUAL ABUSE

We recently developed a model for addressing religious and spiritual issues in trauma-focused CBT for children and adolescents (Walker et al., 2010). This spiritually oriented approach to trauma-focused CBT (TF-CBT) incorporates aspects of personal religiousness, including reference to sacred texts for clients from any world religious and spiritual tradition. Although we encourage psychotherapists to address a range of religious and spiritual issues (with religiously committed clients) across TF-CBT modules, we focus on the use of sacred texts in specific TF-CBT treatment modules here.

Overview of Trauma-Focused Cognitive–Behavioral Therapy

The secular version of TF-CBT has a number of treatment components, summarized by Cohen, Mannarino, Deblinger, and Berliner (2009) using the PRACTICE acronym. According to Cohen et al., this acronym stands for *psychoeducation*, *parental treatment*, *relaxation*, *affective expression and modulation*, *cognitive coping skills*, *trauma narrative and cognitive processing of the trauma*, *in vivo desensitization to trauma reminders*, *conjoint parent–child sessions*, and *enhancing safety and future development*. Psychotherapists typically begin treatment with one or more assessment sessions before proceeding with the manualized treatment. The treatment components are presented in a session-by-session manner in theory but are intended to be flexibly applied so that psychotherapists can engage in any single component at any point in time during psychotherapy.

Application of Sacred Texts Within Spiritually Oriented Trauma-Focused Cognitive–Behavioral Therapy Modules

Throughout this section, we begin by briefly reviewing each TF-CBT module as well as secular treatment interventions within each module. Then, we present ways in which sacred writings can be incorporated into the secular version of each TF-CBT module.

Affective Expression and Modulation

Within the standard TF-CBT manual, affective expression and modulation involves teaching clients feeling identification, techniques to engage in thought interruption, and positive imagery. The standard protocol for this module also involves teaching affective expression to parents of children who have been abused. Feeling identification is typically done using a therapeutic intervention such as the color-your-life technique (O'Conner, 1983), in which children choose different colors to represent different feelings and then color in the outline of a human figure with the colors that they have chosen. Thought interruption is usually done either verbally (telling a thought to go away) or nonverbally (such as snapping a rubber band on one's own wrist). Unwanted thoughts are then replaced with positive imagery in the form of a special event, place, or experience. For example, children sometimes replace unwanted thoughts with the memory of their most recent birthday.

Elsewhere, we have argued that techniques such as thought stopping, positive imagery, and coping self-talk might be more powerful treatment elements if the client was encouraged to use stories, songs, or passages from sacred writings from their personal religious and spiritual tradition as part of TF-CBT (Walker et al., 2010). For example, one of us (Donald F. Walker) treated a Christian teenage girl who had been raped and had intrusive, unwanted thoughts that she was a sinner and that it was her fault for flirting with the boy who had raped her after a party at a friend's house. In this case, Walker helped her to stop her thoughts by singing the first few lines of "Jesus Loves Me," a Christian hymn. She was then instructed to recite a verse from Romans that says that there is no condemnation for those who are in Christ (Romans 8:1).

In addition to suggesting that psychotherapists use sacred writings, songs, and images for thought stopping, we have also suggested that if clients are unable to generate these writings, songs, or images on their own, they can be encouraged to consult with a nonoffending clergy member from their personal faith tradition. In doing this, they can ask for assistance without telling the clergy member their specific reason for asking, if they wish. We have also encouraged psychotherapists to obtain their child clients' and parents' informed assent and consent and to consult with clergy themselves to locate potentially helpful passages from their sacred text to be used in treatment (Walker et al., 2010).

Cognitive Coping and Processing I

This module in the TF-CBT manual involves helping children to see the relationship between their thoughts (reflected in their self-talk) and their behaviors and feelings, an exercise that Cohen et al. (2009) referred to as the *cognitive triangle*. Children and teens are then taught to replace the dysfunctional thoughts contributing to their distress with alternative thoughts that can help them to feel better. Psychotherapists are encouraged at this point in treatment to focus on non–trauma-related cognitions rather than trauma-related thoughts, which are addressed in the second Cognitive Coping and Processing module, which occurs after the client has discussed his or her trauma narrative at length.

In psychotherapy with religiously committed clients, referring to passages from their sacred texts may help them to generate self-talk that will help them to think more rationally and to feel better. For example, in our experience adolescent girls sometimes blame themselves when they have been raped. One of us (Walker) has also seen teenage rape victims who, in blaming themselves, also worry that God will judge them for being raped. Walker has typically directed those clients to biblical passages that speak to God's unconditional love and God's right to judge the person who raped them in helping them to assign blame to the other person and avoid self-condemnation.

Trauma Narrative

In describing one's trauma narrative, Cohen et al. (2009) typically asked children to describe what happened before the event, during the event itself, and afterward. The telling is often done by creating a book with the client about what happened, although any means that is congruent with the client's personality is allowable. Some children prefer to write a song or poem about an abusive event. During this treatment module, Cohen et al. also typically asked children what they were thinking and feeling when the abuse was occurring and concluded by having child or teen clients discuss what was different in their life since the abuse occurred.

Elsewhere, we have suggested that because the chief aim of the first module is to help clients integrate the traumatic experience into their life, psychotherapists should help religiously committed children and teens to explore parallels to their own narrative in stories from the sacred texts of their religious and spiritual traditions (Walker et al., 2010). For example, the biblical story of Job might be particularly beneficial for Jewish and Christian clients to discuss (Pargament, Murray-Swank, Magyar, & Ano, 2005). This story describes an ongoing discussion that occurs between God and Job about Job's suffering after losing his family and his house after a disaster. Although this example uses a story that is familiar to Judeo–Christian clients, we believe that psychotherapists should explore similar stories for clients from various faith traditions. For additional spiritually oriented techniques that one might use in this module, see Walker et al. (2010).

Cognitive Coping and Processing II

In this treatment module, the primary intervention is the exploration and correction of trauma-related cognitive errors. For example, a common cognitive error is the belief that the world will never be safe again (Cohen, Mannarino, & Deblinger, 2006). We have previously encouraged psychotherapists to explore religious and spiritual content when examining trauma-related cognitive errors (Walker et al., 2010). We believe that some religiously committed clients may have maladaptive cognitions that contain religious content (such as believing that God abandoned them or that they committed a sin and were being punished by God in allowing the abuse).

We have also suggested that such cognitions are more likely in situations involving some form of religion-related abuse (Walker et al., 2010). For example, Bottoms, Nielsen, Murray, and Filipas (2003) found that a number of religion-related abusive experiences involved justification for physical or sexual abuse by a parent or religious clergy member in which sacred writings were used to justify the abuse. This is analogous on some level to "the devil quoting scripture for his purpose." Obviously, messages about abuse that have been distorted from sacred texts are, unfortunately, very powerful and damaging to clients' spiritual and emotional lives. However, we also believe that such damage, when rooted in sacred writings, can also be powerfully undone when challenged using other passages from clients' religious and spiritual tradition. For clients practicing from monotheistic religious backgrounds, passages that speak to right conduct on the part of believers (in opposition to the abuse that a perpetrator committed) can be particularly powerful. For example, a child who was sexually abused by a parent who told her that God would send her to hell if she disclosed the abuse could be reassured, by citing passages from the Bible, that God loves her despite what her parent told her.

Summary of Spiritually Oriented Trauma-Focused Cognitive–Behavioral Therapy

Our purpose in this section was not to comprehensively present a model for accommodating client spirituality within the TF-CBT model. We have done that previously and refer the reader to Walker et al. (2010) for a more complete discussion of ways to address spirituality and religiousness within TF-CBT. Instead, we have highlighted ways in which sacred writings may specifically be related to clients' beliefs about abuse that they have experienced. We have also presented methods to confront potentially irrational beliefs related to spirituality using sacred texts as a resource for healing within TF-CBT. We conclude this section with a case study illustrating these concepts.

Case Study: Using Sacred Texts in Trauma-Focused Cognitive–Behavioral Therapy

We recently published an amalgamated case example demonstrating the use of sacred writings in spiritually oriented TF-CBT (Walker et al., 2010). Kristy was a 7-year-old Caucasian girl who was referred for psychotherapy after sexual abuse by her father. Her father was a deacon, a position of lay leadership, in a Baptist church. In an attempt to intimidate Kristy into remaining silent about the abuse, her father told her that she would go to hell and God would hate her if she ever reported the abuse. Afterward, Kristy was removed from her biological parents' home and placed in foster care before being referred for TF-CBT.

As a result of her father's threats, Kristy came to view God as an angry and frightening figure. During psychotherapy, she reported that she feared God would be angry with her and then abandon her if she talked about the abuse with her psychotherapist. Before discussing her trauma narrative, during the first cognitive coping and processing module her psychotherapist addressed her fears by engaging in a collaborative process of identifying and challenging Kristy's beliefs about God. As part of this process, they looked for discrepancies between the God that Kristy had been taught about at church in the Bible and the God described by her father. Eventually, Kristy was able to recognize the inaccurate view of God that her father had threatened her with. This process laid the groundwork for identifying and challenging many other destructive statements Kristy's father had made.

Afterward, when Kristy described her trauma narrative to her psychotherapist, she decided to make a story book. In the book, she drew pictures of what happened while her psychotherapist wrote out the description. During Kristy's telling of the trauma narrative, her psychotherapist asked Kristy where she thought God was when the abuse occurred. Kristy said that God was there, helping her, when it happened. In her picture of the abuse, she depicted God as a star in the sky, helping her in the midst of the abuse.

After discussing the trauma narrative with her psychotherapist, Kristy had some cognitive errors related to God that were not specific to the abuse. At this point in psychotherapy, she was in foster care and did not attend church with her foster family. As a result, she was afraid that God did not know where she was and wondered whether God continued to care for her. To address these fears, her psychotherapist cited passages from the Bible suggesting that God is everywhere and knows everything that people do. Her psychotherapist reminded Kristy that God was with her all of the time. She also told Kristy that she could talk to God anytime by praying. Referring to sacred writings in this fashion helped Kristy to cope with her foster care placement and, ultimately, to resolve her abuse.

CONCLUSION

At the beginning of this chapter, we used a story recommended in Kendall and Hedtke's (2006) Coping Cat manual to illustrate our point that child and adolescent psychotherapists have often used stories to help their clients understand and cope with the challenges of life. We have asserted throughout this chapter that the sacred writings found in various religious and spiritual traditions will be particularly poignant in use in psychotherapy with children and teens from religiously committed families. In keeping with this assertion, we have described the use of sacred texts in the context of several empirically supported psychotherapies for children and teens, including parent training for behavior problems, CBT for depression and anxiety, and TF-CBT for physical and sexual abuse. We view the emerging clinical practice in this area as an exciting crossroads at which empirically supported treatments for children and teens are being informed by a growing, substantial body of literature on the psychology of religion and spirituality. We eagerly anticipate the day when our conceptual models and the case studies illustrating our approach are supplemented by a considerable body of empirical research using sacred texts in psychotherapies with children and adolescents.

REFERENCES

Aesop, R. D. L., Jones, A., & Ashliman, V. S. (2003). *Aesop's fables.* New York, NY: Barnes & Noble Books.

Barkley, R. (1997). *Defiant children* (2nd ed.). New York, NY: Guilford Press.

Barkley, R. (Ed.). (2006). *Attention-deficit/hyperactivity disorder* (3rd ed.). New York, NY: Guilford Press.

Barkley, R. A., Edwards, G., & Robin, A. (1999). *Defiant teens: A clinician's manual.* New York, NY: Guilford Press.

Bottoms, B. L., Nielsen, M., Murray, R., & Filipas, H. (2003). Religion-related child physical abuse: Characteristics and psychological outcomes. *Journal of Aggression, Maltreatment, and Trauma, 8,* 87–114.

Cohen, J. A., Deblinger, E., Mannarino, A., & de Arrellaneo, M. A. (2001). The importance of ethnicity and culture in treating neglected and abused children: An empirical review. *Child Maltreatment, 6,* 148–157. doi:10.1177/107755950100 6002007

Cohen, J. A., Mannarino, A. P., & Deblinger, E. (2006). *Treating trauma and traumatic grief in children and adolescents.* New York, NY: Guilford Press.

Cohen, J. A., Mannarino, A. P., Deblinger, E., & Berliner, L. (2009). Cognitive-behavioral therapy for children and adolescents. In E. B. Foa, T. M. Keane, M. J. Friedman, & J. A. Cohen (Eds.), *Effective treatments for PTSD: Practice guidelines from the International Society for Traumatic Stress Studies* (pp. 223–244). New York, NY: Guilford Press.

De Lange, N. (2000). *An introduction to Judaism*. Cambridge, England: Cambridge University Press.

Eyberg, S. M. (2005). Tailoring and adapting parent-child interaction therapy for new populations. *Education & Treatment of Children, 28*, 163–181.

Garzon, F. (2005). Interventions that apply scripture in psychotherapy. *Journal of Psychology and Theology, 33*, 113–121.

Grimm, B., Grimm, J., Grimm, W., & Dalton, L. E. (2003). *Grimm's fairy tales*. New York, NY: Barnes & Noble Books.

Hood, K. K., & Eyberg, S. M. (2003). Outcomes of parent-child interaction therapy: Mothers' reports on maintenance three to six years after treatment. *Journal of Clinical Child and Adolescent Psychology, 32*, 419–429. doi:10.1207/S15374424JCCP3203_10

Huey, S. J., & Polo, A. J. (2010). Assessing the effects of evidence-based psychotherapies with ethnic minority youth. In J. Weisz & A. Kazdin (Eds.), *Evidence-based psychotherapies with children and adolescents* (pp. 451–465). New York, NY: Guilford Press.

Ibn Pekuda, B. (1996). *Duties of the heart* (Y. Feldman, Trans.). Northvale, NJ: Jason Aronson. (Original work published circa 1080)

Johnson, W. B., Ridley, C., & Nielsen, S. L. (2000). Religiously sensitive rational emotive behavior therapy: Elegant solutions and ethical risks. *Professional Psychology: Research and Practice, 31*, 14–20. doi:10.1037/0735-7028.31.1.14

Kendall, P. C., Choudhury, M., Hudson, J., & Webb, A. (2002). *The C.A.T. project therapist manual*. Ardmore, PA: Workbook.

Kendall, P. C., Furr, J., & Podell, J. (2010). Child-focused treatment of anxiety. In J. R. Weisz & A. E. Kazdin (Eds.), *Evidence-based psychotherapies for children and adolescents* (2nd ed., pp. 45–60). New York, NY: Guilford Press.

Kendall, P. C., & Hedtke, K. (2006). *Cognitive-behavioral therapy for anxious children: Therapist manual* (3rd ed.). Ardmore, PA: Workbook.

Kendall, P. C., Hudson, J. L., Choudhury, M., Webb, A., & Pimentel, S. (2005). Cognitive-behavioral treatment for childhood anxiety disorders. In E. D. Hibbs & P. S. Jensen (Eds.), *Psychosocial treatments for child and adolescent disorders: Empirically based strategies for clinical practice* (2nd ed., pp. 47–73). Washington, DC: American Psychological Association.

Langman, P. F. (1995). Including Jews in multiculturalism. *Journal of Multicultural Counseling and Development, 23*, 222–236. doi:10.1002/j.2161-1912.1995.tb00278.x

Langman, P. F. (1999). *Jewish issues in multiculturalism: A handbook for educators and clinicians*. Northvale, NJ: Jason Aronson.

Lau, A. S. (2006). Making the case for selective and directed cultural adaptations of evidence-based treatments: Examples from parent training. *Clinical Psychology: Science and Practice, 13*, 295–310.

Mahoney, A., Pargament, K. I., Murray-Swank, N., & Murray-Swank, A. (2003). Religion and the sanctification of family relationships. *Review of Religious Research*, *44*, 220–236. doi:10.2307/3512384

Martin, R., & Young, E. (1985). *Foolish rabbit's big mistake*. New York, NY: Putnam.

McCabe, K., & Yeh, M. (2009). Parent-child interaction therapy for Mexican Americans: A randomized clinical trial. *Journal of Clinical Child and Adolescent Psychology*, *38*, 753–759. doi:10.1080/15374410903103544

McCullough, M. E. (1999). Research on religion-accommodative counseling: Review and meta-analysis. *Journal of Counseling Psychology*, *46*, 92–98. doi:10.1037/0022-0167.46.1.92

McDonald, L. M. (2007). *The Biblical canon: Its origin, transmission, and authority*. Peabody, MA: Hendrickson.

O'Conner, K. J. (1983). The color your life technique. In C. E. Schaefer & K. J. O'Conner (Eds.), *Handbook of play therapy* (pp. 251–257). New York, NY: Wiley.

Pargament, K. I., Murray-Swank, N. A., Magyar, G. M., & Ano, G. G. (2005). Spiritual struggle: A phenomenon of interest to psychology and religion. In W. R. Miller & H. D. Delaney (Eds.), *Judeo-Christian perspectives on psychology: Human nature, motivation, and change* (pp. 245–268). Washington, DC: American Psychological Association. doi:10.1037/10859-013

Post, B. C., & Wade, N. G. (2009). Religion and spirituality in psychotherapy: A practice-friendly review of research. *Journal of Clinical Psychology*, *65*, 131–146. doi:10.1002/jclp.20563

Richards, P. S., & Worthington, E. L., Jr. (2010). The need for evidence-based, spiritually-oriented psychotherapies. *Professional Psychology: Research and Practice*, *41*, 363–370. doi:10.1037/a0019469

Rosmarin, D. H., Pargament, K. I., & Mahoney, A. (2009). The role of religiousness in anxiety, depression, and happiness in a Jewish community sample: A preliminary investigation. *Mental Health, Religion & Culture*, *12*, 97–113. doi:10.1080/13674670802321933

Schnall, E. (2006). Multicultural counseling and the orthodox Jew. *Journal of Counseling & Development*, *84*, 276–282. doi:10.1002/j.1556-6678.2006.tb00406.x

Stark, K. D., Streusand, W., Krumholz, L. S., & Patel, P. (2010). Cognitive behavioral therapy for depression: The ACTION treatment program for girls. In A. Kazdin & J. Weisz (Eds.), *Evidence-based psychotherapies for children and adolescents* (2nd ed., pp. 93–109). New York, NY: Guilford Press.

Steinsaltz, A. (2010). *The essential Talmud: An introduction*. Jerusalem, Israel: Koren.

Tan, S. Y. (2007). Use of prayer and scripture in cognitive-behavioral therapy. *Journal of Psychology and Christianity*, *26*, 101–111.

Tan, S. Y., & Johnson, W. B. (2005). Spiritually oriented cognitive-behavioral therapy. In L. Sperry & E. P. Shafranske (Eds.), *Spiritually oriented psychotherapy* (pp. 77–103). Washington, DC: American Psychological Association. doi:10.1037/10886-004

Walker, D. F., & Quagliana, H. (2007). Integrating scripture with parent training in behavioral interventions. *Journal of Psychology and Christianity*, *26*, 122–131.

Walker, D. F., Reese, J. B., Hughes, J. P., & Troskie, M. J. (2010). Addressing religious and spiritual issues in trauma-focused cognitive behavior therapy with children and adolescents. *Professional Psychology: Research and Practice*, *41*, 174–180. doi:10.1037/a0017782

Walsh, M. (2005). *Roman Catholicism: The basics*. London, England: Routledge.

Webster-Stratton, C. (2005). The Incredible Years: A training series for the prevention and treatment of conduct problems in young children. In E. D. Hibbs & P. S. Jensen (Eds.), *Psychosocial treatments for child and adolescent disorders: Empirically based strategies for clinical practice* (2nd ed., pp. 507–555). Washington, DC: American Psychological Association.

Weersing, V. R., & Brent, D. A. (2010). Treating depression in adolescents using individual cognitive behavioral therapy. In J. R. Weisz & A. E. Kazdin (Eds.), *Evidence-based psychotherapies for children and adolescents* (2nd ed., pp. 126–139). New York, NY: Guilford Press.

Zisser, A., & Eyberg, S. M. (2010). Parent–child interaction therapy and the treatment of disruptive behavior disorders. In J. R. Weisz & A. E. Kazdin (Eds.), *Evidence-based psychotherapies for children and adolescents* (2nd ed., pp. 179–193). New York, NY: Guilford Press.

8

PRAYER

DONALD F. WALKER, WILLIAM DOVERSPIKE, SAMEERA AHMED, AVIDAN MILEVSKY, AND JACQUELINE D. WOOLLEY

> Now I lay me down to sleep, The Lord I pray my soul to keep,
> If I should die before I wake, The Lord I pray my soul to take.
>
> —18th-century prayer

In the 18th century, this prayer was often taught to children as a means of coping with the anxiety of the real threat of death as a result of the high childhood mortality rate. In the 20th and 21st centuries, clinical experience and empirical research have consistently found that children of various religious and spiritual traditions often pray when faced with anxiety (Bamford & Lagatutta, 2010). Prayer is also typically considered a fundamental means of becoming closer to God and searching for the sacred in one's life across a range of religious faiths.

In this chapter, we discuss the use of prayer in psychotherapy with children and adolescents. As a backdrop, we begin by providing a rationale for considering prayer as an intervention in child and adolescent psychotherapy. Next, we review several definitions of prayer, discuss ethical recommendations related to its use, and provide clinical recommendations for the use of prayer as an intervention with children and teens. We also provide an overview of prayer practices among people from several major

DOI: 10.1037/13947-009
Spiritual Interventions in Child and Adolescent Psychotherapy, D. F. Walker and W. L. Hathaway (Editors)

world religions, focusing on Christianity, Islam, and Judaism because these are religions that we are more familiar with. We conclude with several case studies involving prayer with child and adolescent clients. Our hope in this chapter (as well as in the others in this book) is to reach both an audience of practitioners who may be more familiar with the body of literature relating psychology to religion and spirituality (e.g., members of the Society for the Psychology of Religion and Spirituality, American Psychological Association [APA] Division 36) and child and adolescent psychotherapists who might be less familiar with that literature but who are interested in learning how to operate in a religiously and spiritually culturally sensitive way with their clients.

We are also aware that prayer is a transcendent experience that defies verbal description and is practiced in countless diverse ways across diverse religious and spiritual traditions. In a real way, any attempt to comprehensively cover the sheer magnitude of prayer practices within the confines of a single book chapter is nearly impossible. Entire books have been written on the subject, and we refer readers who are interested in more in-depth coverage of the practice of prayer from the perspective of various major world religions to, for example, Basit (1997); Foster (1992); Green and Holtz (2006); Iyengar and Menuhin (1995); Keating (2002); Kirzner, Kirzner, and Aiken (2003); Kushner and Polen (2004); Merton (2007); Paramananda (2006); and Zaleski and Zaleski (2005).

RATIONALE FOR PRAYER AS AN INTERVENTION IN CHILD AND ADOLESCENT PSYCHOTHERAPY

Psychologists are ethically bound to treat spirituality, including spiritual practices such as prayer, as aspects of client diversity and with respect (APA, 2010). Furthermore, people of all ages pray for comfort and support when faced with challenging circumstances. As have others, we suggest that psychotherapists consider prayer as an intervention when clients report that they use prayer in their daily life (for reviews, see Beach, Fincham, Hurt, McNair, & Stanley, 2008; Sullivan & Karney, 2008; Worthington, 2008). We also recommend prayer as an intervention under certain clinical conditions, which we describe in detail. Psychologists are ethically obligated and typically want to treat their clients' religious and spiritual beliefs, values, and practices with sensitivity and respect (APA, 2010).

In this chapter, we argue that psychologists should apply this same ethical and clinical ethos to clients of all ages (even children) provided that these conditions apply. In doing so, we acknowledge that younger children, in particular, experience the Divine differently than do adults or even adolescents (see Chapter 4, this volume, for a review). However, we believe that psychologists should (with respect and sensitivity) enter into their clients' inner worlds and discuss prayer in psychotherapy.

DEFINITIONS OF PRAYER AMONG ADULTS AND CHILDREN

Previously, we have found William James's (1902/1936) definition of *prayer* as "every kind of inward communication or conversation with the power recognized as divine" (p. 454) to be very helpful in conceptualizing prayer in its broadest sense outside the context of psychotherapy (see Walker & Moon, 2011). However, when considered specifically in the realm of counseling and psychotherapy, we have found it useful to define *prayer* as an intervention involving communication with the divine for the purpose of meeting a treatment goal that is psychological or spiritual in nature. Prayer in the context of psychotherapy can be commenced by (a) the psychotherapist alone, (b) by the client alone, or (c) by the psychotherapist and client together. Furthermore, interventions involving prayer can occur either in session or out of session. With adults and with children, we believe that interventions involving prayer are dependent on several factors, including the theoretical orientation and practice setting of the psychotherapist, the religious backgrounds of the psychotherapist and client, and the presenting problem of the client.

Interventions involving prayer with children and teens are more complicated than those using prayer with adults, for several reasons. First, parents and guardians maintain the legal right to provide consent for treatment for their children, including prayer. Second, the potential application of prayer in psychotherapy is also more complicated with children and adolescents because of the inherent spiritual and emotional intimacy associated with prayer that is coupled with a somewhat more explicit power differential between an adult psychotherapist and a child or adolescent client. We discuss ways to address these ethical concerns in the next section. Finally, children understand prayer to varying degrees depending on their developmental level.

One of the earliest studies to address children's understanding of prayer was conducted by Goldman (1964). This research demonstrated that children between the ages of 6 and 16 held strong beliefs regarding the efficacy of prayer. However, their conceptions of prayer seemed to be different; children younger than age 9 were found to conceive of prayer as similar to magic or, as Goldman relayed, like "shouting one's requests up the chimney to Santa Claus" (p. 185). Later work by Long, Elkind, and Spilka (1967) also assessed young children's understanding of prayer and found a stagelike progression, with 5- to 7-year-olds displaying a very vague sense of prayer and God, 7- to 9-year-olds conceiving of only the behavioral aspects, and children age 9 and older finally conceiving of prayer in an adultlike manner, as a private conversation with God.

More recent research on prayer concepts, however, has revealed that children understand various important aspects of prayer quite early. For example, Woolley and Phelps (2001) assessed the prayer concepts of 3- to 8-year-old children from primarily Christian families. By age 5, close to 90% of the children reported that they knew what it meant to pray and that they themselves had prayed. Children's understanding of various facets of prayer was found to undergo additional development during the preschool and early elementary years. For example, preschoolers appeared to have a fairly rigid and limited concept, believing that, for example, one can only pray at specific times and in specific places. Young elementary-age children understood that people can pray at any time. Preschool-age children also seemed somewhat unsure about the efficacy of their own prayers, although they often agreed that others' prayers would be answered. As children got older, they became more confident that their own prayers would be answered. Woolley and Phelps also documented children's development in the importance that they placed on various aspects of prayer. Preschool-age children valued the physical components (e.g., closing one's eyes) most, whereas 5- to 6-year-olds considered mental and physical components as equally as important. Children age 7 and older gave more weight to the mental aspects (e.g., thinking of God).

Given that this research has indicated that children as young as age 4 have a concept of prayer, it is important to consider children's beliefs about when someone might engage in prayer and what functions prayer might serve. Do young children, as do older children and adults, understand that engaging in prayer can be an effective means of coping with stress and anxiety? Some studies (Mooney, Graziano, & Katz, 1985; Rew, Wong, & Sternglanz, 2004) have shown that children age 8 and older understand that praying can make them feel better during difficult times. Studies with younger children are rare. However, Bamford and Lagattuta (2010) examined these issues in 4- to 8-year-olds. They found an intriguing age-related development in understanding of the reasons for prayer. Whereas adults primarily believed people would pray when experiencing negative emotions, younger children claimed that people would be more likely to pray when experiencing positive emotions. The critical shift appeared to occur between 6 and 8 years of age, with 8-year-olds claiming that positive and negative emotions motivated prayer equally. Being scared was the first emotion that children understood as motivating prayer. There was also development in children's understanding of prayer between the ages of 6 and 8 regarding how a person would feel after praying. Four- to 6-year-olds claimed that people would feel better after praying if they prayed after experiencing a positive emotion, and older children believed that people would feel better if they prayed after experiencing a negative emotion. So it seems that not until 7 or 8 years of age do children fully understand that prayer can serve as a strategy for dealing with negative emotions.

ETHICS GOVERNING THE USE OF PRAYER WITH CHILDREN AND TEENS

In this section, we briefly review ethical considerations that apply to the use of prayer regardless of the age of the client while also more thoroughly elaborating on ethical principles involved in the use of prayer. When considering the use of prayer in psychotherapy with children and adolescents several ethical standards should be taken into account. These standards include attaining competence, obtaining consent, maintaining boundaries, respecting differences, and avoiding harm.

Attaining Competence

Putting ethics into practice begins with practicing within one's scope of competence as defined by one's education, training, and experience. As Canter, Bennett, Jones, and Nagyn (1994) pointed out, "Merely having an interest in a particular area does not necessarily qualify one to practice in that area" (p. 34). In the APA (2010) "Ethical Principles of Psychologists and Code of Conduct" (hereinafter referred to as the APA Ethics Code), Standard 2.01 (Boundaries of Competence) states, "Psychologists provide services, teach, and conduct research with populations and in areas only within the boundaries of their competence, based on their education, training, supervised experience, consultation, study, or professional experience" (p. 5). APA Ethics Code Standard 2.01(e) further states that in those areas in which generally recognized standards for preparatory training do not yet exist, psychologists take reasonable steps to ensure the competence of their work and to protect clients or patients from harm.

Elsewhere, we have noted that one difficulty encountered when considering the use of prayer in psychotherapy is that so few psychotherapists have received any kind of education or training on which to base such an intervention (Walker & Moon, 2011). In the absence of formal training, psychologists are likely to use their own personal experiences as the basis for spiritual interventions used in psychotherapy (Walker, Gorsuch, & Tan, 2005; Walker, Gorsuch, Tan, & Otis, 2008). Previously, we have suggested that competence can be attained through formal training (e.g., enrolling in a graduate course that focuses on psychology and spirituality), continuing education (e.g., attending workshops or reading peer-reviewed journals such as *Psychology of Religion and Spirituality*), and consultation with other psychologists who have training and experience in the use of spiritual interventions such as prayer (Walker & Moon, 2011). Psychologists may also wish to consult with religious leaders associated with a client's specific religious tradition.

Obtaining Consent

When treating children and adolescents specifically, psychotherapy essentially becomes an ethical balancing act, with the psychotherapist's ethical duties toward the minor client balanced against the legal rights of the parents or guardians. In most states, for a minor to enter into a psychotherapeutic relationship, it is necessary for a parent or guardian to give informed consent (Lawrence & Kurpius, 2000). The definition of a minor differs from state to state, ranging from an upper limit of 18 to 21 years of age in some states to a lower limit in some states that allows 16-year-olds to consent to their own health care in some circumstances (Barnett & Johnson, 2010). Psychotherapists have a responsibility to be familiar with the laws in their state pertaining to minors (Barnett, Hillard, & Lowry, 2001).

APA (2010) Ethics Code Standard 3.10(b) states,

> For persons who are legally incapable of giving informed consent, psychologists nevertheless (1) provide an appropriate explanation, (2) seek the individual's assent, (3) consider such persons' preferences and best interests, and (4) obtain appropriate permission from a legally authorized person, if such substitute consent is permitted or required by law. When consent by a legally authorized person is not permitted or required by law, psychologists take reasonable steps to protect the individual's rights and welfare. (p. 6)

In accordance with this standard, establishing informed consent when working with minor clients involves the dual process of obtaining legal consent from the parents while attaining voluntary assent from the minor client. Assent to treatment implies that psychotherapists involve minors in decisions about their own care and that they agree to participate in their treatment (Welfel, 2006). Consent (from a legal perspective) can be given only by parents, guardians, or custodians of minor children, whereas assent (agreement and cooperation with interventions) may be given by minors themselves. This twofold process begins at the initial session, with all decision makers involved, and continues as an ongoing process as the need arises over the course of treatment.

When minors and their parents or guardians are in agreement with psychotherapy goals, objectives, and interventions (including prayer), few conflicts are likely to emerge when establishing informed consent. However, several potential conflicts may be encountered when there are discrepancies regarding the use of prayer. First, situations arise in which parents request that prayer be used as an intervention contrary to the requests of the child or adolescent client. Lack of assent on the part of the client is likely to render the use of any intervention ineffective and, possibly, unethical. Therefore, in such situations, we recommend against forcing such an intervention on a child or adolescent client. We also advise psychotherapists faced with this sort of potential conflict regarding an intervention to process their internal conflict with both the minor-age client and the parent or parents present in session. For example, one of us (Donald F. Walker) had a male teenage client present for psychotherapy who was struggling with feelings of same-sex attraction. This referral was generated by the teen's parents to an explicitly Christian private practice. The teen's parents were theologically conservative Christians who were alarmed at their teen's expression of same-sex attraction. The parents requested psychotherapy to assist the teen in processing his feelings of same-sex attraction, with their explicitly stated hope that the teenager would stop experiencing such feelings. The teen, however, reported not wanting to give up his gay identity and objected to the parents' goal. As part of the teenager's psychotherapy, the parents requested that Walker join them in prayer in session to pray away the teen's feelings of same-sex attraction. This case illustrates the ethical conflict involved when the goals and means of psychotherapy differ between one or more parents who have a legal right to consent to treatment and a minor child from whom assent should be attained. In this case, Walker had the family meet in a family psychotherapy session and acknowledged the discrepancy between the goals of the parents and the goals of the teen. In this family's case, they chose to proceed with family therapy with the goals of improving communication between both parents and the teen and improving the level of differentiation within the family.

Conversely, a psychotherapist may encounter an ethical dilemma in a situation in which an adolescent client requests prayer to which the parent or guardian has not given consent. Prudent psychotherapists generally do not use interventions for which informed consent has not been properly established. As a general rule, parents who object to their child's participation in psychotherapy probably have a legal right to do so (Remley & Herlihy, 2010). Thus, we recommend obtaining the permission of the child client's parent or legal guardian in such situations. This is less difficult to do when the parent and the child are of the same religious background and the parent is supportive of the child's attempts to make use of religious resources (such as prayer) to cope with his or her presenting issue. For example, Walker treated an African American teenage sex offender who was in the custody of the state at the time of treatment. In processing the teen's cognitions related to his history of sexual offenses, the teenager reported wanting to repent of his sins and receive forgiveness. As part of this process, he reported frequently praying and wanting reassurance that his sins would be forgiven and that he could enter into heaven. As his psychotherapist, Walker assessed the teen's religious background and his understanding of it. The teenage client functioned in the range of borderline mental retardation and did not appear to have a clear understanding of religious doctrine in his tradition, which he reported as Christian. As his psychotherapist, Walker scheduled a meeting with his legal guardian, a caseworker from the Department of Child and Family Services. During that meeting, he informed the caseworker of the client's fears about going to hell and his desire for repentance. She supported his desire to explore his own religious beliefs related to salvation and to seek forgiveness from God. She referred the client to a clergy member from his own tradition and granted Walker permission to make this a focus of treatment for a limited time. During this time, Walker explored the client's beliefs about going to heaven and listened to the content of his prayers to God asking for forgiveness. He also explored with him what it meant to him to be forgiven by God and assisted him in further processing this with his minister.

A third area of potential conflict arises when the parents themselves disagree on the use of spiritual interventions such as prayer. Proceeding with an intervention despite parental disagreement is likely to result in a therapist quandary such as splitting or triangulation. Walker treated an 8-year-old girl whose parents were divorcing in an explicitly Christian private practice. The child's father brought the girl to psychotherapy, wanting to help her process feelings of anxiety related to the divorce and indicating that prayer helped the client to feel calm when she is at home. Her father also made statements to the psychotherapist explicitly blaming the other parent for the child's anxiety because of the way that his ex-wife parented the girl when the client was in her custody. The client's mother came to psychotherapy to express to Walker that she did not want the child to receive counseling. In this instance, Walker scheduled a meeting with both parents present (without the child in session) and provided them both with his recommendations for treatment. During this session, he also encouraged them to consider the best interests of their daughter and to express any concerns about treatment at that time. As a result, all were able to agree on boundaries related to discussing the other parent in treatment, part of which involved allowing both parents to have separate family sessions with their daughter periodically. As a result, treatment continued. In treatment, Walker encouraged the girl to continue her practice of prayer at home when she felt anxious as part of a cognitive–behavioral therapy intervention to reduce her anxiety. We discuss the use of prayer as part of cognitive–behavioral therapy to reduce anxiety in more detail later in this chapter.

Finally, potential conflicts may arise when there are discrepancies in the expression of spirituality between psychotherapist and client, particularly when these discrepancies involve differences in religious background or culture. In such situations, psychologists at a minimum respect such differences, and they avoid imposing their values or beliefs on others.

Maintaining Boundaries

Boundaries can be defined in terms of competence (e.g., scope of education, training, supervision), role (e.g., evaluation, intervention, supervision), time (e.g., extended sessions, cancelled appointments), context (e.g., individual psychotherapy, family therapy, group therapy), place (e.g., office, school, house of worship), and disclosure (e.g., professional vs. personal information).

When considering the use of prayer with clients, psychotherapists may ask themselves several questions concerning boundaries: How well is the psychotherapist managing clear boundaries related to his or her role? If a psychotherapist is having trouble managing boundaries, the use of prayer may further blur them. How intact are the client's ego boundaries, including reality-testing abilities? If the client has weak ego boundaries or distorted perceptions of reality, the use of explicitly spiritual interventions such as prayer could result in confusion, distortion, or misinterpretation on the part of the client. When considering context, where does the use of prayer occur on the continuum between privacy and publicity? Engaging in a community prayer in the context of a group process (e.g., participating in the serenity prayer at the conclusion of a substance abuse group for teenagers) is less likely to be misinterpreted by the client or others, whereas engaging in prayer in the privacy of a psychotherapy session has greater potential to blur role boundaries. In psychotherapy with children and teens, the context is a substantially greater interpersonal power differential between psychotherapists and children and teens. This power differential is even greater when the context involves client presenting issues that are inherently related to difficulties with interpersonal boundaries, such as when a child has been abused, is dealing with an extremely debilitating condition such as psychotic symptoms, or has personality traits that are consistent with a developing personality disorder. When considering place, psychotherapists should ask themselves if prayer is an appropriate intervention in their specific treatment context. For example, one of us (Walker) worked in a community mental health center that actively discouraged prayer as a specific intervention, even though the agency encouraged consideration of religious and spiritual factors during an initial intake assessment. Prayer is certainly an inappropriate intervention in a public school treatment setting, although it may be appropriate in a parochial school (Richards & Bergin, 2005).

For example, one of us (Walker) treated a boy from a Roman Catholic faith background in a school setting. This boy reported having psychotic symptoms in which God told him to hurt other people. The boy felt that these voices were a form of prayer (communication from God). This communication from God confused him because it involved telling him to do something antithetical to God's nature. The boy also questioned whether he was going to hell for having feelings of wanting to hurt others. In this case, Walker contacted the client's parents and got the client a referral to see a psychiatrist before returning to the school setting. When the client returned, having been stabilized, Walker reassured him that the voices that he heard were not from God. Walker then contacted the boy's parents again and referred the client to their priest to further process his fears about going to hell and wanting to pray about the experience.

Respecting Differences

As one of the five foundational ethical principles of the APA (2010) Ethics Code, Principle E (Respect for People's Rights and Dignity) states,

> Psychologists are aware of and respect cultural, individual, and role differences, including those based on age, gender, gender identity, race, ethnicity, culture, national origin, religion, sexual orientation, disability, language, and socioeconomic status and consider these factors when working with members of such groups. (p. 3)

When considering the use of prayer in psychotherapy, psychotherapists may ask themselves several questions concerning multicultural considerations: What are the multicultural implications of using prayer with a client? In other words, what is the significance of using prayer with respect to the client's age, sex, race, ethnicity, religion, national origin, indigenous heritage, or sexual orientation? What is the prevailing practice in the client's local community, organization, or institution? Magaletta and Brawer (1998) advised psychologists to be sensitive to the real and ascribed differences in power between themselves and the clients whom they serve. Diversity-sensitive psychotherapists are aware of the inequity of power, particularly with respect to differences in the intellectual and emotional maturity levels that exist between them and their minor clients.

Whether done explicitly or implicitly, *value imposition* refers to a psychotherapist's attempts to influence a client to adopt the psychotherapist's values, attitudes, beliefs, or behaviors (Richards & Bergin, 2005). Culturally sensitive psychotherapists know their own values, attitudes, and beliefs, and they avoid imposing their values and beliefs on clients. Hage (2006) maintained that psychologists have a responsibility to monitor themselves so that they do not impose their values pertaining to spirituality on clients. Avoiding imposing one's values on a client may at times involve subtle behaviors that go beyond the psychotherapist's disclosures. For example, asking a client to pray during psychotherapy sessions may represent an imposition of the therapist's values rather than reflecting a respect for the client's values. In contrast, Magaletta and Brawer (1998) reported that one psychotherapist they knew demonstrated respect for Muslim clients by learning about the ritual prayers than Muslims offer five times a day and by avoiding scheduling Muslim clients during these times. Such an approach demonstrates respect for clients while strengthening the therapeutic alliance.

Avoiding Harm

When considering the use of prayer in psychotherapy, questions arise concerning contraindications or circumstances that might result in a client being harmed or feeling exploited in the psychotherapeutic relationship. Contraindications against the use of prayer include psychotherapist competencies and client characteristics.

With regard to psychotherapist competencies, a psychotherapist should use prayer in psychotherapy only if he or she possesses competence in using prayer and other spiritual interventions. Magaletta and Brawer (1998) suggested that psychologists be aware of ways in which a client's religious or cultural group engages in prayer before attempting to do so with clients. More recently, Worthington (2008) went further to suggest that a psychotherapist should avoid using prayer with clients when the psychotherapist does not know enough about a client's religion to do so psychotherapeutically. Later in this chapter, we review in detail specific client characteristics that contraindicate the use of prayer.

While considering ways of avoiding harm to clients, it can be argued that a strict risk management approach that prevents psychotherapists from doing any harm may also prevent psychotherapists from doing any good (Zur, 2007). For example, a survey of primary care physicians indicated that 91% of respondents considered prayer an important treatment modality, yet 50.6% rarely or never discussed prayer with patients (Wilson, Lipscomb, Ward, Replogle, & Hill, 2000). In a related vein, a national survey of more than 1,000 clinical psychologists conducted by Hathaway, Scott, and Garver (2004) found that the majority of respondents believed a client's spirituality is an important aspect of functioning. However, this survey also revealed that the majority of psychologists do not routinely include spirituality in their treatment of clients. Hathaway et al. concluded that spirituality may be a neglected domain in clinical practice. As Corey, Corey, and Callanan (2010) pointed out, "This omission might well limit the effectiveness of therapy for some clients, which involves a clear ethical concern" (p. 94).

CLINICAL RECOMMENDATIONS RELATED TO PRAYER IN PSYCHOTHERAPY

Walker and Moon (2011) suggested that the use of prayer in psychotherapy should be tied to an assessment of both the client (including factors related to the client's presenting problem as well as contraindications to the use of prayer) and oneself as a psychotherapist (e.g., one's training related to using spiritually oriented interventions and one's religious cultural competence with a particular client). We discuss these factors, as well as the process of gaining informed consent for treatment, in greater detail in this section. Throughout this discussion, where applicable, we draw on material from Walker and Moon because a number of principles related to the use of prayer apply with clients of any age. However, throughout this dialogue, we focus on the application of these more general principles related to the use of prayer to the practice of child and adolescent psychotherapy specifically.

Client Assessment

McMinn (1996) suggested that psychotherapists consider "which forms of prayer should be used with which clients under which circumstances" (p. 81). According to McMinn, psychotherapists should consider (a) whether using prayer in psychotherapy will help establish a healthy sense of self for the client in question, (b) whether using prayer with a particular client will help that client foster a healthy relationship with God at a particular point in psychotherapy, and (c) whether using prayer in psychotherapy with a particular client will help establish a healing psychotherapeutic relationship.

McMinn (1996) also conceptualized the use of prayer as involving a continuum of risk ranging from low risk (involving assigning prayer as an out-of-session homework assignment) to high risk (praying together repeatedly over a number of sessions). In a related vein, Richards and Bergin (2005) suggested that psychotherapists and clients should probably pray together during sessions only when three circumstances converge: (a) competent psychological care is being provided, (b) in-session prayer is specifically requested by the client, and (c) thorough psychological, spiritual, and religious assessment have convinced the psychotherapist that engaging in prayer is not likely to lead to confusion in psychotherapeutic role boundaries.

Worthington (2008) emphasized the need for psychotherapists to be aware of their clients' specific religious traditions before using prayer in psychotherapy. He made the point that although psychologists often consider spirituality a broad construct that is independent of a person's religious traditions, clients do not. Instead, most religiously committed clients want their psychotherapist to help them incorporate aspects of their personal spirituality (including prayer) from within their particular religious tradition.

Developmentally, as we discussed earlier in the chapter, children younger than ages 7 or 8 may not be able to understand that prayer can be used as a coping mechanism. Therefore, we recommend that psychotherapists assess children's developmental understanding of prayer when considering prayer as an intervention with preschool- and school-age children. In addition, psychotherapists are encouraged to carefully consider the content of children's prayers when they pray. Grossoehme et al. (2010) published a content analysis of more than 800 children's written prayers in a pediatric hospital over a 6-month time period. Their linguistic analysis suggested that there was a balance between prayers that were focused on causation (asking the Divine to change the child's circumstance) and insight (helping the child to understand it). In a related vein, prayers tended to be evenly split between attending to the present moment and understanding the past. As a result, Grossoehme et al. recommended that psychotherapists carefully avoid changing the focus of children's prayers when children are praying. For example, they suggested that psychotherapists should avoid moving child clients from immediate concerns focused on feeling better about a stressful situation (when praying) to promoting insight about the event before children are ready to make those transitions.

Contraindications to the Use of Prayer in Psychotherapy

Previously, we have made the overarching recommendation against incorporating prayer in psychotherapy when the client either (a) does not pray as part of his or her regular spiritual life or (b) does not want to include prayer in his or her psychotherapy at this particular time (Walker & Moon, 2011). We extend this recommendation to psychotherapy with children but also note that psychotherapists should discuss with both parent and child situations in which a parent requests prayer as part of the child's therapy and the child does not want it, or vice versa. We have also previously emphasized that prayer may be inappropriate at some secular clinical sites and is undoubtedly inappropriate in the public school setting because of regulations related to the separation of church and state (Walker & Moon, 2011).

In addition to these broad recommendations regarding the client's faith system and the setting for psychotherapy, we also encourage psychotherapists to consider the function of prayer within the faith system and psychological functioning of their child and adolescent clients. For example, a child who is highly anxious might be in a religiously committed family and be religiously committed him- or herself. He or she might report praying (or wanting to pray) frequently, but in a manner that would serve to reinforce maladaptive psychological functioning. If prayer is incorporated in psychotherapy without addressing the child's presenting symptoms, then prayer could become a rote experience that serves to reduce anxiety without helping the child to address it. Conversely, prayer could be used as a spiritually oriented intervention that addresses the child's presenting symptoms while also being used by the client to enhance his or her spirituality. A healthy way to use prayer as an intervention with such a client could involve, for example, encouraging the client to pray for the strength to endure his or her anxiety while being careful to avoid praying for his or her fears to simply go away. We would also suggest to an anxious client (and his or her parents) that the client also maintain prayer as a spiritual practice during times when he or she is not anxious so as to preserve the spiritual significance of prayer.

A second specific presenting problem in which prayer as a psychotherapeutic practice is contraindicated carte blanche involves situations in which the client has been diagnosed with obsessive–compulsive disorder and prays compulsively. Garcia (2008) reported a case study involving a college-age adolescent Catholic girl who prayed the rosary compulsively when she had sexual thoughts or when she felt unclean because she had heard someone close by swearing. Her psychotherapist addressed her compulsive practice of prayer by prescribing the times and places during the day when she was to pray. In this case, her psychotherapist also engaged in the unusual practice of exposing her to swearing and offensive, blasphemous language in the psychotherapy office followed by response prevention to her praying. Although we believe that her psychotherapist could have achieved a similar objective in a more religiously sensitive manner, we would also engage in response prevention of prayer if prayer was being done in a compulsive manner by such a client. In particular, we encourage psychotherapists to consider prescribing times for a client dealing with religious scrupulosity to pray. We also encourage psychotherapists to obtain a parental release of information and child assent to collaborate with the child or teenage client's religious leader. We believe that encouraging the child client to consult with his or her clergy member can help the client to keep sight of the spiritual significance of prayer within his or her religious and spiritual faith tradition.

A third presenting problem in which prayer is contraindicated, at least initially, involves situations in which clients are psychotic. On more than one occasion, we have talked with psychotic clients who, in either an assessment or in the context of regular psychotherapy, believed that they were having or had just experienced an actual discussion with God. Depictions of God by psychotic clients are frequently quite vivid and often involve them believing that they have seen parts of heaven. We would discourage any form of prayer as an intervention with such clients, at least until they have been stabilized on antipsychotic medication. Moreover, we also encourage psychotherapists to actively confront these clients' belief that they have talked to God when they are psychotic, during the episode and afterward. Depending on their age, their family's religious background, and the degree to which they have been provided with religious instruction, such clients may need further psychoeducation as well as religious education about prayer and mystical experiences within their faith tradition. In these instances, we have typically provided psychoeducation about psychosis to those clients in an age-appropriate way and then referred them to get further instruction about their faith tradition's understanding of how people experience God from their clergy member. Before referring such clients to their religious leader, we typically schedule a family session in which one or both parents are present as well and have the client process the psychotic experience with his or her parents so that they can also discuss their understanding of how people experience God within their faith tradition.

In addition to psychological problems in which prayer is contraindicated as a psychotherapeutic practice, we also believe that there are several religious and spiritual contraindications to prayer in psychotherapy as well. First, we discourage prayer as an intervention when the client's presentation involves parental pressure to conform to a particular way of being religious—either implicitly or explicitly. Second, we also discourage using prayer to cope with any psychological problem in which the use of prayer is only to pray that the problem itself goes away. We believe that praying in this fashion reinforces poor religious and nonreligious coping methods and also devalues the experience of prayer as a spiritual discipline or practice.

Informed Consent for Prayer With Children and Adolescents

Before using prayer as an intervention, psychotherapists should obtain parental informed consent and child assent. As Walker and Moon (2011) suggested, clients should be informed of the psychotherapist's familiarity with their religious and spiritual tradition regarding prayer. Clients should also be informed of their psychotherapist's comfort with using prayer as part of psychotherapy. The parent and child should be informed of any potential risks involving prayer. For example, clients should be reminded that prayer does not guarantee that God will respond to them in the way that they are asking. They should also be told that the locus of change in psychotherapy ultimately rests on them. Finally, clients should also be informed of their right to choose alternative treatment methods that do not include prayer and given information about what those methods might be. Informed consent and assent should be continually updated throughout the treatment process, and the psychotherapist should routinely check that prayer is meeting the client's goals for psychotherapy.

PRAYER PRACTICES OF MEMBERS OF SPECIFIC RELIGIOUS TRADITIONS

In this section, we review various ways in which members of diverse spiritual and religious affiliations practice prayer. We focus on Christian, Jewish, and Islamic approaches to prayer because we are most familiar with these approaches personally and professionally. Across traditions, we provide an overview of forms of prayer within each faith tradition, then describe the application of prayer in psychotherapy using one or more case examples.

Christian Approaches to Prayer

Christianity is a monotheistic religion based on the life and teachings of Jesus of Nazareth as described in the New Testament. Although Christianity is a monotheistic religion, Christians view God as consisting of one person with three essences—the Father, Son, and Holy Spirit. A number of diverse Christian denominations exist that can be broadly categorized as Orthodox, Roman Catholic, and Protestant sects. Protestant beliefs can be categorized along a continuum ranging from fundamentalist to conservative, evangelical, mainline, and theologically liberal. Across denominations, a core belief is that Jesus is the Son of God and that belief in his death and resurrection is a basis for salvation.

Among Christians, *prayer* is "an act of worship, experience, and communication with any or all members of the Trinity" (Walker & Moon, 2011, p. 155). However, prayer is a multifaceted experience, and Christians of various denominations experience prayer differently outside the context of psychotherapy. For example, Roman Catholics are typically taught to pray to saints or angels to make intercessions for them, whereas Protestants are usually taught to pray directly to God. For additional information on different sects within Christianity, we refer the reader to Richards and Bergin (2000).

Application to Psychotherapy

Foster (1992) identified 21 different ways for Christians to pray. When presenting case examples, we focus on two forms of Christian prayer: simple prayer and contemplative prayer. What Foster referred to as *simple prayer* seems to be a logical way to incorporate prayer into psychotherapy with Christian children and teens. The practice of simple prayer involves, as it implies, talking to God without incorporating liturgy or a structure to the conversation. One of us (Walker) has worked in both secular and explicitly religious clinical settings in which a child or teen simply talked to God as part of his or her treatment, both in and outside of the session. There are several presenting problems for which simple prayer seems appropriate, including dealing with traumatic grief, coping with anxiety, managing anger, or fostering forgiveness among family members.

According to Foster (1992), *contemplative prayer* involves becoming quiet and then focusing on God, perhaps by repeating the word *God* or *love* or a phrase such as the "Jesus prayer" found in the New Testament: "Lord Jesus Christ, son of God, have mercy on me" (Luke 18:10–14). The use of contemplative prayer as a spiritual discipline is intended to help the person praying to become more aware of the presence of God in his or her life. As an additional psychotherapeutic benefit, this practice also tends to help the individual praying to become more calm and relaxed as well.

Case Study: Simple Prayer for a Young Girl's Traumatic Grief

One of us (Walker) has worked with several children of various ages dealing with traumatic grief in a secular setting. The following case example has been amalgamated from several such cases. Identifying and presenting information have been changed to protect client confidentiality. A 7-year-old Caucasian girl, Jane, was brought to psychotherapy by her mother after the murder of her father. Her initial presentation to therapy was precipitated by an increase in defiant behavior at home and at school in which she refused to follow directions and engaged in angry outbursts. She also exhibited some signs of depression, including difficulty sleeping and irritability. She was diagnosed with an adjustment disorder with mixed disturbance of emotions and conduct.

During the early stages of therapy, in separate adjunct sessions with her mother, Walker explored the extent to which Jane had been informed of the circumstances of her father's death. Her mother reported that she herself had been told of her husband's murder by a policeman while Jane's grandmother was present. Her mother believed that Jane had not heard how the murder occurred. Subsequent therapy sessions with Jane made it clear that she had overheard her mother talking with her grandmother about the circumstances of her father's murder. Although Jane did not meet formal diagnostic criteria for posttraumatic stress disorder, her anger and depression were clearly precipitated by her learning of her father's death.

Recent writing on traumatic grief (e.g., Cohen, Mannarino, & Deblinger, 2005) has emphasized the need for traumatic grief–focused work in which the child's trauma narrative is heard by the therapist and integrated into the client's experience. In addition to more secular trauma-focused cognitive–behavioral therapy, Walker also incorporated Jane's talks with God about her father's death into her trauma narrative. Specifically, Walker provided Jane with paint and paper on an easel and encouraged her to paint whatever came to mind. During these sessions, Jane often painted her idea of heaven. Walker asked Jane what she thought of heaven and whether she had talked with God about what had happened. She often asked God why he had taken her daddy. She also said that she frequently talked with her dad, believing that he could hear her when she talked to him in heaven.

Walker conceptualized his role as a psychotherapist as fostering these conversations between Jane, God, and her father, and he encouraged Jane to paint and discuss her feelings about the murder, God, and her father during therapy. He also viewed his role as honoring her relationship with her father and her grief and as bearing witness to her suffering. During the psychotherapy sessions, rather than trying to tell Jane how to grieve or what to believe about her suffering, Walker attempted to bear witness to her pain and be with her in it.

Case Study: Contemplative Prayer With a Christian Parent

Walker also provided family therapy to a single mother, Anna, with three children, of whom the middle child (preteen) was the identified patient. Diagnosed with oppositional defiant disorder, Billy often got into fights with his younger brother, frequently refused to comply with his mother's requests, and would yell back at his mother when she attempted to redirect him during fights. Anna had become increasingly concerned because he was getting bigger and he knew it, and he was subtly threatening her when she tried to get control of him. Her family was very poor and often had difficulty attending therapy because of lack of funds for transportation. In addition, she was dealing with depression herself. As a result, when Billy fought with his siblings, she often threw her hands up and left the room, allowing them to resolve it themselves (which they often did by screaming at each other, then separating, with Billy slamming the door shut behind him and going to play basketball). After encouraging Anna to seek treatment for her own depression (which she did), one therapy goal was to get her to reengage in the family and to mediate disputes and enact discipline whenever there were fights between Billy and his siblings. One of the questions that Walker asked her was what helped her to feel calm during those moments when she felt overwhelmed. Anna said that sometimes when she prayed, she felt calm and centered. She also said during this time of centering that she found it helpful to focus on

God. Without labeling it as such, she was engaging in a process that Foster (1992) referred to as *contemplative prayer*. Walker encouraged her to step back when she first became overwhelmed, pray and get centered, and then engage Billy and his siblings.

During the course of family psychotherapy over the next several months, Anna reported that during times of conflict at home between Billy and his brothers, she would frequently remove herself from the situation initially and then pray a centering prayer before returning to the conflict to mediate it. Combined with the strides that she made in her own individual psychotherapy as a result of dealing with her depression, she was able to gradually improve in her role as a family disciplinarian. As her sons came to the realization that she was able to monitor their behavior and discipline them as necessary, their behavior gradually improved.

Jewish Approaches to Prayer

Clinicians working with Jewish populations are encouraged to understand the substantial differences that exist between members of various denominations of Jews (Bilu & Witzum, 1993; Langman, 1995, 1999). The three primary denominations of Jews are Orthodox, Conservative, and Reform. Orthodox Jews "accept that G-d gave the Torah, the Hebrew Bible, to the People of Israel at Mount Sinai, along with a divinely ordained interpretation of its commands" (Schnall, 2006, p. 277). Orthodox Jews apply the teachings of the Bible and the Talmud to all aspects of life, including daily routines, personal interactions, family life, and business matters. Conservative and Reform Jews, however, practice a more egalitarian Judaism and emphasize the need to view Jewish law in the context of modernism (Schlosser, 2006). Conservatives Jews may be more likely to ascribe divinity to the Bible than Reform Jews. However, both denominations view the Talmud as discussions with historical value but with little legislative authority (De Lange, 2000).

Differences between these denominations of Jews also exist in terms of approaches to prayer. Traditionally, prayer in the Jewish faith is practiced communally. A quorum of at least 10 Jewish males age 13 or older, called a *minyan*, is required to engage in the ideal form of prayer. Furthermore, the prayers chanted are meticulously scripted and are organized in a prayer book called a *siddur*. However, prayer can also be recited privately if an individual cannot attend the communal prayer in the synagogue. The prayers recited individually are identical to the scripted and organized prayer recited communally minus several sections that can only be recited with a minyan. With changes to the tradition emblematic of more egalitarian Jewish denominations, such as Conservative and Reform, prayer has evolved in these groups to include more female representation in communal prayer and the incorporation of nonscripted individualistic prayer.

Integrating Prayer in Psychotherapy With Jews

Several considerations need to be taken into account when attempting to integrate prayer in psychotherapy with Jewish clients. First, religiously committed Jews may view mental health professionals with distrust, especially if the therapist is a non-Jew (i.e., Strean, 1994). Therapists are strongly encouraged to obtain informed consent from their clients to consult with the family's rabbi to ensure that the clients are comfortable that the intervention is religiously sanctioned (Schnall, 2006).

Second, considering the traditional focus on communal and scripted prayer, Orthodox Jews may view private, in-session prayer as inappropriate. As such, instead of actually engaging in prayer during sessions, therapists may want to discuss in treatment the client's experiences and thoughts when praying communally (Miller & Lovinger, 2000). Religious Jewish clients should be open to discussing the thoughts they may have during their prayers considering the importance placed on focusing and concentrating during prayer in traditional laws of prayer. Referred to as *kavanah,* this aspect of prayer necessitates that individuals engaged in prayer have proper thoughts during prayer and focus on the words and meaning of the prayers uttered. In addition to the traditional reasons for the importance of having kavanah, such as the magnitude of the conversation between man and God and the need to make sure that the proper thoughts accompany the conversation, engaging clients in a discussion about having proper kavanah during prayer can serve a therapeutic benefit as well. Having clients focus on the words uttered during prayer may create a relaxed state during prayer similar to the relaxation experienced during meditation (Kaplan, 1985). In many meditative traditions, relaxation entails focusing on an object of meditation. This object can be a sensation, such as a smell or feeling, or it can be a specific word. Encouraging clients to have kavanah during prayers can help create a meditative state that has been used in prior work as a technique to reduce anxiety and other disturbances in well-being (Marlatt & Kristeller, 1999).

For more egalitarian Jews, some form of prayer during the actual psychotherapy session may be beneficial. The type of prayer and the method of praying should be discussed with the client to produce a product that is both meaningful and sensitive to the prayer tradition of the client. Some of these clients may have felt alienated or distant from prayer in the past as a result of a disconnection with tradition. Hence, prayer in psychotherapy with these clients needs to be approached cautiously because the experience may reignite the alienation or may result in a religious reawakening (Miller & Lovinger, 2000).

Case Study: Prayer With a Jewish Adolescent to Deal With Loss

This case involved Maya, a 16-year-old Jewish girl whose family was seeing a psychotherapist (Milevsky) to deal with difficulties the family was experiencing with Maya's younger sister. The 14-year-old sister had been adopted as an infant and had recently experienced pervasive behavioral disturbances. During this time, the sister's biological mother resurfaced and offered to take back her child. Although reluctant to give up their child, the adopted parents agreed to transfer custody back to the biological mother, considering the family turmoil created by the adopted child. Maya was very disturbed by the fact that her parents were giving her sister back to her biological mother and experienced a profound sense of loss. Maya was also fearful that her sister's biological mother was not a good influence on her and that something bad might happen to her sister after she moved in with her biological mother.

Milevsky suggested that the family organize a departure ceremony that would include the recital of the traditional traveler's prayer, which is a prayer for a safe journey recited at the onset of every intercity journey. He encouraged the family to focus the prayer on the journey their daughter was about to embark on with her biological family, producing the following amalgamated prayer:

> May it be Your will, God and the God of our ancestors, that You lead her toward peace, guide her footsteps toward peace, and make her reach her desired destination for life, gladness, and peace. May You rescue her from the hand of every foe, ambush along the way, and from all manner of punishments that assemble to come to earth. May You send blessing in her handiwork, and grant her grace, kindness, and mercy in Your eyes and in the eyes of all who see her. May You hear the sound of our humble request because You are God who hears prayers and supplications. Blessed are You, Adonai, Who hears prayer.

The ceremony and prayer were conducted in session with the therapist and family. Maya recited the traveler's prayer. The experience was profoundly moving for the family, and Maya reported in a follow-up session that the experience was a turning point in her acceptance of her sister moving away from home. This case provides an example of the multifaceted ways in which prayer can be used with Jewish clients within the psychotherapeutic process.

Muslim Approaches to Prayer

In Islam, prayer is considered an integral part of a Muslim's life and consists of two main forms: *salah* and *du'a*. *Salah* comes from the Arabic work *silah*, which means "connection." The purpose of salah is to remind the individual of God through regular connection, meditation, and reflection during specific times of the day. Salah is a ritual prayer that involves prescribed movements of standing, bowing, and prostrating oneself before God. During the prayer, verses from the Qur'an and supplications in praise of God are recited and are associated with specific movements of the prayer. Muslims are required to pray five times a day, during specified time periods: dawn, midday, late afternoon, after sunset, and in the evening. Some Muslims may pray more than the five specified prayers, and others may choose not to uphold the religious requirements of prayer. The length of prayer will depend on the specific prayer, Qur'anic verses recited, and the individual. Prayers may be performed individually or collectively, although collective prayer is encouraged. Although prayer is not religiously required of an individual until he or she has reached puberty, children are encouraged to pray at a young age.

Du'a is a supplication that consists of communicating or talking with God (e.g., asking for assistance, direction, and thanking). Making du'a is not a required act, but it is encouraged, and it is a method to develop and maintain a personal connection with God. There are no mandatory guidelines for making du'a (as is the case with salah). Muslims may use specific du'as in Arabic that were used by the Prophet Muhammad for different activities in the day (e.g., waking up, putting on clothes, before eating) and are meant to help remind individuals of their Creator. Du'as can be made on any topic or issue, in any language, at any time, in a group or by oneself, in any location. There is no specific movement attached to du'as, which can be done while the individual is simultaneously involved in other activities.

Integrating Prayer in Psychotherapy With Muslim Clients

Incorporating Salah Into Therapy. The power and strength of prayers comes in understanding what the individual is saying and the implications of the movements as he or she attempts to connect with God. Depending on the child's age and religious knowledge, he or she may not be familiar with the meanings and implications of what he or she is reciting in prayer. As such, clinicians may need the parents or religiously knowledgeable individuals to assist the client in learning the meaning of prayers. For individuals dealing with anxiety and feelings of loneliness, prayer can be a powerful tool, if the individual is able to connect with God in a spiritual manner. In every salah, the individual is required to recite the opening chapter (*Al-Fatiha*), which is a direct plea to God for general guidance. After reciting these verses from the opening chapter, clients can be encouraged to reflect on the meaning and implications of what was recited and to talk to God about their specific needs, which can decrease the individual's feelings of loneliness. After completing the recitation of the *Al-Fatiha*, the client can be encouraged to recite verses that have personal meaning to his or her struggles. The personalization of the prayer can help to connect the individual more strongly to God, which can have a destressing impact. Throughout the prayer and in between the required actions of salah, the client can be encouraged to supplicate to God, that is, make du'a (in Arabic or in their native language) after each action. In addition to the required five daily prayers, Muslim clients can be encouraged to use the Prayer for Guidance, known as *Salah-tul-Istikhara*, an optional prayer that the individual can do to seek guidance from God on an important decision. The guidance can be for a specific item (e.g., whether to engage in a specific activity) or a general one (e.g., how to deal with bullies). The Prayer of Need, known as *Salah-tul-Hajah*, an optional prayer, can also be encouraged when the individual is in need of assistance from God (e.g., money, children, job).

For religiously minded clients, salah can be used to help cope with anxiety and decrease stress levels. In addition, the fact that prayers are at five specific times within the day can help divide the day into more manageable units or time frames, particularly for young children.

Incorporating Du'a Into Therapy. Du'a can be used to help verbalize the individual's thought, feelings, and concerns and channel them to God, who is all powerful and able to control all matters. This can be a cathartic emotional experience for the client. Therefore, making du'a, much like making salah, can help to reduce the anxiety, stress, and tension experienced because of the cathartic impact of sharing one's problems with a higher authority. This form of prayer may be particularly helpful for Muslim clients experiencing various forms of anxiety.

Case Study: Prayer With a Muslim Teen to Cope With Anxiety

One of us (Ahmed) worked with Hussain, a 14-year-old boy living in the United States. He was referred for treatment because of symptoms of generalized anxiety disorder, namely, excessive anxiety, restlessness, difficulties concentrating, and sleep disturbance. According to Hussain's mother, he had always been an anxious child; however, during the few months before he was referred he had stopped going out, watching television, surfing the Internet, and interacting with his family. Although his parents did not attach great importance to their religious beliefs, Hussain indicated that his religious beliefs were extremely important to him, and he would like them to be incorporated into treatment.

Ahmed began by exploring the underlying issues related to his anxiety. Hussain attributed his anxiety to not wanting to cause additional problems for his parents, who had a tumultuous marriage that was fraught with screaming and yelling. However, there had been no change in his parents' relationship. Exploration of other sources of stress revealed that Hussain had increasingly felt anxious about being the only Muslim in his new high school. He reported that the recent wave of Islamophobia in the media made him worried that other students might pick on him because of his faith.

Ahmed augmented conventional anxiety treatment with spiritual resources to assist Hussain. During Hussain's daily prayers, he was encouraged to express his feelings to God, particularly when he was in the position of *sujud*, prostrating before God, with his forehead, nose, both hands, knees, and toes touching the ground. This position within the prayer is considered the position in which a person is closest to God, and the ability to tell God all his problems would help Hussain express his feelings to a higher authority without fearing interpersonal consequences. Ahmed worked with Hussain to understand the themes of negative self-talk and channeled that knowledge to help Hussain identify and develop du'as that were spiritually and personally meaningful that he could repeat to counter his negative self-talk in anxiety-provoking situations. With each therapeutic success Hussain encountered, he would offer the prayer of thankfulness, *salahtul-shukr*, to become close to God.

CONCLUSION

At the beginning of this chapter, we asserted that prayer is a spiritual intervention that can be used with child and adolescent clients. We have discussed ethical and clinical considerations for psychotherapists to reflect on before using prayer as an intervention. Psychotherapists should consider contraindications to prayer involving clients' presenting problems. However, when done in a developmentally sensitive way that is congruent with a client's religious tradition, prayer can be spiritually meaningful and therapeutic at the same time. We are honored to have witnessed the power of prayer in several case studies involving clients whom we have seen. We look forward to the day when clinical practice involving prayer is increasingly informed by both spiritual tradition and empirical research demonstrating the efficacy of prayer in psychotherapy with children and teens.

REFERENCES

American Psychological Association. (2010). *Ethical principles of psychologists and code of conduct (2002, amended June 1, 2010)*. Retrieved from http://www.apa.org/ethics/code/index.aspx

Bamford, C., & Lagattuta, K. H. (2010). A new look at children's understanding of mind and emotion: The case of prayer. *Developmental Psychology*, *46*, 78–92. doi:10.1037/a0016694

Barnett, J. E., Hillard, D., & Lowry, K. (2001). Ethical and legal issues in the treatment of minors. In L. VandeCreek & T. Jackson (Eds.), *Innovations in clinical practice* (pp. 257–272). Sarasota, FL: Professional Resources Press.

Barnett, J., & Johnson, W. B. (2010). *Ethics desk reference for psychologists*. Washington, DC: American Psychological Association.

Basit, A. (1997). *The essence of the Quran*. Chicago, IL: ABC International Group.

Beach, S. R., Fincham, F. D., Hurt, T. R., McNair, L. M., & Stanley, S. M. (2008). Prayer and marital intervention: A conceptual framework. *Journal of Social and Clinical Psychology*, *27*, 641–669. doi:10.1521/jscp.2008.27.7.641

Bilu, Y., & Witzum, E. (1993). Working with Jewish ultra-orthodox patients: Guidelines for a culturally sensitive therapy. *Culture, Medicine and Psychiatry*, *17*, 197–233. doi:10.1007/BF01379326

Canter, M., Bennett, B., Jones, S., & Nagyn, T. (1994). *Ethics for psychologists: A commentary on the APA Ethics Code*. Washington, DC: American Psychological Association. doi:10.1037/10162-000

Cohen, J. A., Mannarino, A. P., & Deblinger, E. (2006). *Treating trauma and traumatic grief in children and adolescents*. New York, NY: Guilford Press.

Corey, G., Corey, M. S., & Callanan, P. (2010). *Issues and ethics in the helping professions* (8th ed.). Belmont, CA: Brooks/Cole.

De Lange, N. (2000). *An introduction to Judaism*. London, England: Cambridge University Press.

Foster, R. J. (1992). *Prayer: Finding the heart's true home*. San Francisco, CA: HarperSanFrancisco.

Garcia, H. A. (2008). Targeting Catholic rituals as symptoms of obsessive compulsive disorder: A cognitive-behavioral and psychodynamic, assimilative, integrationist approach. *Pragmatic Case Studies in Psychotherapy*, *4*, 1–38.

Goldman, R. (1964). *Religious thinking from childhood to adolescence*. London, England: Routledge & Kegan Paul.

Green, A., & Holtz, B. W. (2006). *Your word is fire: The Hasidic masters on contemplative prayer* (4th ed.). Woodstock, VT: Jewish Lights.

Grossoehme, D. H., VanDyke, R., Jacobson, J., Cotton, S., Ragsdale, J. R., & Seid, M. (2010). Written prayers in a pediatric hospital: Linguistic analysis. *Psychology of Religion and Spirituality*, *2*, 227–233. doi:10.1037/a0020035

Hage, S. M. (2006). A closer look at the role of spirituality in psychology training programs. *Professional Psychology: Research and Practice*, *37*, 303–310.

Hathaway, W. L., Scott, S. Y., & Garver, S. A. (2004). Assessing religious/spiritual functioning: A neglected domain in clinical practice? *Professional Psychology: Research and Practice*, *35*, 97–104. doi:10.1037/0735-7028.35.1.97

Iyengar, B. K. S., & Menuhin, Y. (1995). *Light on yoga: The Bible of modern yoga*. New York, NY: Schocken Books.

James, W. (1936). *The varieties of religious experience*. New York, NY: Random House. doi:10.1037/10004-000 (Original work published 1902)

Kaplan, A. (1985). *Jewish meditation: A practical guide*. New York, NY: Random House Digital.

Keating, T. (2002). *Foundations for centering prayer and the Christian contemplative life: Open mind, open heart, invitation to love, mystery of Christ*. London, England: Continuum International.

Kirzner, Y., Kirzner, Y., & Aiken, L. (2003). *The art of Jewish prayer*. New York, NY: Judaica Press.

Kushner, L., & Polen, N. (2004). *Filling words with light: Hasidic and mystical reflections on Jewish prayer*. Woodstock, VT: Jewish Lights.

Langman, P. F. (1995). Including Jews in multiculturalism. *Journal of Multicultural Counseling and Development, 23*, 222–236. doi:10.1002/j.2161-1912.1995.tb00278.x

Langman, P. F. (1999). *Jewish issues in multiculturalism: A handbook for educators and clinicians*. Northvale, NJ: Jason Aronson.

Lawrence, G., & Kurpius, S. (2000). Legal and ethical issues involved when counseling minors in a non-school setting. *Journal of Counseling and Development, 78*, 130–136. doi:10.1002/j.1556-6676.2000.tb02570.x

Long, D., Elkind, D., & Spilka, B. (1967). The child's conception of prayer. *Journal for the Scientific Study of Religion*, 6, 101–109. doi:10.2307/1384202

Magaletta, P. R., & Brawer, P. A. (1998). Prayer in psychotherapy: A model for its use, ethical considerations, and guidelines for practice. *Journal of Psychology and Theology, 26*, 322–330.

Marlatt, G. A., & Kristeller, J. L. (1999). Mindfulness and meditation. In W. R. Miller (Ed.), *Integrating spirituality into treatment: Resources for practitioners* (pp. 67–84). Washington, DC: American Psychological Association. doi:10.1037/10327-004

McMinn, M. (1996). *Psychology, theology, and spirituality in Christian counseling*. Wheaton, IL: Tyndale House.

Merton, T. (2007). *New seeds of contemplation*. New York, NY: New Directions.

Miller, L., & Lovinger, R. J. (2000). Psychotherapy with conservative and reform Jews. In P. S. Richards & A. E. Bergin (Eds.), *Handbook of psychotherapy and religious diversity* (pp. 259–286). Washington, DC: American Psychological Association. doi:10.1037/10347-011

Mooney, K. C., Graziano, A. M., & Katz, J. N. (1985). A factor analytic investigation of children's nighttime fear and coping responses. *Journal of Genetic Psychology, 146*, 205–215. doi:10.1080/00221325.1985.9914448

Paramananda. (2006). *Change your mind: A practical guide to Buddhist meditation*. Birmingham, England: Windhorse.

Remley, T. P., Jr., & Herlihy, B. (2010). *Ethical, legal, and professional issues in counseling* (3rd ed.). Upper Saddle River, NJ: Pearson.

Rew, L., Wong, Y. J., & Sternglanz, R. W. (2004). The relationship among prayer, health behaviors, and protective resources in school-age children. *Issues in Comprehensive Pediatric Nursing, 27,* 245–255. doi:10.1080/01460860490884156

Richards, P. S., & Bergin, A. E. (Eds.). (2000). *Handbook of psychotherapy and religious diversity.* Washington, DC: American Psychological Association. doi: 10.1037/10347-000

Richards, P. S., & Bergin, A. E. (2005). *A spiritual strategy for counseling and psychotherapy* (2nd ed.). Washington, DC: American Psychological Association. doi:10.1037/11214-000

Schnall, E. (2006). Multicultural counseling and the orthodox Jew. *Journal of Counseling & Development, 84,* 276–282. doi:10.1002/j.1556-6678.2006.tb00406.x

Schlosser, L. Z. (2006). Affirmative psychotherapy for American Jews. *Psychotherapy: Theory, Research, Practice, Training, 43,* 424–435.

Strean, H. (1994). *Psychotherapy with the Orthodox Jew.* Northvale, NJ: Jason Aronson.

Sullivan, K. T., & Karney, B. R. (2008). Incorporating religious practice in marital interventions: To pray or not to pray? *Journal of Social and Clinical Psychology, 27,* 670–677. doi:10.1521/jscp.2008.27.7.670

Walker, D. F., Gorsuch, R. L., & Tan, S. Y. (2005). Therapists' use of religious and spiritual interventions in Christian counseling: A preliminary report. *Counseling and Values, 49,* 107–119.

Walker, D. F., Gorsuch, R. L., Tan, S. Y., & Otis, K. E. (2008). Use of religious and spiritual interventions by trainees in APA-accredited Christian clinical psychology programs. *Mental Health, Religion, and Culture, 11,* 623–633.

Walker, D. F., & Moon, G. W. (2011). Prayer. In J. D. Aten, M. R. McMinn, & E. L. Worthington Jr. (Eds.), *Spiritually oriented interventions for counseling and psychotherapy* (pp. 139–167). Washington, DC: American Psychological Association. doi:10.1037/12313-006

Welful, E. R. (2006). *Ethics in counseling and psychotherapy: Standards, research, and emerging issues* (3rd ed.). Belmont, CA: Brooks/Cole.

Wilson, K., Lipscomb, L. D., Ward, K., Replogle, W. H., & Hill, K. (2000). Prayer in medicine: A survey of primary care physicians. *Journal of the Mississippi State Medical Association, 41,* 817–822.

Woolley, J., & Phelps, K. E. (2001). The development of children's beliefs about prayer. *Journal of Cognition and Culture, 1,* 139–166. doi:10.1163/156853701316931380

Worthington, E. L., Jr. (2008). Prayer and marital intervention: Can it be long and strong enough to matter? *Journal of Social and Clinical Psychology, 27,* 686–692. doi:10.1521/jscp.2008.27.7.686

Zaleski, P., & Zaleski, C. (2005). *Prayer: A history.* Boston, MA: Houghton Mifflin.

Zur, O. (2007). *Boundaries in psychotherapy: Ethical and clinical explorations.* Washington, DC: American Psychological Association. doi:10.1037/11563-000

9

GOD IMAGES

LYNN OLSON, VICKEY MACLIN, GLEN MORIARTY, AND HEATHER BERMUDEZ

Many readers may be familiar with the Christian story of the prodigal son (Luke 15:11–32) found in the New Testament section of the Bible. The story begins with the youngest son asking his father for his inheritance, which some read symbolically to mean that the son was wishing his father were dead (Hultgren, 2002). At the least, the son demanding his inheritance while his father is living is seen as arrogant and insulting. The father grants his son his wish and gives his son his portion of wealth. The son then goes to a faraway city and burns through the money, spending it on wild living. Shortly thereafter, the son has wasted all of his money and is now very poor. The city then goes into a deep famine. The son is forced to work as a laborer who looks after pigs. He is miserable, starving, and humbled. He begins to reflect on the differences between his past and present fortunes. He recalls that his father's servants have a much better life than he does. His father's servants have plenty of food to eat and are very comfortable. He is chronically

DOI: 10.1037/13947-010
Spiritual Interventions in Child and Adolescent Psychotherapy, D. F. Walker and W. L. Hathaway (Editors)

hungry and very uncomfortable. The prodigal decides to head back to his family home. He thinks through what he will tell his father to try to persuade him to take him back as a servant or hired hand. After a long walk back, he finally nears his father's house. His father squints and sees him in the distance. Luke (15:20–24) captures it:

> But while he was still a long way off, his father saw him and was filled with compassion for him; he ran to his son, threw his arms around him and kissed him. The son said to him, "Father, I have sinned against heaven and against you. I am no longer worthy to be called your son." But the father said to his servants, "Quick! Bring the best robe and put it on him. Put a ring on his finger and sandals on his feet. Bring the fattened calf and kill it. Let's have a feast and celebrate. For this son of mine was dead and is alive again; he was lost and is found." So they began to celebrate.

The father is incredibly gracious and overflowing with love and generosity. The son is trying to get his speech out, but his father is already upon him, hugging him and welcoming him home. He is overcome with joy and orders a fattened calf to be readied; the fattened calf is the choicest cow the father owns.

This story is replete with meaning. Broadly, within a Christian narrative, the son represents the fallenness of humanity, and the father represents the graciousness of God. In this context, humans make poor decisions and alienate themselves from one another and from God. God, however, demonstrates his unconditional love for his children, celebrating their return and redemption.

We have chosen this story because it nicely illustrates the difference between a person's experience of God and his or her beliefs about God and faith. Clearly, the prodigal son was imagining a different scenario. He was imagining that his father would be distant and shaming. Instead, his father was warm and forgiving. Many people identify with this tale because they have difficulty experiencing God as loving. They intellectually believe that God is loving, but they do not experience God as loving. They cognitively hold to this idea of grace—God's unmerited favor—but still feel as though they have to earn God's love. Similarly, they believe they are forgiven, but they often feel unforgiven—as though God is still mad at them.

Although we used a Christian narrative as an illustration, this gap between what a person believes about God and what he or she feels about God—or stated another way, the gap between a person's head understanding of God and his or her heart understanding of God—is not a phenomenon that is restricted to any one faith. Rather, this space between what is known or believed and what is felt or experienced by people occurs across the world religions.

In this chapter, we explore intervention strategies with children and adolescents whose experience of God may be affecting their spiritual and overall development. Although there is limited research on the use of God-image treatment with children, initial research has pointed to a few factors as important indicators of assessment and treatment. Furthermore, our God image work with other populations (see Moriarty & Davis, 2012) has significantly influenced our understanding of how God-image interventions may be used to help children experiencing difficulties in their relationship with God. Indeed, the theoretical backdrop and research are very similar; however, the application and adaptation for children is what sets this chapter apart (see Moriarty, 2006; and Moriarty & Davis, 2012). We begin by defining relevant terms, then outline the theoretical basis of the God image before providing an overview of the research literature reviewing factors influencing God image in children. Additionally, we explore how theory and research inform interventions that can be used to help children and adolescents struggling with maladaptive God images. We follow this with a practical discussion of how to specifically use God-image interventions in child and adolescent psychotherapy. Finally, we present a series of case examples to illustrate the use of these interventions in psychotherapy.

DEFINITIONS

The term *God* used throughout this chapter is a global reference and is meant to refer to all divine attachment figures across theistic religious and spiritual traditions (Davis, 2010; Granqvist & Kirkpatrick, 2008). However, a true understanding, especially in a physical sense, of an intangible and ethereal divine being is not possible. As a result, humans create different representations of God with which they interact. Several authors have delineated among the natures of these different representations. Specifically, *God images* refer to the internal representations of the personal, subjective relationship individuals have with God. God images usually operate at an unconscious level of awareness to influence the individual's affective and physiological experiences of God (Moriarty & Davis, 2012; Rizzuto, 1979). In a related vein, Gibson (2006) posited that the God image is the individual's emotional experience, or *heart knowledge*, of God. This heart knowledge is the internal working model that entails the feelings and beliefs about the relationship and also guides the individual's behavior within that relationship. Gibson's (2007) work also provides examples of the potential for multiplicity of God images, indicating a working God schema that may reveal different perceptions of God during different experiences in life.

God concepts are another mental representation of God. In contrast to God images involving heart knowledge, God concepts are an individual's cognitive understanding of God (or head knowledge) and are based on the theological teachings the individual has received (Gibson, 2006). As such, God concepts include beliefs about how individuals should relate and interact with God, how God interacts with the individual, and the doctrinal understanding of God's character. In short, God images relate to feelings and emotions, whereas God concepts relate to cognition and thinking.

FACTORS INFLUENCING GOD IMAGE IN CHILDREN

Given that the theoretical precursors of the God image have been reviewed in other works (e.g., Moriarty & Davis, 2012), the more specific aspects of those theoretical concepts provide more insight into the inclusion of the God image in the treatment of childhood difficulties. We review two primary lines of research that have provided guidance about the development of God image in children: child development, especially as it relates to cognitive development, and parent–child attachment.

Developmental Influences on God Image

One particular issue that emerges relative to children is the developmental progression of God images in children. Generally, the view that a child's spiritual development occurs in a developmental progression is not new. Our early understandings of spiritual development (see Fowler, 1981, 1996) as well as contemporary views (see Johnson & Boyatzis, 2006) hinge on the assumption that a developmental process underlies people's spiritual and faith development and, more specifically, their understandings and representations of God. Early theoretical formulations suggested that the development of the God concept occurs around age 6 (Williams, 1971) with a progression toward a more mature understanding paralleling Piaget's cognitive development model (Nye & Carlson, 1984). However, the recognition of an earlier formation of both the concept of God (Barrett & Richert, 2003) and the image of God has been reported in children younger than age 6 (Goldman, 1964; Harms, 1944; Wilber, 1996). Furthermore, these experiences can exist during childhood apart from an advanced, cognitively developed understanding of God and may not follow a developmental progression as once believed (Barrett & Keil, 1996; Barrett & Richert, 2003; Dillon, 2000).

A more challenging question has been not whether a God image exists in early childhood but rather how it exists. That is, whether this occurs in linear stages or categorically has yet to be determined. Initial research suggested linear stage models. For example, Harms (1944) was one of the earliest researchers to investigate this issue. Harms analyzed drawings of children's experiences of God among more than 4,000 children ages 3 to 18 and found predictable differences in content. He subsequently identified three stages of religious experience. In the first, fairy-tale stage (ages 3–6), God is viewed as a "king" or "daddy." During the second, realistic stage (ages 7–12), children emphasize a specific characteristic such as symbols of God or Christ or religious figures (e.g., priests). Finally, during the individualistic stage (adolescence), students' representations tend to cluster into one of three groups: (a) dogmatic representations; (b) more emotional expressions of personal symbolism; and (c) aspects of ancient, philosophical, or mystic experiences of God. Subsequent research (e.g., Nye & Carlson, 1984), as noted earlier, continued investigating the linear model of development, paralleling God images or representations, cognitive development, Piaget's theory of cognitive development, or all of these.

In more recent work, however, several have questioned this linear-stage model of development, especially as related to God image, linking stage models or such perceptions to cognitive development (see Barrett, 2001; T. Hart, 2006). Other research lines have pointed to categorical models of development. For example, in his work, T. Hart (2003, 2006) identified four types of experiences of or capacities for spiritual experience in children: *wonder* (awareness, experience, and attitude), *wondering* (epistemological questioning), *wisdom* (accessing profound insight and guidance), and *between you and me* (relational capacities). In his approach, T. Hart (2006) suggested that the experience of God may be an inherent element of rather than a result of spiritual and cognitive development in children.

Others have investigated the symbolic or anthropomorphic aspects of God representations in children (Barrett & Richert, 2003; Goldman, 1964; Richert & Barrett, 2005). Early studies emphasized that early understandings of God focused on the human traits (Goldman, 1964). However, others (e.g., Tamminen, 1994) suggested that children's conceptualizations go beyond human physical traits. As a result, the preparedness hypothesis illustrates that God images emerge from perceptual and relational mechanisms that exist internally, resulting in the young child's capacity for a representation of, and attachment to, God outside of the constraints of cognitive development (Barrett & Richert, 2003; Richert & Barrett, 2005).

Taken together, it is clear that there is much to be learned about the developmental experience of God image in children. What it means to form a God image through the process of development within and across domains (e.g., cognitive, spiritual) has yet to be determined. Therefore, we consider other factors such as the quality of one's attachment to parents.

Attachment and God Image

Bowlby's (1969/1982, 1973, 1980) pioneering work on attachment theory provided another framework for conceptualizing and studying God-image tendencies (Granqvist & Kirkpatrick, 2008; Kirkpatrick, 2005; Noffke & Hall, 2007). *Internal working models* are mental expectations people develop that predict how others will respond to them, and they are initially learned through early relationships with primary caregivers. However, they remain open to revision across the life course, through subsequent experiences in attachment relationships (Badenoch, 2008; Davis, 2010; Siegel, 1999). According to Bowlby (1973), internal working models provide mental representations that underlie people's feelings, thoughts, behaviors, sensations, and motivations in any type of relationship, including relationships with divine attachment figures. Internal working models include representations of both the other and the self (Bowlby, 1973).

In recent literature (see Moriarty & Davis, in press, for a review), four attachment-based models have emerged for describing the role of parental attachment in shaping one's image of God. The internal working model correspondence hypothesis (Kirkpatrick, 1992; Kirkpatrick & Shaver, 1990) states that the relationship with God corresponds to experienced human attachments. The emotional compensation hypothesis (Kirkpatrick, 1992; Kirkpatrick & Shaver, 1990) suggests that the relationship with God compensates for "an insecure global attachment style with humans" (Moriarty & Davis, 2012, p. 8). The socialized correspondence hypothesis (Granqvist, 1998, 2002; Granqvist & Hagekull, 1999) suggests that considerable childhood experiences of secure religious caregivers lead to a secure relationship with God. Finally, the implicit relational knowledge correspondence hypothesis (Hall, 2004; Hall, Halcrow, Hill, & Delaney, 2005) suggests that the relationship with God reflects implicit emotional experiences with others but is distinct from "people's explicit religious/spiritual functioning" (Moriarty & Davis, 2012, p. 9). It is important to note that the implicit relational knowledge model explains the seeming incongruity observed in the compensatory framework. That is, compensatory individuals often seem as though they have an intimate relationship with God, as measured by frequency of church attendance or religious commitment and so forth; however, this behavior is often motivated by underlying anxiety. The implicit relational knowledge model explains how these individuals may seem explicitly close to God but are implicitly insecure in their relationship with God. Preliminary research with adults has supported the implicit relational knowledge correspondence hypothesis (Hall et al., 2005; Moriarty & Davis, 2012).

More specifically, parent–child attachments appear to be particularly important in the God image. Gerkin's (1994) essential conclusion was that the infant–mother relationship serves as the foundation for the development of an image reflecting deity. The developing perception of God is dynamic through the individual development of the child and through the progression of relational experiences between the parent and child (Dickie et al., 1997; Kirkpatrick, 1992, 1997). In addition, the perception being developed is unique to the specific child and parent (Gerkin, 1994). That is, two children in one family may perceive the same parent differently on the basis of the unique experiences between individual parent and individual child. The common thread between the God image of siblings in a family, or of children of a similar age from different families, lies in the certainty of the process-oriented quality of the development of the God image (Gerkin, 1994) and the tremendous influence of parenting and the dynamics of the parent–child relationship on the God image (Hertel & Donahue, 1995).

TREATMENT DIRECTION FOR CHILDREN AND ADOLESCENTS

When working with clients to address or change perspectives of God images, different theoretical orientations and corresponding techniques can be used (see Moriarty & Hoffman, 2007, for a review). Art therapy, cognitive–behavioral therapy (CBT), and object relations therapy are highlighted here because they have been shown to be helpful in transforming children's thoughts, attitudes, and behaviors (K. J. Hart & Morgan, 1993; Reinecke, Dattilio, & Freeman, 1996; Waller, 2006).

Norcross and Goldfried (2005) proposed a psychotherapy integration approach that Moriarty and Davis (2012) applied to the task of deliberately integrating diverse theoretical orientations or techniques in facilitating God-image change. In child and adolescent psychotherapy, children and teens often require multiple approaches to treating presenting problems that are themselves multidimensional (Ollendick & King, 2004). We believe that this approach would also prove beneficial when working with children and adolescents to specifically help them further develop their internalized God images. Thus, in this section, we present the application of God-image interventions within art therapy, CBT, and object relations therapy and from an integrative psychotherapy perspective using interpersonal therapy as a foundation while incorporating cognitive–behavioral techniques.

It may not be appropriate to use the interventions we discuss next—the Draw a God and the GIATR interventions—with clients of certain religious faiths and ethnic cultures. Some religions, such as Islam, find it inappropriate to draw pictures or even imagine God. "Rendering images of God in Islam is an impossibility, and amounts to disbelief, as God tells us in the Quran that nothing resembles Him: 'There is nothing like Him, but He is All-Hearing,

All-Seeing'" (Qur'an 42:11). Additionally, in some Asian and American Indian cultures, it is not respectful to look someone in the eye. So, for these exercises it is important to make necessary adjustments depending on the person's religious faith and cultural background.

Art Therapy

Art was used in therapy as early as 1940 by Edith Kramer (Waller, 2006). Kramer saw art as having the ability to bring healing and help in dealing with emotions that were difficult to process. Art therapy can be particularly beneficial by helping children identify and express feelings in a symbolic manner (Waller, 2006). This nonverbal process can be especially helpful in working through God-image difficulties. Art therapy provides a safe place for children to identify and process God-image challenges without fear of judgment. This symbolic process allows children to begin to name and process difficulties in their relationship with God.

The Draw a God art therapy exercise (Moriarty, 2006; Moriarty & Davis, 2012) involves the drawing of three pictures. This exercise can help children and adolescents differentiate between their God image and their God concept, or between a heart understanding and a head understanding of God. For the first picture, clients are asked to "draw a picture of you and God," which typically displays themes of love and kindness. For the second picture, clients are instructed to "draw a picture of how you feel you and God look after you have done something wrong. Draw what you feel, not what you think." This second picture often encompasses feelings of detachment and anger from God. Psychotherapists then follow up this picture with questions assessing closeness to and distance from God. If clients report feeling distant, then the psychotherapist inquires about what steps they take to help themselves feel close to God again. For the final picture, the client is encouraged to "draw a picture of how you would like to feel you and God look when you do something wrong." The aim of this last picture is to engage the individual's own faith tradition in understanding of and belief about God. When doing this exercise, the goal is to help the child understand that God is present even when the child makes mistakes or fails. This can be emphasized with the child by noting that God may be different in the first two pictures. The difference in the second picture is often a good way to explore how caregivers have shaped and influenced the child's God image, especially as it relates to discipline. The third and last picture gives the child the opportunity to imagine and experience God in a way that is more in keeping with the child's faith tradition. Requiring only three pieces of paper and a pencil, this exercise is a simple, inexpensive assessment.

Cognitive–Behavioral Approaches

CBT techniques have been supported by research for being both efficacious and effective in treating such disorders as attention-deficit/hyperactivity disorder, depression, anxiety, and certain phobias (Ollendick & King, 2004; Spirito & Kazak, 2006; Wolfe & Mash, 2006). When CBT is used with children, it is important that the child's developmental and cognitive levels of functioning be taken into consideration. Younger children tend to have different ways of processing information, and older children have better abilities to think, evaluate, and process information (Evans & Sullivan, 1993; Pellegrini, Galinski, Hart, & Kendall, 1993). Thus, older children are better able to engage in an exercise like the God Image Automatic Thought Record (GIATR; Moriarty, 2006; Moriarty & Davis, 2012), which we recommend using with children ages 10 and older.

God Image Automatic Thought Record

The GIATR (see Table 9.1) is a cognitive–behavioral tool that can be used to help clients make adjustments in their thinking processes as related to their God images and self-images (Moriarty & Davis, 2012). The concept of the GIATR can be beneficial in helping children learn to challenge the automatic thoughts that can impede their image and experience of the true God of their faith. The primary goal of the GIATR is to teach children how to question maladaptive thoughts about God because the maladaptive thoughts affect their ability to experience the God of their faith in a meaningful way. Because children have the opportunity to complete the GIATR on paper several times, they are able to see how their negative emotions and thoughts influence the way they relate to God. As children work through and complete this exercise a number of times, they begin to make a habit of challenging irrational thoughts and beliefs rather than continuing to focus on them. Subsequently, it is hoped that the children will eventually begin to experience more positive emotions (e.g., love, happiness, peace, kindness, safety, closeness) in their relationship with God (Moriarty & Davis, 2012). In our use of the GIATR in therapy with clients (primarily with adults), we have found that clients benefit from the exercise and have left the experience having changed not only how they think of God but also how they experience God in their day-to-day lives.

TABLE 9.1
God Image Automatic Thought Record

Situation	Feelings	Automatic thought(s)	Real God response	Outcome
Briefly describe an actual event that made you feel like God was probably having negative thoughts about you and/or negative feelings toward you.	Any negative feelings that you felt as a result—Rate the strength of each feeling, 0 to 100.	Any negative thoughts and/or feelings you felt like God was probably having about you or toward you in that moment—Rate the degree to which you believed God was thinking/feeling that way toward you at that time, 0 to 100%.	Knowing what you know about the Real God, as described by your scriptures, teachings, or leaders, what do you think God was perhaps more realistically thinking and feeling toward you in that moment—Rate the degree to which you believe that the Real God response is probably how God *really* thought and felt toward you at that time, 0 to 100%.	Relist the negative emotions that you originally felt as a result of the situation—Now rate the strength of each feeling, after imagining God thinking/feeling the Real God response, 0 to 100.

Note. From *Pastoral Care of Depression: Helping Clients Heal Their Relationship With God* (p. xx), by G. L. Moriarty, 2006, Binghamton, NY: Haworth. Copyright 2006 by Haworth/Routledge Press. Reprinted with permission.

The GIATR is designed to provide a way to recognize and change automatic thoughts that prevent individuals from having a positive emotional experience of God (or another divine attachment figure). Following are abbreviated instructions for the administration of the GIATR (adapted from Moriarty & Davis, 2012):

1. The therapist instructs the child to describe an incident in which the child felt as though God had negative thoughts and feelings about the child.
2. The therapist gives the child a list of feeling words and asks the child to list all the feelings he or she had as a result of the incident (e.g., sadness, shame, rejected, anxious, angry). The therapist has the child rate the feelings on a scale ranging from 0 to 100, with 0 = *total absence of the emotion* and 100 = *overwhelming presence of the emotion*.
3. The therapist has the child list any negative thoughts or feelings the child believes God has about or toward him or her when the incident happened. The therapist again has the child rate the degree to which he or she believes God was thinking or feeling the identified way on a scale ranging from 0 to 100, with 0 = *I was not at all certain that God was thinking/feeling that way toward me* and 100 = *I was 100% certain that God was thinking/feeling that way toward me*.
4. The therapist then asks the child, on the basis of what the child knows from his or her experience of the Real God from scriptures, spiritual teachings, or spiritual leaders, what he or she thinks God was really (realistically) thinking about and feeling toward the child when the incident happened. The therapist has the child write out the more likely response from the Real God and then has the child rate the degree to which the Real-God response is more likely to be how God really thought and felt toward the child, on a scale ranging from 0 to 100, with 0 = *I am not at all positive that the Real God was thinking/feeling that way toward me* and 100 = *I am 100% positive that the Real God was thinking/feeling that way toward me*.
5. The therapist then instructs the child to close his or her eyes and get a mental picture of the Real God—whatever God may look like to the child, whether a person or a mythological figure such as Aslan from *The Chronicles of Narnia*. The therapist asks the child to imagine looking into the eyes of the Real God and asks the child to allow him- or herself to experience the Real God responding to him or her in the way that

was previously described. The therapist instructs the child to remain in the experience for a minute or two and then to slowly open his or her eyes.

6. After the child opens his or her eyes, the therapist has the child do the final step of relisting the negative emotions that were initially felt as a result of the incident. Then the child rates the strength of each feeling after imagining the Real God's thoughts or feelings toward him or her on a scale ranging from 0 to 100, with 0 = *total absence of the emotion* and 100 = *overwhelming presence of the emotion*.

The GIATR is an exercise we have seen benefit our clients when they have engaged in it for several weeks to challenge the irrational thoughts that can lead to any number of emotions, such as anger, frustration, resentment, and depression. Although our experience in using the technique with children is limited, we believe that when a psychotherapist spends time working with a child consistently using the GIATR, the child can experience some of the same positive outcomes that we have seen with our adult clients.

Interpersonal Therapy and Object Relations Therapy

Object relations theory and the concepts associated with treating individuals using this theory tie closely to early childhood events. A clinician using object relations therapy considers human beings the objects (St. Clair, 2000). The psychotherapist works with clients to identify ways in which events early in life have affected and influence the ways in which individuals engage with others and interpret events that happen in their relationships. In using object relations with children, it is important to consider their developmental and verbal capabilities. Melanie Klein pioneered the use of object relations therapy with children by incorporating play therapy in her work with them. She believed that the child's core sense of self is fully tied to the first and most influential object relationship with his or her mother (St. Clair, 2000). As such, when a clinician is working with a child or adolescent using object relations theory, it is imperative to consider early childhood relationships, in particular that with the mother figure in the child's life.

Object relations therapy is part of a broader school of interpersonal psychotherapies that have in common the central importance of conceptualizing client difficulties as being rooted in relational problems with parents and/or other significant figures in a child's life (for a more complete discussion, see Teyber & McClure, 2010). With older children and adolescents, psychotherapists can allow the child to talk about his or her relationships with the parents in a nonthreatening, nonjudgmental, and nonevaluative setting. As part of an interpersonal psychotherapy approach, psychotherapists sometimes use process comments to highlight maladaptive ways in which the client is relating to them. Afterward, psychotherapists typically help their clients reflect on and alter these maladaptive relationship patterns.

Summary of Integrative Psychotherapy Approaches

An integrative psychotherapy approach can be helpful in addressing God-image challenges among children and adolescents. Additionally, psychotherapists should be mindful of the child's developmental and cognitive level of functioning. When object relations theory is used as a conceptual framework, psychotherapists can incorporate the Draw a God exercise or the GIATR in the treatment of the child. Using these previously mentioned techniques, the child is able to make connections between how the relationship with his or her caregivers influences how he or she relates to God when different events happen in the child's life.

CASE EXAMPLES

To further flesh out these strategies, we provide case examples that highlight an integrative approach with CBT, interpersonal therapy, and art therapy influences. Each of the cases has been deidentified to protect the confidentiality of the individuals who were seen by Vickey Maclin (art therapy and object relations therapy cases) or Glen Moriarty (integrative psychotherapy case using CBT and interpersonal therapy concepts).

Addressing God Images Using Art Therapy

Jauri Tan Bee, an amalgamated client based on several clients who were seen by Maclin, was a 9-year-old third-generation Chinese American who was raised in a home with her parents and grandparents. Jauri and her parents had a Christian faith, but they also acknowledged the traditional faith of their extended family, which was Buddhism. Jauri's parents were both physicians, and she was their only child. Jauri was raised attending church and acknowledged that she had adopted a Christian faith in God at a very young age. Ten months before coming in for a psychotherapy session, Jauri's mother and father were called to school by the guidance counselor, who informed them that Jauri had reported being touched in her "privates" by an older boy at the school. The guidance counselor informed the parents that Jauri had told her that she felt as though God had not protected her from the boy and that she no longer wanted to have anything to do with God. Jauri's parents were referred for psychotherapy with Jauri, but they delayed taking Jauri in because they felt that they could work with their daughter and help her to return to their expressed Christian faith. The parents decided after several weeks of not seeing any change in Jauri's attitude, and in fact seeing her become more anxious and depressed, to take her to see a psychotherapist.

During the intake, Jauri's parents expressed to Maclin that they wanted their daughter to return to the Christian beliefs she had before the incident. They also indicated that they wanted help in knowing how to deal with the psychological problems that were probably factoring into Jauri's decision to not want anything to do with their faith. In the first session with Jauri, Maclin learned that Jauri liked to draw and asked her to draw some pictures. Using art therapy, she established a good rapport with Jauri, and through the drawing helped her to begin to feel comfortable enough to consider drawing pictures that expressed how she saw and felt about herself since the boy at school had touched her. In addition to getting her to draw pictures about herself, Maclin also helped Jauri to begin to write stories about some of the feelings she had since the incident. Maclin saw the psychotherapy with Jauri as a twofold process, in that she wanted to work to alleviate the anxiety and depression as well as help Jauri with how the incident had influenced her relationship with her God, which had before the molestation provided her some meaning.

After several sessions with Jauri, Maclin asked her to draw a picture of how she saw her relationship with God before the boy touched her in ways that made her feel uncomfortable. When Jauri completed that picture, Maclin gave her another piece of paper and asked her to draw a picture of how she thought God saw her after the incident with the boy. Jauri was able to talk about the pictures as well as her feelings about what the boy did to her. After drawing the two pictures and talking about the experience, Jauri was able to express some of the feelings that she had about and toward God. Some of what she stated about her relationship with God before the boy touched her was that she felt close to him and that he cared about her. However, after the incident she indicated that she had been angry toward God, and because she was angry she did not think he would want to be close to her. Jauri was later able to draw pictures that she felt depicted how her relationship with God was before the touching incident and was also able to draw a picture of what she thought needed to happen for the relationship to return to what it was before she had been touched in ways that made her feel uncomfortable. When Jauri had come for several sessions and worked on this area through artwork, she was able to begin to feel more positive toward God and was also able to begin to deal with the negative feelings she had about herself as a result of what the boy had done to her. As she was able to see her relationship with God more positively and talk about the molestation, she had an increase in positive feelings about herself and a decrease in anxious and depressive episodes.

Addressing God Images Using Integrative Psychotherapy

Sarah Newberry, an amalgamated client based on several actual psychotherapy clients of Moriarty's, was a 16-year-old Pentecostal (Assemblies of God) Christian. She presented with mild anxiety surrounding growing away from her parents and her level of commitment to her faith. Sarah was going through the initial stages of differentiating from her parents. She was beginning to deidealize them and become more aware of their personal weaknesses and limitations. More specifically, she began to question some of their life and financial decisions and how those decisions affected her life and the lives of her siblings. Finally, Sarah expressed anxiety about her relationship with God. She stated that she believed God loved her unconditionally but that, at the same time, God felt distant and hard to please. She wondered whether she was "doing enough spiritual devotions" and questioned whether she was "losing the fire."

Sarah grew up in a two-parent, traditional home with three older siblings. Her mother stayed in the home and her father was self-employed, doing odd jobs whenever someone happened to call. Sarah considered herself to have had a fairly positive childhood and early adolescence. She perceived her mother to be loving, present, and very religious. Sarah also thought her mother was easily overwhelmed and had trouble managing the home. Her father was frequently gone from the home because participating in sports was his main priority. When he was home, he was affectively available as long as Sarah agreed with him and did not complain or question how he chose to spend his time or his money. When Sarah brought up concerns or requests for nicer clothes, her mother would respond by suggesting that she should be happy with the clothes she had. In a similar way, her father would respond by emotionally withdrawing and suggesting she was greedy for desiring nicer things.

Sarah started treatment because she was anxious and confused about her relationships with her parents and God. She participated in 15 sessions of integrative psychotherapy. As treatment progressed, Sarah's anxiety decreased and her confusion about her relationships with her parents and God also decreased.

The early stages of treatment focused on assessment and on building the therapeutic alliance. Moriarty conducted a clinical interview that was augmented with specific God-image questions. Additionally, after the first session, Sarah completed several God-image measures to further differentiate her God images and God concepts. She completed a few self-report measures, an adjective checklist that compared parental attributes with God attributes, and the Draw a God exercise (outlined earlier). These tools were helpful in differentiating the intellectual and affective components of her God image.

In the next few sessions, Sarah began to open up about some of the issues she had with her parents. At first, her criticisms were minor. It seemed as though she was testing Moriarty to see whether she could be honest about her struggles. Gradually, Sarah opened up more about her frustration with her parents and their hippie, nonplanning lifestyle. Sarah began to articulate how she was different from her parents; she embraced being proactive and conscientious rather than being ashamed of these characteristics. A similar process occurred with her relationship with God. Sarah's faith tradition emphasized the emotional experience of God. Sarah participated in many affective church experiences on Sunday and Wednesday nights at youth group. For example, she would lift her hands in worship and regularly participate in altar calls to seek prayer and more intimate encounters with God. These aspects of her faith continued to be important to her, but she no longer felt that she had to be that way all the time. Rather, she began to value the intellectual components of her faith. The shifts in her understanding of herself and her relationships with her parents also played out in her relationship with God.

In the middle stages of psychotherapy, Moriarty stayed the course and further explored Sarah's relationships with her parents and God. Sarah owned more of her own strengths and realized that her way of being was not wrong, just different from her parents' primary way of navigating life. Her anxiety decreased as she accepted her sense of ambition and desire to have mastery. Exploration of her God images also continued. Sarah had been on several mission trips and had observed suffering firsthand. Previously, she had been hesitant to look at the pain and chaos she observed—it seemed too scary and somehow incongruent with her faith. On an emotional level, Sarah did not feel as though it was okay to think about the problem of evil. Her fear was that God would become upset with her. She feared that it was a signal that she did not have enough faith. As psychotherapy progressed, Sarah felt more confident in exploring these issues with God and even her pastor. Sarah's pastor helped her make sense of her struggles from a theological perspective. She realized there were no easy answers, but she no longer felt as though she had to shirk from the conundrum that puzzles many Christians—if God is all good and all loving, then why is there suffering? Gradually, Sarah's God image shifted from one that was distant if she questioned or was less emotional in worship to one that was present, even in times of doubt and reflection.

During this same period of treatment, Moriarty introduced the GIATR. Sarah felt as though God was distant from her if she was not as emotionally activated in service as her peers. Similarly, she felt as though God was far away when she initially began to look at the real suffering others experienced. Through the use of the GIATR, Sarah began to realize that God valued her whole person, not just the emotional aspects. Additionally, through looking at examples in the Bible, she recognized that many characters and saints doubted and struggled with aspects of their faith. She was able to see that God was present even in these hard times.

Moriarty also drew on interpersonal psychotherapy's technique of using immediacy in the therapeutic relationship to help Sarah see how this pattern of acquiescence plays out in multiple relationships. The following excerpt is an example of immediacy in therapeutic relationship:

> Sarah, it seems that there were times in the recent past where you struggled to express your thoughts to your parents [past relationships]. Similarly, when you talk about your friends, I sometimes get the impression that you just kind of go along with them, even though you have good thoughts and points that would add to the conversation [present relationships]. Also, I see this same thing happening in your relationship with God [God-image relationship]. You have thoughts and questions about your religious faith, but it seems you hesitate to consider them or bring them up to God. Finally, in here with me [therapeutic relationship], I know you are smart and sometimes question things I say. You usually share your thoughts with me, but only after I prompt you. Do you see how this is a pattern?

These types of interpersonal exchanges, looking at patterns that played out across relationships, were used to help Sarah gain the confidence to begin to express herself in therapy. Initially, she was hesitant to share her thoughts. As psychotherapy progressed, she became more and more confident. She no longer minimized her viewpoint but shared it willingly—without being encouraged. These interpersonal shifts in psychotherapy colored her experiences with God. God was not an insecure being that became distant when engaged; rather, God was present and enjoyed an authentic, real relationship with her, even in times of doubt and struggle.

The last weeks of treatment reinforced the changes that Sarah had made during the early and middle stages of therapy. Her psychotherapist focused on helping Sarah see that there are multiple approaches to life and that her approach was not wrong, just different from the path her parents chose. Similarly, there were multiple ways to engage her faith and her relationship with God. Sarah realized that she was not less "on fire" for God because her faith had transitioned and opened to one that was more reflective. She had space in the relationship to be honest and authentic. She no longer felt as though she had to minimize her questions; rather, she could embrace them and find support with others, her pastor, and even in her relationship with God.

Addressing God Images Using an Object Relations Approach

Malik Foster, an amalgamation of several adolescent clients seen by Maclin, was a 16-year-old African American boy who lived with his parents and two younger sisters. Malik had spent most of his life in the church and had been actively involved in his youth group until approximately 6 months before coming in for psychotherapy. Malik's parents were concerned because Malik had begun to display negative behaviors at home and at church and his grades had begun to drop. During the intake session, Malik told his parents that he did not want to go to church and that he no longer believed that God was a loving God. He stated that he started doing what he wanted to do because it did not matter anymore what God thought. Furthermore, he told them that he did not really care what they wanted him to do because they did not always demonstrate that they cared about him, because they either were just not around or did not seem to be invested in him anymore.

After individual sessions started with Malik, he informed Maclin that 8 months earlier two of his closest friends had been killed in two separate car accidents, a close family friend had moved to another state, and his girlfriend had informed him that she was pregnant by another boy and she was breaking up with him. Malik further stated that he blamed his parents' God for all the bad things that had happened. He said, "If God was a loving God, he would not have allowed so many bad things to happen. So, I just don't believe that God loves or cares about me."

Upon further investigation by Maclin, Malik reported that he had grown up going to church because he knew that it pleased his parents. He stated that he had actually enjoyed going, too, but his attitude toward church had really begun to change after his girlfriend told him that she was pregnant and breaking up with him. He indicated that he could no longer believe that God was in control and that if he was, then he just did not care about Malik because of all the painful things that had happened to him.

It seemed to Maclin that Malik had ascribed to both his relationship with God and his relationship with his parents that they were either all good or all bad, and he had difficulty believing that they could be both at the same time. Given this conceptualization, she used object relations theory to challenge the fragmented and frustrated internalized experiences (St. Clair, 2000) that had likely developed through Malik's early relationships with his mother and father.

Malik's psychotherapist began the process by exploring with Malik some of his early experiences in his relationship with his parents. Malik's father was away during much of his growing-up years, and Malik said he consequently developed a really close relationship with his mother. Malik reported that he recalled spending many of his hours as a child with his mother and believed that she loved him and enjoyed spending time with him on a regular basis. However, when he was 6 years old, his mother went back to school and was not as available to him and his sisters as she had once been. Malik remembered this being a difficult time because he loved his mother but he was also mad at her for leaving him with several different babysitters. He stated that he never let his mother know that he was mad because he wanted her to still love him. During the intake session, he further reported that when he told his parents that they did not care about him, it was the first time he had ever said anything like that to them. Malik indicated that he did not know how his parents could say that they loved him but then not be there to spend time with him as his mom had done when he was younger. When Maclin asked him whether it was possible for his parents to be good and bad at the same time, he gave an emphatic reply of "no." Malik said that he had felt angry toward his mom but had never expressed that anger until the session.

After several sessions, Maclin processed with Malik his perceptions and images of himself and his parents and how his expectations of his parents had greatly influenced his relational patterns with others, including God. After helping him to better understand his relational patterns, she began to delve into the image and concept that he had developed about God. Using the Draw a God exercise, Malik was able to engage in a critical examination of his own beliefs. He was able to challenge the concepts that he had learned and adopt a more personal and self-critical perspective that did not have him viewing his parents or God as being either all good or all bad. In addition to the Draw a God exercise, Maclin asked Malik to read the popular book *The Shack* (Young, 2007) so that he could gain a visual picture of someone else's struggle with a negative view of God on the basis of painful experiences and losses that happen in a person's life.

Several weeks after talking about the structures that had developed as a result of his early relationship with his mother, Malik was able to acknowledge that there had been a time in his life when, just as he was not able to let his mother know that he was angry, he had also not been able to show anger toward God. Since taking time in psychotherapy to talk about his early relationships and being able to make the connection to how he also related to God in similar ways, he was able to give his parents the room to be human and allow himself the room to be human with God as he worked on renewing his previous relationship with God. In light of Malik's view and perspective of God and his early experiences with his mother, he had developed a belief system that did not allow him the opportunity to have negative experiences of people that he loved and to whom he wanted to be close.

As a result of reaching a place of conflict and confusion over feeling let down, Malik began to display maladaptive behaviors as a way of dealing with the pain and confusion. Before the external display, he had learned to internalize bad or frustrating things in his environment and had decided to be bad himself. He had also made God bad and rejected God rather than try to deal with the difficult situations that happened. Using God-image work, Maclin was able to work with Malik to better establish a view of how he thought about the God that he grew up learning about, as well as to engage with both God and his parents in a more authentic and less anxiety-provoking manner. Maclin helped him examine what he had learned over the years about what the true God was like so that he could learn to express his anger, frustration, resentment, and any other feelings without internalizing or redirecting those feelings toward God, such that God was either good or bad. After several sessions, Malik was able to acknowledge his feelings without having to distance himself from God out of fear and realize that God could handle his bad feelings and still be in relationship with him.

CONCLUSION

In this chapter, we have discussed God-image theoretical contributions, factors affecting God-image development, and clinical approaches to addressing client God images in child and adolescent psychotherapy. We began by defining God images and God concepts. In brief, God images are the emotional, heart-based, implicit understandings of God, whereas God concepts are the cognitive, head-based, explicit understandings of God. We then outlined clinical approaches with a particular emphasis on art therapy, CBT, and interpersonal (specifically object relations) therapy. We closed with three case examples highlighting how God-image theory and research can influence religious and spiritual work with children and adolescents. In the future, we anticipate that our understanding of the implications of God image in children, practically and theoretically, will continue to guide spiritually oriented interventions with children.

REFERENCES

Badenoch, B. (2008). *Being a brain-wise therapist: A practical guide to interpersonal neurobiology*. New York, NY: Norton.

Barrett, J. (2001). Do children experience God as adults do? In J. Andresen (Ed.), *Religion in mind: Cognitive perspectives on religious belief, ritual, and experience* (pp. 173–190). New York, NY: Cambridge University Press.

Barrett, J. L., & Keil, F. C. (1996). Conceptualizing a non-natural entity: Anthropomorphism in God concepts. *Cognitive Psychology*, *31*, 219–247. doi:10.1006/cogp.1996.0017

Barrett, J. L., & Richert, R. A. (2003). Anthropomorphism or preparedness? Exploring children's God concepts. *Review of Religious Research*, *44*, 300–312. doi:10.2307/3512389

Bowlby, J. (1969). *Attachment and loss: Vol. 1. Attachment.* New York, NY: Basic Books.

Bowlby, J. (1973). *Attachment and loss: Vol. 2. Separation.* New York, NY: Basic Books.

Bowlby, J. (1980). *Attachment and loss: Vol. 3. Loss, sadness and depression.* New York, NY: Basic Books.

Bowlby, J. (1988). *A secure base: Parent-child attachment and healthy human development.* New York, NY: Basic Books.

Davis, E. B. (2010). *Authenticity, inauthenticity, attachment, and God-image tendencies among adult evangelical Protestant Christians* (Unpublished doctoral dissertation). Regent University, Virginia Beach, VA.

Dickie, J. R., Eshleman, A. K., Merasco, D. M., Shepard, A., Vander Wilt, M., & Johnson, M. (1997). Parent-child relationships and children's images of God. *Journal for the Scientific Study of Religion, 36*, 1, 25–43. Retrieved from PsycINFO database.

Dillon, J. J. (2000). The spiritual child: Appreciating children's transformative effects on adults. *Encounter: Education for Meaning and Social Justice, 13*(4), 4–18.

Evans, H. L., & Sullivan, M. A. (1993). Children and the use of self-monitoring, self-evaluation, and self-reinforcement. In A. J. Finch Jr., N. W. Michael III, & E. S. Ott (Eds.), *Cognitive-behavioral procedures with children and adolescents: A practical guide* (pp. 67–89). Needham Heights, MA: Allyn & Bacon.

Fowler, J. W. (1981). *Stages of faith: The psychology of human development and the quest for meaning.* New York, NY: HarperCollins.

Fowler, J. W. (1996). *Faithful change.* Nashville, TN: Abingdon Press.

Gerkin, C. (1994). Projective identification and the image of God: Reflections on object relations theory and the psychology of religion. In B. H. Childers & D. W. Waanders (Eds.), *The treasure of earthen vessels: Explorations in theological anthropology in honor of James N. Lapsley* (pp. 52–65). Louisville, KY: Westminster John Knox Press. Retrieved from PsycINFO database.

Gibson, N. J. S. (2006). *The experimental investigation of religious cognition* (Unpublished doctoral dissertation). University of Cambridge, Cambridge, England. Retrieved from http://divinity.npsl.co.uk/prrg/people/staff/staff.acds?context=1609849&instanceid=1609850

Gibson, N. J. S. (2007). Measurement issues in God image research and practice. In G. L. Moriarty & L. Hoffman (Eds.), *God image handbook for spiritual counseling and psychotherapy: Research, theory, and practice* (pp. 227–246). Binghamton, NY: Haworth Press.

Goldman, R. (1964). *Religious thinking from childhood to adolescence.* London, England: Routledge Kegan & Paul.

Granqvist, P. (1998). Religiousness and perceived childhood attachment: On the question of compensation or correspondence. *Journal for the Scientific Study of Religion, 37*, 350–367.

Granqvist, P. (2002). Attachment and religiosity in adolescence: Cross-sectional and longitudinal evaluations. *Personality and Social Psychology Bulletin, 28*, 260–270.

Granqvist, P., & Hagekull, B. (1999). Religiousness and perceived childhood attachment: Profiling socialized correspondence and emotional compensation. *Journal for the Scientific Study of Religion, 38*, 254–273. doi:10.2307/1387793

Granqvist, P., & Kirkpatrick, L. A. (2008). Attachment and religious representations and behavior. In J. Cassidy & P. R. Shaver (Eds.), *Handbook of attachment: Theory, research, and clinical applications* (2nd ed., pp. 906–933). New York, NY: Guilford Press.

Hall, T. W. (2004). Christian spirituality and mental health: A relational spirituality framework for empirical research. *Journal of Psychology and Christianity, 23*, 66–81.

Hall, T. W., Halcrow, S., Hill, P. C., & Delaney, H. (2005, August). *Internal working model correspondence in implicit spiritual experiences.* Paper presented at the 113th Annual Convention of the American Psychological Association, Washington, DC.

Harms, E. (1944). The development of religious experience in children. *American Journal of Sociology, 50*, 112–122. doi:10.1086/219518

Hart, K. J., & Morgan, J. R. (1993). General issues in cognitive-behavioral treatment of children and adolescents. In A. J. Finch Jr., W. M. Nelson III, & E. S. Ott (Eds.), *Cognitive-behavioral procedures with children and adolescents: A practical guide* (pp. 1–24). Boston, MA: Allyn & Bacon.

Hart, T. (2003). *The secret spiritual world of children.* Makawao, HI: Inner Ocean.

Hart, T. (2006). Spiritual experiences and capacities of children. In E. C. Roehlkepartain, P. E. King, L. M. Wagener, & P. L. Benson (Eds.), *The handbook of spiritual development in childhood and adolescence* (pp. 163–177). Thousand Oaks, CA: Sage.

Hertel, B. R., & Donahue, M. J. (1995). Parental influences on God images among children: Testing Durkheim's metaphoric parallelism. *Journal for the Scientific Study of Religion, 34*(2), 186–199. doi:10.2307/1386764

Hultgren, A. J. (2002). *The parables of Jesus: A commentary.* Grand Rapids, MI: William B. Eerdmans.

Johnson, C. N., & Boyatzis, C. J. (2006). Cognitive-cultural foundations in spiritual development. In E. C. Roehlkepartain, P. E. King, L. M. Wagener, & P. L. Benson (Eds.), *The handbook of spiritual development in childhood and adolescence* (pp. 211–223). Thousand Oaks, CA: Sage.

Kirkpatrick, L. A. (1992). An attachment-theory approach to the psychology of religion. *International Journal for the Psychology of Religion, 2*, 3–28. doi:10.1207/s15327582ijpr0201_2

Kirkpatrick, L. A. (1997). A longitudinal study of changes in religious belief and behavior as a function of individual differences in adult attachment style. *Journal for the Scientific Study of Religion, 36*, 207–217. doi:10.2307/1387553

Kirkpatrick, L. A. (2005). *Attachment, evolution, and the psychology of religion*. New York, NY: Guilford Press.

Kirkpatrick, L., & Shaver, P. (1990). Attachment theory and religion: Childhood attachment, religious beliefs, and conversion. *Journal for the Scientific Study of Religion, 29*, 315–334. doi:10.2307/1386461

Moriarty, G. L. (2006). *Pastoral care of depression: Helping clients heal their relationship with God*. Binghamton, NY: Haworth Press.

Moriarty, G. L., & Davis, E. B. (2012). Client God images: research, theory and practice. In J. Aten, K. O'Grady, & E. Worthington Jr. (Eds.), *Psychology of religion and spirituality for clinicians: Using research in your practice* (pp. 131–160). New York, NY: Routledge.

Moriarty, G. L., & Hoffman, L. (Eds.). (2007). *God image handbook for spiritual counseling and psychotherapy: Research, theory, and practice*. Binghamton, NY: Haworth Press.

Noffke, J. L., & Hall, T. W. (2007). Attachment psychotherapy and God image. In G. L. Moriarty & L. Hoffman (Eds.), *God image handbook for spiritual counseling and psychotherapy: Research, theory, and practice* (pp. 57–78). Binghamton, NY: Haworth Press.

Norcross, J. C., & Goldfried, M. R. (2005). The future of psychotherapy integration: A roundtable. *Journal of Psychotherapy Integration, 15*, 392–471. doi:10.1037/1053-0479.15.4.392

Nye, W. C., & Carlson, J. S. (1984). The development of the concept of God in children. *Journal of Genetic Psychology, 144*, 137–142.

Ollendick, T. H., & King, N. J. (2004). Empirically supported treatments for children and adolescents: Advances toward evidence-based practice. In P. M. Barrett & T. H. Ollendick (Eds.), *Handbook of interventions that work with children and adolescents: Prevention and treatment* (pp. 3–25). New York, NY: Wiley.

Pellegrini, D. S., Galinski, C. L., Hart, K. J., & Kendall, P. C. (1993). Cognitive-behavioral assessment of children: A review of measures and methods. In A. J. Finch Jr., W. M. Nelson III, & E. S. Ott (Eds.), *Cognitive-behavioral procedures with children and adolescents: A practical guide* (pp. 90–147). Boston, MA: Allyn & Bacon.

Reinecke, M. A., Dattilio, F. M., & Freeman, A. (Eds.). (1996). *Cognitive therapy with children and adolescents: A casebook for clinical practice*. New York, NY: Guilford Press.

Richert, R., & Barrett, J. (2005). RESEARCH: Do you see what I see? Young children's assumptions about God's perceptual abilities. *International Journal for the Psychology of Religion, 15*, 283–295. doi:10.1207/s15327582ijpr1504_2

Rizzuto, A. (1979). *The birth of the living God*. Chicago, IL: University of Chicago Press.

Siegel, D. J. (1999). *The developing mind: How relationships and the brain interact to shape who we are*. New York, NY: Guilford Press.

Spirito, A., & Kazak, A. (2006). *Effective and emerging treatments in pediatric psychology*. New York, NY: Oxford University Press.

St. Clair, M. (2000). *Object relations and self psychology: An introduction* (3rd ed.). Belmont, CA: Brooks/Cole.

Tamminen, K. (1991). *Religious development in childhood and youth: An empirical study*. Helsinki, Finland: Suomalainen Tiedeakatemia.

Tamminen, K. (1994). Religious experiences in childhood and adolescence: A viewpoint of religious development between the ages of 7 and 20. *International Journal for the Psychology of Religion, 4*, 61–85. doi:10.1207/s15327582ijpr0402_1

Teyber, E., & McClure, F. H. (2010). *Interpersonal process in therapy: An integrative model* (6th ed.). Pacific Grove, CA: Brooks/Cole.

Waller, D. (2006). Art therapy for children: How it leads to change. *Clinical Child Psychology and Psychiatry, 11*, 271–282. doi:10.1177/1359104506061419

Wilber, K. (1996). *The Atman Project: A transpersonal view of human development*. Wheaton, IL: Quest.

Williams, R. (1971). A theory of God-concept readiness: From the Piagetian theories of child artificialism and the origin of religious feeling in children. *Religious Education*, 66, 62–66.

Wolfe, D. A., & Mash, E. J. (Eds.). (2006). *Behavioral and emotional disorders in adolescents: Nature, assessment, and treatment*. New York, NY: Guilford Press.

Young, W. P. (2007). *The shack*. Newbury Park, CA: Windblown Media.

10

FORGIVENESS INTERVENTIONS WITH CHILDREN, ADOLESCENTS, AND FAMILIES

FREDERICK A. DIBLASIO, EVERETT L. WORTHINGTON JR., AND DAVID J. JENNINGS II

Love and forgiveness are values that have commonly been associated through the centuries with close interpersonal relationships. Children, adolescents, and their parents will have their normal share of hurts and conflicts, and sometimes more serious offenses will bring them to the door of a psychotherapist. Sometimes forgiveness interventions become necessary to assist children in forgiving their parents for the pain of family life situations created by parental decisions—for example, a decision to divorce. Clinicians may also find that helping children to forgive is necessary in resolving abuse inflicted by parents. Alternatively, clinical forgiveness intervention may be the vehicle of treatment in cases in which children with behavioral disruptive disorders have inflicted the pain and hurt and need to seek the forgiveness of parents and siblings whom they have offended.

Research and practice experience have revealed that forgiveness work is an effective healing intervention that restores emotional and spiritual health

DOI: 10.1037/13947-011
Spiritual Interventions in Child and Adolescent Psychotherapy, D. F. Walker and W. L. Hathaway (Editors)

and promotes reconciliation in relationships (Worthington, Jennings, & DiBlasio, 2010). However, little is known about how to apply forgiveness interventions directly to children and families who are in psychotherapy. The purpose of this chapter is to provide professional clinicians with a greater understanding of forgiveness and practice techniques when working with children, adolescents, and families.

We start by taking a brief look at the literature on forgiveness theory and research, and we then focus on three forgiveness models: process (Enright, 2001), REACH (Worthington, 2006b), and decision based (DiBlasio, 2000). From these models, we identify several therapeutic concepts and suggest a few specific interventions that might benefit children and adolescents—either through individual psychotherapy or through family psychotherapy. Two case examples—a 9-year-old and a 14-year-old and their families—are presented. Throughout the chapter, we use the words *child* and *children* to represent both children and adolescents unless specifically delineated. Relevant personal information was changed in all case material to protect client confidentiality.

EMOTIONAL AND DECISIONAL FORGIVENESS

Two types of forgiveness were noted by Worthington (e.g., Worthington, 1998, 2003, 2006b). *Emotional forgiveness* is the emotional replacement of negative unforgiving emotions (i.e., hurt and anger) by positive other-oriented emotions, such as empathy, sympathy, compassion, or love. When people forgive, their negative emotions subside. They are less motivated to seek revenge or avoid the transgressor, and if forgiving is complete, they may feel love, compassion, sympathy, or empathy for the transgressor. People may also grant *decisional forgiveness*, which applies to their behavioral intentions toward the offender. They decide to steer clear of revenge, not to avoid the transgressor (unless continued interaction is potentially dangerous), and to treat the transgressor as a person of worth even though they may still have negative emotions. Essentially, decisional forgiveness is a sincere intention statement about controlling one's future behavior (DiBlasio, 2000; Worthington, 2006b). Forgiveness may be initiated by reasoning; simply experiencing positive other-oriented emotions toward the transgressor; acting kindly toward the transgressor; and/or having the transgressor act contritely or in a way that provokes empathy, sympathy, compassion, or love.

We view forgiveness as described as beneficial for the forgiver. However, is forgiveness appropriate in all situations? If someone does not want to embark on an intervention that might lead to forgiveness, professionals are ethically obligated to respect client self-determination. Clients' values and beliefs play a significant role in whether they believe forgiveness is appropriate. Client beliefs will also drive the answers related to whether, when, and how a forgiver communicates forgiveness to an offender. Whereas psychotherapists may give their opinions about these issues, it is ultimately a client decision. However, in the discussion it is important to help family members understand that forgiveness can coexist with setting boundaries to protect oneself and with various forms of reconciliation. For example, a child may be forgiving of an abusive parent, but the abuse may lead to a type of reconciliation in which the child and parent must always have outside supervision when together.

DEVELOPMENT OF FORGIVENESS IN CHILDREN

The first step in learning how forgiveness works for children is to view it from a developmental perspective. A well-established principle in developmental psychology is that children become capable of certain thought processes as the brain matures. For example, a young child might think that the moon is like a person that follows her as she rides in a car. However, in her teen years, not only does the child understand the science of the earth's and moon's orbits, but she may also have more abstract thoughts about God's divine nature that created a light-reflecting heavenly body that has a predictable orbit. Enright and colleagues (Enright, 1991; Enright & Fitzgibbons, 2000) illustrated the maturation of cognition by presenting a six-stage model illustrating how children move from conditional to unconditional forgiveness.

We assume that children first learn forgiveness at a very early age as parents instruct them to seek forgiveness from and grant it to family members (Worthington, 2006a). Forgiveness is likely conditional in the early stages. Therefore, out of obedience and perhaps concern with displeasing parents or incurring negative consequences or punishment, children learn the mechanics of forgiveness by articulating forgiveness language taught by parents. Much as a child at age 3 can count to 10 and not comprehend the true mathematical operations of what 10 really means, so too can a child learn the procedure of forgiveness but not fully understand and feel the depth of its meaning as an internal state. As the brain and speech develop, children begin to recognize that mandated requirements do not always correlate with their decision or emotional state. Parents begin to notice that children will communicate forgiveness words, but at times their unforgiving attitudes are reflected in their nonverbal communication. For example, an 8-year-old son was asked to request forgiveness of his mother, and the boy grudgingly said, "Sorry." The father intervened and instructed his son to make the request in a full sentence. The father began to reprimand his son after the son snidely responded, "I'm sorry." The son made the argument that the phrase "I'm sorry" was a full sentence complete with subject and verb and therefore met the technical requirements, but he obviously missed the heartfelt repentance that the father expected.

Many factors are involved in understanding the dynamics of forgiveness with children, such as the parent–child relationship, the child's temperament, emotion-regulation capability, parental meta-emotional philosophy, cognitive development of the ability to reason about justice and forgiveness, repertoire of stress-coping strategies, and religious and spiritual environment (Worthington et al., 2010). Forgiveness interventions that account for these contextual factors, the decisional and emotional aspects of forgiveness, and children's developmental stage hold potential for promoting healthy forgiveness in the family unit.

OVERVIEW OF FORGIVENESS RESEARCH

A review of the literature produced only a small number of forgiveness intervention studies with children, adolescents, parents, and families. We found only a few studies that had been published in refereed journals. A search for recorded dissertations produced slightly more, but overall our search showed a paucity of research studies specific to children and adolescents. In addition, none of the intervention studies involving children tested actual psychotherapy encounters; instead, they were group educational and experiential interventions. We found no studies of family therapy that included children and forgiveness interventions.

Forgiveness group interventions have been shown to be effective, particularly with adolescents. Overall, it appears that forgiveness gains are modest but that forgiveness interventions can be applied across cultures with some substantial beneficial effects. The interventions seem to mostly affect attitudes and ratings of forgiving, and sometimes behavioral changes are noted as well (see Worthington et al., 2010, for a comprehensive review and citations). Only one study has been conducted specifically to help teach parents how to forgive and how to promote forgiveness in their children (Keifer et al., 2010). Using Worthington's (2006b) forgiveness and reconciliation through exploring empathy model, parents were trained in how to forgive their children for disappointments and how to forgive their coparenting partners when misunderstandings occur over parenting. Forgiveness of a target offense and overall forgiveness showed significant increases after treatment and at 3-week follow-up.

In contrast to the research on children and family members, research on interventions to promote forgiveness in adults, especially within couple relationships, is much more robust. Overall, forgiveness interventions with several different models have consistently been found to be effective with adults and couples (see Worthington et al., 2010). These findings show promising possibilities for extending forgiveness interventions to family psychotherapy with children, but more research would be needed to show its efficacy in this context.

INTERVENTION MODELS TO PROMOTE FORGIVENESS

Next, we present three models that are found in the literature that we believe show promise for application to individual and family psychotherapy with children. Although only a brief introduction to the models is possible, we encourage practitioners to further investigate them in building a forgiveness practice theory for assisting children and families.

Process Model

Enright and colleagues (Enright & Fitzgibbons, 2000; Freedman, Enright & Knutson, 2005) have proposed a process model of forgiving. The model has 20 units, which are arrayed in four phases. The first eight units make up the *uncovering phase*. During uncovering, the person gets in touch with personal pain, which can become very distressing. Anger is the chief negative emotion experienced and, once processed and discussed, can lead to the beginning of healing.

Units 9 through 11 involve the *decision phase*. Forgiveness is defined, and the person considers what is involved before committing to forgive. The person considers the possibility of making a positive change toward healing and commits to giving up thoughts of revenge toward the offender. In this stage, the offended person commits to taking the first steps toward forgiveness.

Units 12 through 15 make up the *work phase*. In the work phase, people try to understand the offender and the context of the transgression, followed by accepting and absorbing the pain. This phase includes developing new ways to think about the offender and attempting to understand the offensive behavior in the context of the problems faced by the offender throughout his or her life. An effort is made to view the offender as a member of the human community. A moral commitment is made to respond with moral love and mercy to the offender.

In the *outcome phase*, Units 16 through 20, the person develops a sense of healing and as a result gives a gift of forgiveness to the offender. In the process, the forgiver finds emotional relief and increased empathy and compassion. This forgiving stance tends to generalize and becomes the basis of becoming a better person.

The process model has been tested mostly with adults with various presenting problems and with populations. Examples include incest survivors, people struggling with substance abuse and dependence, and men whose partners had experienced an abortion. It has also been tested with people with physical health problems such as cancer and cardiovascular disorders (for reviews, see Baskin & Enright, 2004; Freedman et al., 2005).

REACH Forgiveness Model

Worthington (2006b) developed five steps to reach forgiveness, in which memory of the five steps is cued by the acronym REACH. To begin, *R*, for the recall of the hurt, is when the offender recalls the event in a way different from the usual ruminative recall. Namely, the person recalls without blaming the offender or self-pitying. After a conscious attempt to decide to forgive, an attempt at *E* (*empathize to emotionally replace*) is made during the longest portion of the method. Emotional replacement can substitute empathy, sympathy, compassion, or love for the unforgiving emotions of resentment, bitterness, hostility, hatred, anger, and fear. *A* is an *altruistic gift of forgiving* in which, through humility and empathy, the person decides to forgive and emotionally experiences forgiveness. *C* stands for *commit to the forgiveness experienced*. The person makes a public commitment (which could be to others or just a letter or note to him- or herself) to solidify the experience of deciding to forgive and emotionally forgiving. The commitment is intended to help the person *H*, *hold onto forgiveness*. Detailed manuals are publicly available at http://www.people.vcu.edu/~eworth (Worthington, 2010) and can be downloaded and modified for local use without financial cost.

The REACH model is designed for psychoeducational group settings; however, the concepts hold significance for designing therapeutic strategies for children and adolescents. Worthington's (2006b) model has been applied, tested, and found effective in numerous spiritual and secular settings and populations (e.g., see Lampton, Oliver, Worthington, & Berry, 2005; Stratton, Dean, Nooneman, Bode, & Worthington, 2008; Worthington et al., 2010).

Decision-Based Model

DiBlasio (1998, 2000) has offered willing clients an opportunity to explore the offense and understand why it occurred and given them an opportunity to seek and grant forgiveness in a lengthy step-by-step therapeutic session. The steps include the following:

- Definitions of forgiveness are discussed.
- The focus on each person having the opportunity to seek forgiveness for his or her wrongful actions is established.

- The forgiveness treatment is introduced, and a decision is made whether to participate.
- A statement of the offense is made.
- The offender provides an explanation.
- Questions are asked and answers are given about the offense.
- The offended person gives emotional reactions.
- The offender shows empathy and remorse for the hurt he or she caused the other.
- The offender develops a plan to stop or prevent the behavior.
- The offended person shows empathy for the offender's hurt.
- The choice and commitment involved in letting go are emphasized.
- A formal request for forgiveness is made.
- A ceremonial act is planned.

Additional details about the treatment can be found in DiBlasio (1998, 2000); for application to Christian clients, see Cheong and DiBlasio (2007), DiBlasio (1999, 2010), and DiBlasio and Benda (2008).

The initial focus of this model is decision-based forgiveness; consequently, cognitive (decisional) forgiveness is highlighted. However, it is important to note that the model also promotes emotional forgiveness and behavioral communication of one's forgiveness in the session as well. A particular advantage of this model is that DiBlasio has successfully applied it since 1980 (cases reported in the literature since 1990; see Worthington & DiBlasio, 1990) in psychotherapy situations involving adults, couples, adolescents, families, and family-of-origin situations. Empirically, the model has been shown to be effective with marital couples in a major control group study (DiBlasio & Benda, 2008), and it emphasizes steps that include well-tested forgiveness intervention variables, such as creating insight into offense behavior, expression of emotional hurt, empathy of the offender and offended toward each other, commitment to hold on to the forgiveness decision, and so forth. It is hoped that more researchers will test the decision-based model and compare it with ones that unfold over time.

CLINICAL APPLICATION AND INTERVENTION TECHNIQUES

Undoubtedly, clinicians value theory and research. Nevertheless, we assume they also want to know "What do I do with Gloria in the next session?" and "How can I help promote forgiveness during psychotherapy with the Smith family?" Early research on the clinical use of forgiveness demonstrated that psychotherapists want to learn more about specific application of techniques (DiBlasio & Proctor, 1993). Despite the fact that the research on forgiveness has expanded rapidly over the past two decades, practice literature still remains lacking in regard to child and family psychotherapy. Next, we present an initial effort to take models that are documented in the literature and derive selected concepts and suggest clinical application.

The REACH and the Enright (2001) process models, if applied to the psychotherapy room, would likely take place over the course of several weeks (e.g., the process model might require 20 weekly sessions). These models highlight the differences between emotional and decisional forgiveness and would likely involve a progressive unfolding of both over the course of the psychotherapy. The decision-based model would, interestingly, do the same thing, but DiBlasio (2010) found that clients rarely desire an unfolding process over time when they are given the direct choice of a forgiveness session at any point they determine during the psychotherapy (most choose for the clinician to conduct the session in the beginning of psychotherapy). The decision-based model shows that 1-day forgiveness sessions with clients not only culminate in forgiveness decisions but also produce emotional and behavioral forgiveness that lasts over time. Forgiveness sessions are often followed by additional psychotherapy sessions, but sometimes the forgiveness session is enough to establish lasting forgiveness (see DiBlasio, 2010). In either case, all three models embrace therapeutic healing of children and families throughout weeks of psychotherapy, regardless of when decisional forgiveness occurs.

Making the Models Spiritually Relevant

Is forgiveness a spiritual process? The answer to that question will depend on the spiritual orientation of the responder. Hence, making forgiveness relevant would require the psychotherapist to explore and understand clients' faith perspectives and, where possible, to follow their desires on the matter. It is well-known that forgiveness is central to many religious beliefs. In the United States, only 15% of people are atheist, agnostic, or have no religion (U.S. Census Bureau, 2012). Therapists who approach forgiveness as primarily a generic or secular concept will miss the mark with many religious families. However, to reduce forgiveness to some general spiritual approach would be to filter out enough religious content so that it meets the lowest common spiritual denominator of all theistic and nontheistic religions and forms of spirituality. Psychotherapists are encouraged to understand their clients' spiritual perspectives and, where possible, attempt to tailor the interventions mentioned in this chapter in a spiritually relevant fashion. For example, in the United Sates 76% of people are affiliated with a Christian religion or a nondenominational Christian faith (U.S. Census Bureau, 2012). Forgiveness is central to the Christian faith because it is founded on Jesus' death, resurrection, and atonement for the forgiveness of sins (e.g., John 3:16). Moreover, the teachings of Jesus emphasize that his followers must forgive others (e.g., Matthew 8:14–15). Consequently, for clients who desire the therapy to be Christian focused, the psychotherapist may discuss the love of the Father, the teachings of Jesus, and the power of the Holy Spirit. However, this is not as easy as it sounds because of psychotherapists' faith perspectives. Sometimes making forgiveness intervention spiritually relevant to clients is not entirely possible for some psychotherapists because by doing so they violate their own spiritual convictions. Where these gulfs exist between clients' and psychotherapists' spiritual beliefs, sound therapeutic contracting and understanding in the beginning is helpful.

Application of Forgiveness Practice Concepts

Each psychotherapist is faced with formulating a practice theory about forgiveness strategies, applied concepts, and timing of interventions. In reality, forgiveness intervention is often just one part of the presenting problems. However, forgiveness is a key that will usually unlock major therapeutic doors to resolving embittered relationships, child acting-out behaviors, self-destructive behavior that often accompanies long-term anger, depression, anxiety, and many other interrelated mental health disorders. Therefore, we recommend that psychotherapists offer, and be fully prepared to engage in, some type of forgiveness intervention with all willing clients when presenting problems directly or indirectly involve unresolved offenses. At times, forgiveness will become the main focus of psychotherapy, and at other times it will be needed as a tool to free or assist clients to therapeutically address other issues.

Following are brief descriptions of practice concepts (among others) that are constant across the three models. When used in practice, each concept needs to be tailored to the context of each family and to the developmental stage of children. Individually, the concepts are likely to be familiar to advanced psychotherapists, and clinicians have established methods to address them. However, what might be innovative is considering them all at once as building blocks drawn from the research to assist in the building of a systematic forgiveness approach.

Offenses against children have a wide range of severity from mild to the most devastating and heinous acts of violence. Likewise, children commit offenses that vary on a spectrum of severity. Whereas the practice application found here can be applied to various severity levels, each practice concept and application should be evaluated for its goodness of fit to the problem and the context of the people involved.

Using Developmentally Appropriate Forgiveness Interventions

Meaningful interventions are tailored to fit children's developmental stage. Interventions with young children often include techniques that are metaphorical or representative. Much as adults, older teens usually respond to therapeutic content that is direct. However, because of the egocentrism that is common in the teen years, therapeutic approaches need to be relevant and contextual and help teens to move from overfocus on self to consideration of others. Enright, Knutson, Holter, Baskin, and Knutson (2007) in particular have addressed the developmental issue by unfolding an innovative forgiveness curriculum for kindergarten through Grade 12 that has been conducted in Wisconsin and in Belfast, Ireland.

Recognizing and Working Through the Hurt

It is essential for children and adults to emotionally connect with what happened to them (or if they offended against someone, to recognize the harm they inflicted). Offenses often lead to temporary or perhaps permanent consequences that involve a need for personal and interpersonal recovery. A sense of loss and grieving is created when offenses take away something that was valued. For example, a son whose college money was secretly spent by his father may forgive and restore the father–son relationship, but the son's image of the parent is permanently altered.

Promoting Insight

Children and adults gain an informed perspective through an understanding of the context of the situation, the history and perception of the offender (whether family member or person outside of the family), and the amount of intended (or unintended) harm. Exploration into the factors that are involved in the offense usually reveals that family members have not inflicted hurt on one another out of pure malice. Insight usually involves both the offender and the offended searching for all the ways they contributed to the problem. When children are offended against by their parents or other adults, great therapeutic care, sensitivity to, and consideration of developmental appropriateness are used when examining their participation.

Releasing Negative Emotions

Children often act out negative emotions or internalize them (e.g., inappropriate anger outbursts, self-destructive behaviors, depression). Psychotherapy provides a place for the release of negative emotions in a safe environment that paves the way for therapeutic resolution.

Encouraging Empathy

Offenses within families involve significant hurts for both the offender and the offended. Promoting empathy helps offenders understand and relate to the hurt they inflicted, which in turn gives the person offended a positive experience of being understood by the offender. Empathy (and remorse) from the transgressor improves the chances for successful granting of forgiveness. Similarly, when offended children and adults achieve empathy, it aids them in conceptualizing the hurts and pain that occurred in the offender's life that factor into the offense. Moreover, they experience the shame and guilt offenders often go through for having brought pain to a loved one. The realization and humility that all humans have made mistakes contribute to an ability to be empathetic.

Conducting Forgiveness Sessions

When children and parents are willing, they benefit by processing the offense in one or more therapeutic sessions in a fashion that could lead to seeking or granting decisional forgiveness. Each session is carefully defined beforehand so clients can make an informed decision about whether to participate. Forgiveness sessions work best when they are thorough, structured, and focused. Who participates becomes a matter of therapeutic judgment and negotiation with family members. Whether over several weekly sessions or in one long session, the forgiveness intervention should account for concepts discussed in this section.

Using Role Play

In some situations, children meeting directly with an offender is not possible, feasible, or therapeutically indicated (see, e.g., the later case example). Use of role play allows the psychotherapist to take the role of either the offender or, if a child is the offender wanting to seek forgiveness, the offended person. Psychotherapists have a vista of opportunity in such roles because they can alternate between representing what an offender would have said or should have said, and they can provide potential explanations in the process. Psychotherapists might also consider using an empty chair so children and family members can talk to the person who hurt them or the person whom they offended (for more information, see Worthington, 2010). If transgressors and the offended person meet for a forgiveness session, children might benefit from preparing by role-playing with the psychotherapist beforehand.

Creating Plans for Stopping and Preventing Hurtful Behaviors

Although forgiveness is possible regardless of the behaviors, repentance, or remorse of offenders, psychotherapists should encourage offenders to stop offensive behaviors and to set up plans that will prevent them from offending in the future. Commitment to well-spelled-out and specific items by the offender is necessary (some items include the agreement and commitment of the offended). Therapeutic diligence is required to check on the progress of the plan and whether clients are putting forth sufficient effort over the course of the psychotherapy. Plans should create accountability with a person outside the immediate family (see the next section) and protect children from future hurt. When the child is the offender, setting up self-control and outside controls makes the offense difficult to repeat, thereby making his or her forgiveness request meaningful.

Creating Accountability

Forgiveness work with children and parents is enhanced when they willingly give permission to a psychotherapist to help them stay focused and follow through on decisions and commitments made in treatment. Additionally, outside accountability is often encouraged through the use of trusted relatives and other adults. Religious environments typically provide a plethora of trustworthy adults who are eager to be of service. Regular meetings and phone contacts between the offender and the accountability person create a deterrence to future offenses and provide an encouraging role model. They also bring comfort to the offended person because the offender is receiving help and is monitored for accountability.

Understanding Forgiveness as a Gift

Enright (2001) stated, "Forgiveness is an act of mercy toward an offender, someone who does not necessarily deserve our mercy. It is a gift to our offender for the purpose of changing the relationship between ourselves and those who have hurt us" (p. 25). Helping children and family members who have been offended to connect to the gift aspect of forgiveness promotes the concept that forgiveness is something that they choose to give as a gift or withhold.

Committing to Forgiveness

On occasion, psychotherapy with children is not effective because the clinician does not have the child client's full commitment to the process. It is interesting to note that children are skilled at achieving goals as they develop and master epigenetic developmental tasks and are willing to take on challenges. Encouraging them to decide whether to commit to a forgiveness effort is helpful because it enhances their participation and internal locus of control. If the child is old enough, creating and signing an agreement that highlights the aim of making a good effort to forgive may be appropriate (Worthington, 2010).

Holding on to Forgiveness

When children and parents decide to forgive and move forward, hurtful feelings may emerge later on the subject of the forgiven offense and can lure them into doubting their forgiveness or, worse, returning to resentful and bitter behaviors. The psychotherapy becomes a safe haven to sort through hurt feelings, and at the same time it provides children and parents encouragement that forgiveness can coexist with a time of emotional healing. Relating to offenders, psychotherapy helps the forgiven person to work through the feelings of shame and guilt while fully embracing the forgiveness that was granted by others and possibly accepting permanent divine forgiveness for the transgression.

Involving Parents

Parental involvement is highly valued when it is safe to do so. Much of the work surrounding forgiveness may not only involve parents but also be led by them with the assistance of the psychotherapist. Many configurations of how parents are involved are determined by the nature of the offense, for example, whether the offense was committed by a parent or someone outside of the family.

Making the Formal Request

Each situation will have its unique issues, but either directly through a forgiveness session or indirectly through role play, children and parents benefit from formal requests for forgiveness. Much healing can take place for an offended child just hearing a heartfelt request from the one who inflicted the pain. In regard to children who offended others, a request for forgiveness after a thorough reflection allows them to feel restored enough to move forward without shame and guilt.

Examples of Intervention Techniques

Five selected concepts from those listed earlier are highlighted briefly in this section to provide practitioners with examples of how to move from the forgiveness concepts to specific treatment. We do not attempt a comprehensive treatment of each area here; instead, our goal is to stimulate creative therapeutic thought by offering a few suggestions. Many possible configurations and treatment options exist for using any one of the concepts listed earlier. We hope that readers will explore the literature on the models to understand the concepts more fully and to design a practice theory that accounts for all of these concepts for each case.

Promoting Insight: Difficult Parent Personalities

Seldom do family members intend to inflict hurt on each other, especially parents toward their children. In some cases, parents have difficult personalities or personality disorders that complicate forgiveness for their children because they often take defensive rather than accountable and humble positions on their offensive behaviors. Some parents continue offending despite countervailing treatment efforts, making forgiveness a difficult challenge for children who suffer hurtful behaviors. The offensive behaviors are particularly confusing for children of spiritually oriented parents because these offenses are incongruent with love, peace, and humane treatment of others.

If the cumulative percentages of prevalence of personality disorders within the normal population found in the *Diagnostic and Statistical Manual of Mental Disorders* (4th ed., text rev; American Psychiatric Association, 2000) are correct, more than 20% of adults have a personality disorder. Common practice knowledge has revealed that a number of offenses occurring within families (especially those offending children) are the result of parents with mild to severe personality problems. If adults accept the diagnostic assessment, or at least accept that they have a series of symptoms that cause pain to others, forgiveness work is enhanced. For example, DiBlasio (2001) referred to personality disorders such as narcissistic, borderline, histrionic, and antisocial as identity problems that may involve emotional and relational dyslexia. Although the etiology of personality disorders is unknown (see Sadock & Sadock, 2007), DiBlasio suggested that personality disorders may be a result of learning problems in the brain, much as with someone with an academic learning disability. When offenses toward children occur, it is important for psychotherapists to assist children and parents to grasp that the offense is wrong and never justified regardless of whether the offender has a personality disorder. Psychotherapists walk a delicate line in such cases because, on the one hand, it is often helpful for children to understand that their parents' dysfunction may be brain related, but, on the other hand, the psychotherapist does not want to alienate the parents. At the same time, if psychotherapists present the dysfunction in a loving fashion that capitalizes on the parents' strengths (thus promoting healthy identity), inroads are made into helping adults with personality disorder not depend on certain negative emotions and thoughts as being reliable enough to follow through with behavior. One client who accepted this theory as being true for him improved between sessions. This client was diagnosed as having narcissistic personality disorder, a disorder that typically does not respond well to routine psychotherapy. When asked by the psychotherapist for details of how he applied the concept, he simply reported, "I now send myself to my room to calm down when my kids do something wrong, and when I return I find that it is easy to use my diplomacy skills to handle the problem." The strength-based approach of the psychotherapy in the previous session was to elaborate on his outstanding diplomacy, as demonstrated in his job as an attorney. This admiration from the psychotherapist helped to facilitate the client's reception of the challenge to use these skills in the home.

A second example comes from a case in which the mother was diagnosed as having borderline personality disorder. After the initial diagnosis was presented in a loving and strength-based fashion, Mrs. Jones agreed to set more reasonable expectations for her children. Her psychotherapist focused on her strengths, such as deep devotion to her family, ability to communicate with others outside the family, creative thinking, and insightful ideas that the psychotherapist was even applying at home. However, when it came to her assessment of the children and their failures to live up to her expectations (and, worse, their failure to do so because of a lack of respect toward her), Mrs. Jones committed to viewing her thoughts and emotions as not fully reliable. Instead, she adjusted her expectations down a few notches. Although she was a very dutiful mother, when it came to being patient with the mishaps and disobedience of her children, she could no longer trust that her negative emotional and cognitive reactions were commensurate with the reality of the problem (psychotherapy helped her set a more accurate reality). Mrs. Jones and her children accepted that her brain was not to be trusted in this area, especially when she was emotionally angry and hurt. This promoted more behavioral self-control by the mother, allowing other treatment to have positive effects. Forgiving parents is easier for children when they see their parents admitting to problems, seeking help in psychotherapy, being accountable to someone for follow through, and refusing to rely on old negative thought patterns.

Conducting a Forgiveness Session: Selected Considerations

Although clinicians may vary in the timing of a session that focuses on forgiveness, many would agree that in most cases such a session is profitable at some point during the course of treatment (whether it occurs in one long session or over several sessions). When sessions involve bringing transgressors and the offended together, such as family members seeking forgiveness from one another, it is important to encourage culpability. As a hypothetical example, when asked to put his offense into words, a child might say, "I want to seek forgiveness for the mean things I say to my mom because she always is getting on my case." The psychotherapist should call attention to the less-than-adequate culpability by saying, "In this statement of your offense, I hear the statement of your offense and what you believe your mother is doing wrong; can you be clearer about your offense only?"

The psychotherapist works with children and parents during the session to spell out and commit to a plan to stop or prevent offensive behaviors. The plan incorporates a few items that the offender willingly agrees to be accountable for. As a hypothetical example, three items (among others) for a Christian teen who when angry is verbally harsh with his younger sister may be to agree to go to his room to calm down when he is upset with her, go weekly to a community anger management group for teens, and memorize and regularly recite his choice of scripture related to controlling anger. Weekly reports to a nearby trusted uncle who also checks in with parents and the sister could become outside accountability.

Releasing Negative Emotions: Metaphorical "Releasing" Exercise

Although originally designed for groups of adults in psychoeducational settings, the REACH releasing exercise (adapted from Worthington, 2010) has the potential to support children as they pair a physical experience with an internal process in a psychotherapy setting. Use of active psychotherapy techniques that involve movement, drawing, play, and other activities is important in shifting children from the externalized experience to an internal spiritual and psychological process. The positive subliminal and metaphorical benefits that result make this technique helpful for children even if they are not at an abstract cognitive developmental stage.

The psychotherapist asks a willing child client who was offended by a parent to stand up, hold his or her arms out in front of the body, and imagine holding a grudge that he or she may have against the parent (to facilitate the following discussion, we will say the forgiveness exercise involves a young boy and his mother). A young child may need an age-appropriate explanation of what it means to hold a grudge. The therapist asks the child to prepare to squeeze his hands tightly together to represent how tightly he is holding on to the grudge and prepares him that when the therapist says "go," he is to squeeze hard and try to hold the grudge as long as he can. The psychotherapist might say, "You can feel the weight of the grudge growing, and you want to let go of the grudge because you can feel that it is hard to keep squeezing it and it is heavy." However, the psychotherapist would encourage the child to keep holding the grudge (if he releases early, the psychotherapist would ask him to try again). The idea is to let the child feel the weight and pressure of tightly squeezing his hands together, which becomes a metaphor for the weight and burden of holding onto unforgiveness. After an age-appropriate amount of time, the psychotherapist says:

> Hold the grudge for a few more seconds until I count down and say let go. If you are ready to make a decision to forgive and you are going to try to treat your mother as a valuable person whom God loves despite the

fact that she hurt you, then get ready to let go of the grudge. Don't do it until I say so. Imagine that the grudge is a bird that has been kept captive. When I say "Let it go," I want you to release it. Even if you do not make a full commitment to decide to forgive at this moment, I want you to let it go anyway and feel the freedom that comes with making a decision to forgive. Three, two, one—now let go.

The therapist asks the child what it felt like to relax his arms and not be squeezing any longer. Last, the therapist helps the child to make connections among holding on to a grudge, unforgiveness, and the release that is felt when he lets it go and forgives. Worthington (2010) gave helpful information on forgiveness strategies with religious clients, and he also provided guidance for more secular situations.

Using Role Play: Missing Person

Whenever possible and therapeutically appropriate, family members should represent themselves in psychotherapy sessions. However, in some cases a parent may no longer be involved in the child's life or may be deceased. At times, it is appropriate for another family member or the psychotherapist to take on the role of the missing parent.

When psychotherapists play the role of a missing parent, they can use therapeutic judgment and alternate between what the parent might have said (given the description provided by the family) and shift to what might had been said if the parent were thinking clearly and taking responsibility. Children are encouraged to ask questions. Psychotherapists have an opportunity to supply direct answers that provide insight into the hurtful behavior. In addition, psychotherapists can validate children who have not received sufficient validation from the missing parent.

Conversely, some children feel the need to process their own wrongs and seek forgiveness of a parent who is now deceased. When psychotherapists play the role of the parent in these situations, they ought not be too quick to dismiss children's sense of guilt for their offenses. Children who are allowed to take appropriate responsibility for their wrongdoing are freed to reap the benefits of the proxy forgiveness granted by the role-playing psychotherapist.

Developmentally Appropriate Forgiveness Interventions: Processing Hurt Through Play Psychotherapy and Mutual Storytelling

Certain projective techniques, such as play psychotherapy and mutual storytelling, help young children process hurt and work through anger issues. Although play psychotherapy is well understood by psychotherapists, less known is the technique of mutual storytelling (see Gardner, 1971). *Mutual storytelling* is a technique in which children tell original, made-up stories that are followed by the psychotherapist using the same or similar characters in telling a corrective story. Children usually project their struggles and issues subliminally in the context and characters of a story. The protagonist often represents the child, and other characters symbolically represent others in the child's family, peer group, or both. Usually, the stories contain offenses committed against the protagonist, and the outcomes of the stories are usually dismal. After the child tells the story, psychotherapists use the same context and characters to tell a corrective story. Psychotherapists place emphasis on the thoughts and feelings of the protagonist, which makes available indirect pathways to connect to the hurts of child clients. Young children frequently tell stories involving animals. Although it is beyond the scope of this chapter, interested psychotherapists should review Gardner's (1971) work in detail.

CASE STUDIES

Two case studies were selected to reflect two developmental stages. The first is a case study of a 9-year-old that was provided by Donald F. Walker, the first editor of this book. The second reflects a case involving a 14-year-old who was seen for psychotherapy by Frederick A. DiBlasio.

Case 1: Loss and Found

John was a 9-year-old boy of mixed African American and Caucasian ethnicity whose father had left his family, divorced his mother, and moved out of state several years before John came to psychotherapy. John was referred for psychotherapy because of repeated physical fights with his younger brother and his older sister and for often talking back to his mother and to teachers at school. The clinician completed an initial assessment by separately interviewing John and his mother. After interviewing both of them individually, it was clear that John qualified for a diagnosis of oppositional defiant disorder.

Initially, the clinician engaged John's mother in parent training in behavioral interventions. She self-identified as a Christian client, and biblical references were therefore used to encourage her to tie John's privileges to his behavior at home (see Chapter 7). Although this intervention was successful in changing his behavior, John continued to be angry. Although over time he no longer expressed his anger overtly in the form of explosive verbal outbursts, at times he remained passive aggressive and displayed some general irritability.

In exploring John's irritable mood, a continuing theme that emerged was his anger toward his father. In the process of examining his anger, John eventually articulated that he was angry that his father had left and that he blamed himself for his father leaving. He also expressed anger that his mother would not forgive him for his past misbehavior and for her belief that there was something inherently wrong with him that made him act the way he did. In conceptualizing his anger, the psychotherapist viewed John's anger toward his father as a defense against his more painful feelings of being hurt, rejected, and even abandoned by his father. In addition, his anger toward his mother may have been a defense, to some degree, against painful feelings of rejection from her, as well as against facing feelings of inadequacy when tasked with assignments at school that he sometimes felt unable to complete.

John was in need of forgiving his parents and himself and receiving forgiveness from his mother. Enright (2001) referred to these three dimensions of forgiveness as the *forgiveness triad* and suggested that each might have differential sources of healing for a person. In John's case, addressing all three had significant implications for his recovery and healing.

Each of these aspects of forgiveness required a somewhat different intervention, given the referent (others, self, or receiving another's forgiveness). In helping John work through the process of forgiving his father, the clinician reflected back to him that there must have been many things that he had wanted to learn from his father. John agreed and mentioned several sports, including football and basketball, as things that he had wanted to learn from his father but no longer had the opportunity to do so. John's anger was, in part, a way to keep his father involved in his thought life. Although very young, John was able to realize through the psychotherapy that in staying angry with his father, he was trying to hold onto him somehow. In helping John to forgive his father, the psychotherapist framed the idea that John's hurt and anger could be let go but that he could replace this with the positive things that he remembered from his involvement with his father.

Over time, John was able to acknowledge the deep hurt that he experienced when his father left the family, while more fully acknowledging the role that he believed that he had played in his father's choice to leave. For instance, John admitted that he had not always been good when his father was at home and that he sometimes talked back to his father or fought with his siblings. He stated that he believed that his father might have left because John had been bad or because he was not very cool for his father to hang out with. In helping John to forgive himself, the psychotherapist explored alternative reasons for why John's father might have left. During this process, John was able to identify several other causes for his father leaving. First, he said that his father had a difficult time finding work in the area in which they lived and that his father had told him he was leaving for a better paying job. Second, he indicated that his father had frequently had verbal arguments with his mother and that he might have left because he was unhappy with her rather than being unhappy just with John. Third, he said that his father was difficult to live with because he had a bad temper. Identifying each of these reasons and determining the role that they might have played in his father's leaving allowed John to take appropriate responsibility for his part in his family's conflict (his defiance toward his parents and his past fighting with his siblings). This lowered the amount of anger that he directed toward himself (lessening his depression) while also setting the stage for John to engage in the process of forgiveness and reconciliation with his mother.

In discussing John's relationship with his mother, the clinician reflected to John that it seemed as though he wanted to be forgiven by her and to be given a second chance. John agreed that this was so and also expressed that although he recognized that he had hurt her for some time with his defiant behavior, he did not know how to change things with her. The psychotherapist reframed his mother taking John to psychotherapy as a sign that she also wanted things to change and be better between the two of them, and John was asked whether he would be willing to have joint sessions with his mother in which they talked about how things were going between them. John reluctantly agreed, and the clinician set up regular joint sessions between the two of them.

During the initial phase, with the clinician's help, mother and son were able to identify that they wanted things to be different between them. A goal in the beginning was to achieve a basic level of empathy between them. John revealed his feelings about what it was like not having a father around and the loss it caused to not have his father to help him learn things such as sports and how to become a man. The mother shared her joy of having John as a baby but now being fearful of the problems that could develop for him for the future.

Mother and son also seemed to find a mutual point of empathy concerning what it was like to be a mixed-race family. John's mother identified the prejudices that she and her husband faced as a biracial couple, and John shared the adversity he faced in school as a biracial child. Through this and other moments of receiving empathy, John was able to acknowledge how difficult it was for his mother to cope with his negative behaviors. When his mother offered forgiveness to John, the clinician helped John to understand the process by asking him what would it look like to be forgiven. John was able to let his mother know that for him, forgiveness meant that he would have his mother's trust and that he would be allowed to do things without someone constantly watching over him. During the forgiveness intervention, John's sense of loss was replaced with a newfound forgiveness of self and a restored forgiving relationship between mother and son.

Case 2: Slaying Dragons

Depression and other marital issues brought Don and Mary (both approximately 24 years old) into psychotherapy with Frederick A. DiBlasio.

Several months previously, Mary had brought her 14-year-old brother, Carl, across country to the East to live with her and her husband. Carl was the youngest sibling to his five older sisters; Mary was second from the oldest. Mary had convinced her father that it was best for all that she and Don have Carl come live with them because of the intense struggles between Carl and their father.

Although the couple was struggling financially, they were doing well at providing a strong faith-based environment, home educating Carl, meeting his emotional and physical needs, and finding ways to cope with his mild attention-deficit/hyperactivity disorder. During a marital counseling session, Mary remarked that Carl had a difficult time with his anger toward their father, prompting DiBlasio to offer individual (and family) psychotherapy for Carl. All three wanted the therapy to be Christian focused.

During the first interview, DiBlasio built rapport with Carl and found him to be very alert, articulate, and intelligent. The interview reflected that he was insightful in comprehending and communicating abstract thinking, and he had no problem focusing during the interview. He stated that he was angry with his father because he was not a loving father toward him. At first his description was vague, focusing mostly on his father's impatience and lack of nurturance. Although Carl was engaged with DiBlasio and talked freely about most things, DiBlasio noticed that he was more reserved when talking about his father. In contrast, his conversation became animated when discussing his mother. According to Carl, his father caught his mother having an affair. Carl explained that because this incident occurred when he was only 2 years old, he did not perceive his mother's behavior as an offense toward him. The mother lost a vigorous legal battle for custody of the children and eventually moved to another state. Although she was reported to be unstable in her personal life, Carl felt positively about her and enjoyed his periodic visits with her. Other than these visits, Carl's mother was not involved in Carl's life.

In the second session, Carl was able to open up more and talk about his feelings toward his father. However, when asked again to explain some specifics of how his father acted toward him, Carl would simply refer to the summary statement that his father was impatient and not nurturing. He was more descriptive about his own behavior, which included disobedience, deception, and manipulation of his father and sisters.

Forgiveness was discussed during this session as a general concept but was not related to his father. DiBlasio believed it best to discuss Carl's thoughts about what forgiveness meant before dealing with specific situations. Carl believed that forgiveness was when a person ceased to be upset with someone for what was done to him or her and started acting normally again toward that person. DiBlasio discussed the differences between emotional hurt and negative thinking about the person. Carl was interested in the concept that people could decide to forgive and attempt to control negative thinking, even though the emotional hurt still existed. Moreover, he was intrigued that people could make the decision to forgive at any point they chose. After careful thought, DiBlasio decided not to invite the father to the upcoming forgiveness session. From Don and Mary's description of the father, it was unlikely that he would make the trip across country for the session. In addition, the father's symptoms as described indicated the possibility of a moderate to serious personality disorder. Given the circumstances, DiBlasio and the clients decided to first work with Carl on forgiveness issues before approaching the father. Mary was asked to join the session as a person who could give insight into the father and assist DiBlasio's role play of the father when necessary during the session.

Following is a brief summary of the 2-hour forgiveness session. Carl and Mary were asked how they defined forgiveness. Carl had, interestingly, absorbed the previous session and decided to adopt the decision-based concept. Both Mary and Carl had a strong belief in Jesus and his teachings about forgiving others. Given their religious commitment, the clients freely embraced and welcomed DiBlasio's suggestion to pray and talk about scripture during the session.

Mary and Carl reported during the statement-of-the-offense step that their father, out of frustration resulting from not being able to control Carl's behaviors, had restricted him to a stool that stood 6 inches off the ground for 2 years from morning to night (from age 12 to age 14). DiBlasio asked a number of questions that confirmed that this statement was not exaggerated. The restriction included that Carl could not talk with his sisters, and it eventually included denial of food. Carl said that when his father was in another room or when he was away from the house that he would get up and sneak food, being careful to get back to the stool to avoid being caught by his father. There was a time of silence as tears came to DiBlasio's eyes, followed by a therapeutic processing of the hurt, isolation, loneliness, and waste of precious time that resulted from such treatment. DiBlasio at one point asked, "What in the world did you do while sitting on that stool for so long?" Carl replied, "I slew many dragons" (meaning he spent his time daydreaming). The session was the longest and most in-depth discussion that Carl had ever had regarding the offense. DiBlasio noted that this experience would require a significant amount of psychotherapy time in subsequent weeks and that it was important within the session to try to figure out an explanation for the father's behavior (realizing that an explanation did not mean justification). Although DiBlasio could not formally make a diagnosis, the description of the father's behavior was overwhelmingly consistent with narcissistic personality disorder. He emphasized to Carl that people with this disorder actually do not learn from, or have, the empathy to understand the pain they inflict on others. However, he pointed out that the father, if he had this disorder, was still fully accountable for his behavior. Mary and Carl were convinced that their father had good intentions and was not acting out of malice, and the discussion provided a framework to make sense out of how good intentions could coexist with maltreatment.

The other steps of the session were enacted, which included Carl fully discussing his emotional hurt (which became the focus of later psychotherapy) and a plan that included commitment to future psychotherapy, implementation of loving boundaries, and how Mary and Carl could protect themselves from possible future offenses. DiBlasio asked permission to role play what the father would say as a request for forgiveness if he were rational and thinking clearly. However, he emphasized that Carl had complete freedom as to whether he wanted to make a cognitive decision to forgive his father. Carl was very touched during the request for forgiveness as tears rolled down his cheek. He understood that his father might never get to the point of fully owning and expressing wrongdoing, but he decided that he wanted to let it go and not harbor unforgiveness any longer. The time and date of the forgiveness session was noted, and at DiBlasio's prompting Mary and Carl came up with a way that they would celebrate the forgiveness (a special night where Carl could ask for his heart's desire regarding dinner, discussion, and activity). The following week, Carl reported that since the forgiveness session his feelings toward his father had changed for the better. He said, "I no longer feel anger toward my father. Now I mourn for what could have been for me and my sisters."

Once he made the decision to forgive, future treatment was enhanced because he was not ensnared in the roots of bitterness, which distract and prevent recovery. After reviewing the road ahead and the therapeutic effort that would be involved, DiBlasio asked, "Are you ready to slay one more dragon?" After an explanation, Carl understood and found the use of his earlier metaphor meaningful: He smiled and gave a firm answer of yes. The forgiveness decision freed Carl to face his internal pain directly during the remaining weeks of psychotherapy.

CONCLUSION

Forgiveness within the psychotherapy encounter helps children and other family members to move forward therapeutically and spiritually. Theory and research have pointed to certain practice concepts that have the potential to promote the seeking and granting of forgiveness. Sufficient research evidence has shown that certain concepts are important in adults' forgiving and seeking forgiveness. As demonstrated in this chapter, these concepts can be applied to children and seem to work in the practice context. However, the research available related to psychotherapeutic interventions using child and adolescent subjects is not sufficient. We hope that this chapter will encourage the development of intervention strategies that can then be quantitatively tested.

We encourage clinicians to use the concepts presented here to design forgiveness interventions and apply them in such a manner that they fit the context of the family and the nature of the offenses. Psychotherapists bring a wealth of practice experience to the table, such as techniques to assist children and family members to gain insight, address anger, and release negative feelings. Organizing a systematic approach so that these interventions lead to forgiveness will help family members slay the dragons of bitterness and resentment that hinder healing and loving relationships.

REFERENCES

American Psychiatric Association. (2000). *Diagnostic and statistical manual of mental disorders* (4th ed., text rev.). Washington, DC: Author.

Baskin, T. W., & Enright, R. D. (2004). Intervention studies in forgiveness: A meta-analysis. *Journal of Counseling and Development, 82*, 79–90. doi:10.1002/j.1556-6678.2004.tb00288.x

Cheong, R., & DiBlasio, F. A. (2007). Christ-like love and forgiveness: A biblical foundation for counseling practice. *Journal of Psychology and Christianity, 26*, 14–25.

DiBlasio, F. A. (1998). The use of decision-based forgiveness intervention within intergenerational family therapy. *Journal of Family Therapy, 20*, 77–94. doi:10.1111/1467-6427.00069

DiBlasio, F. A. (1999). Scripture and forgiveness: Interventions with families and couples. *Marriage and Family: A Christian Journal, 3*, 257–267.

DiBlasio, F. A. (2000). Decision-based forgiveness treatment in cases of marital infidelity. *Psychotherapy: Theory, Research, Practice, Training, 37*, 149–158. doi:10.1037/h0087834

DiBlasio, F. A. (2001). *Effective treatment of personality disorders*. Forest, VA: American Association of Christian Counselors.

DiBlasio, F. A. (2010). Christ-like forgiveness in marital counseling: A clinical follow-up of two empirical studies. *Journal of Psychology and Christianity, 29*, 291–300.

DiBlasio, F. A., & Benda, B. B. (2008). Forgiveness intervention with married couples: Two empirical analyses. *Journal of Psychology and Christianity, 27,* 150–158.

DiBlasio, F. A., & Proctor, J. H. (1993). Therapists and the clinical use of forgiveness. *American Journal of Family Therapy, 21,* 175–184. doi:10.1080/01926189308250915

Enright, R. D. (2001). *Forgiveness is a choice: A step-by-step process for resolving anger and restoring hope.* Washington, DC: American Psychological Association.

Enright, R. D., & Fitzgibbons, R. (2000). *Helping clients forgive: An empirical guide for resolving anger and restoring hope.* Washington, DC: American Psychological Association. doi:10.1037/10381-000

Enright, R. D., & Human Development Study Group. (1991). The moral development of forgiveness. In W. Kurtines & J. Gewirtz (Eds.), *Handbook of moral behavior and development* (Vol. 1, pp. 123–152). Hillsdale, NJ: Erlbaum.

Enright, R. D., Knutson, J. A., Holter, A. C., Baskin, T., & Knutson, C. (2007). Waging peace through forgiveness in Belfast, Northern Ireland II: Educational programs for mental health improvement of children. *Journal of Research in Education, Fall,* 63–78.

Freedman, S. R., Enright, R. D., & Knutson, J. (2005). A progress report on the process model of forgiveness. In E. L. Worthington Jr. (Ed.), *Handbook of forgiveness* (pp. 393–406). New York, NY: Routledge.

Gardner, R. A. (1971). *Therapeutic communication with children: The mutual story telling technique.* Northvale, NJ: Jason Aronson.

Keifer, R. P., Worthington, E. L., Jr., Myers, B. J., Kliewer, W. L., Berry, J. W., Davis, D. E., . . . Hunter, J. L. (2010). Training parents in forgiving and reconciling. *American Journal of Family Therapy, 38,* 32–49.

Lampton, C., Oliver, G., Worthington, E. L., Jr., & Berry, J. W. (2005). Helping Christian college students become more forgiving: An intervention study to promote forgiveness as part of a program to shape Christian character. *Journal of Psychology and Theology, 33,* 278–290.

Sadock, B. J., & Sadock, V. A. (2007). *Kaplan and Sadock's synopsis of psychiatry: Behavioral sciences/clinical psychiatry* (10th ed.). Philadelphia, PA: Lippincott Williams & Wilkins.

Stratton, S. P., Dean, J. B., Nooneman, A. J., Bode, R. A., & Worthington, E. L., Jr. (2008). Forgiveness interventions as spiritual development strategies: Workshop training, expressive writing about forgiveness, and retested controls. *Journal of Psychology and Christianity, 27,* 347–357.

U.S. Census Bureau. (2012). *Statistical abstract of the United States* (131st ed.). Washington, DC: U.S. Department of Commerce.

Worthington, E. L., Jr. (1998). An empathy-humility-commitment model of forgiveness applied within family dyads. *Journal of Family Therapy, 20,* 59–76. doi:10.1111/1467-6427.00068

Worthington, E. L., Jr. (2003). *Forgiving and reconciling: Bridges to wholeness and hope*. Downer's Grove, IL: InterVarsity Press.

Worthington, E. L., Jr. (2006a). The development of forgiveness. In E. M. Dowling & W. G. Scarlette (Eds.), *Encyclopedia of religious and spiritual development in children and adolescence* (pp. 165–167). Thousand Oaks, CA: Sage.

Worthington, E. L., Jr. (2006b). *Forgiveness and reconciliation: Theory and application*. New York, NY: Routledge.

Worthington, E. L., Jr. (2010). *Forgiveness intervention manuals*. Retrieved from http://www.people.vcu.edu/~eworth

Worthington, E. L., Jr., & DiBlasio, F. A. (1990). Promoting mutual forgiveness within the fractured relationship. *Psychotherapy: Theory, Research, Practice, Training, 27*, 219–223. doi:10.1037/0033-3204.27.2.219

Worthington, E. L., Jr., Jennings, D. J., II, & DiBlasio, F. A. (2010). Interventions to promote forgiveness in couple and family context: Conceptualization, review, and analysis. *Journal of Psychology and Theology, 38*, 231–245.

AFTERWORD: REFLECTIONS AND FUTURE DIRECTIONS

DONALD F. WALKER AND WILLIAM L. HATHAWAY

In the Introduction to this volume, we suggested that our rationale for this book was driven by the convergence of two powerful forces within psychology: evidence-based practice within clinical child psychology and the development of spiritual interventions within the psychology of religion and spirituality. The discipline of clinical child psychology of religion and spirituality is still in its infancy, as this text clearly demonstrates. Many, if not all, of the interventions that have been described suffer from a dearth of randomized clinical trials on which to base claims about their efficacy. Instead, evidence for the effectiveness of these interventions comes from the description of clinical case studies in each chapter. In that respect, we are encouraged by the assorted case examples that have been put forth representing a variety of presenting problems, ages, and religious and spiritual traditions.

DOI: 10.1037/13947-012
Spiritual Interventions in Child and Adolescent Psychotherapy, D. F. Walker and W. L. Hathaway (Editors)

REFLECTIONS ON THE FUTURE OF PRACTICE AND RESEARCH

In this Afterword, we reflect on the material that has been presented and on the future of practice and research in this area. We focus on three overarching issues involving practice and research: (a) pretreatment assessment and case conceptualization, (b) spiritually oriented interventions that are used in the context of secular evidence-based practices for children and teens, and (c) religious and spiritual interventions that operate independently of secular empirically supported treatments.

Assessment and Case Conceptualization

Over the past decade, various theorists have alternatively highlighted that spirituality and religion may be a resource for healing within psychotherapy, a barrier to treatment, or an aspect of clients' overall functioning that has been negatively affected by their diagnosed psychological disorder (Hathaway, 2003; Hathaway & Barkley, 2003; Raiya, Pargament, & Magyar-Russell, 2010; Richards & Bergin, 2005). Spirituality and religion also serve as a lens through which parents and their children view the world, understand their presenting problems, and identify ways to resolve their problems (Chapters 3 and 7).

We are excited at the ongoing efforts to better understand and assess the potential role of children's (and their families') spirituality and religion in their presenting problems. We now have several models for understanding and assessing children's spiritual and religious functioning. In Chapter 3, Mahoney et al. offered a practical, clinically useful framework for case conceptualization with their relational spirituality framework. This framework is unique in its focus on the role of spirituality and religion in forming, maintaining, and transforming family relationships. Mahoney et al.'s framework is also distinct in its focus on considering how parental spirituality shapes the expectations that parents have for psychotherapy with respect to goals and the interventions used to meet those goals. As Mahoney et al. acknowledged in their chapter, a great deal of empirical work remains to be done with aspects of the model that they advanced. In particular, work needs to be done to understand the role of parental religion in determining psychotherapy outcomes among clinic-referred families. More broadly, additional research needs to be conducted regarding specific religiously prescribed parenting practices in promoting or disturbing mental health among children. For example, in considering parenting practices such as corporal punishment, we wonder whether exercises such as spanking might produce differential outcomes among clinic-referred versus non–clinic-referred religious parents and the conditions under which they might produce different outcomes.

Hathaway's model for assessment and case conceptualization (Chapter 2) highlights the importance of considering the effects of psychological disorders on the religious and spiritual functioning of children and teens. Hathaway's model is unique in this regard. We both appreciate the need to better understand the spiritual effects of psychological disorders. Hathaway and Barkley (2003) presented a conceptual model for this sort of case conceptualization when they systematically considered the effects of symptoms of hyperactivity, impulsivity, and inattentiveness associated with attention-deficit/hyperactivity disorder on the religious and spiritual functioning of children. Similar attempts have been made to describe the religious and spiritual impairments associated with autistic spectrum disorders (Marker, Weeks, & Kraegel, 2007). These efforts have highlighted, in particular, the difficulties that religiously committed children with neurodevelopmental disorders may have in becoming trained in their religious tradition in the context of their local congregation. As with many of the other models presented in this book, much of the evidence for children's religious and spiritual impairment because of childhood disorders involves published case studies. These conceptual models are useful but would benefit from additional research describing such impairment in children resulting from various psychological symptoms and their associated disorders.

In a somewhat related vein, Richards and Bergin (2005) previously advanced a model for assessing the role of spirituality and religion in a client's presenting problem. Although Richards and Bergin did not develop this model specifically for use with religious children and their parents, we find it clinically useful and have used it in our psychotherapy work with religiously committed children and their families. In their assessment protocol, Richards and Bergin distinguished between what they call a Level 1 versus a Level 2 assessment of client religion and spirituality. According to Richards and Bergin, a Level 1 assessment involves assessing clients' religion and spirituality broadly as part of a larger psychosocial assessment evaluating clients' physical, social, behavioral, cognitive, educational, occupational, and emotional functioning. During Level 1 assessments, psychotherapists typically ask screening questions (e.g., "Is your religious and spiritual faith important to you?" "Do you have a religious or spiritual affiliation?" "Are there any religious or spiritual issues that you want to discuss as part of treatment?").

When clients report that their faith is relevant to their presenting problems, or if it is deemed to be, Richards and Bergin (2005) have encouraged the application of a Level 2 assessment of spirituality and religion. During Level 2 assessments, psychotherapists should assess clinically relevant aspects of clients' spirituality and religion such as their worldviews, value–lifestyle congruence, God images, spiritual identities, doctrinal knowledge, and religious and spiritual health.

We have found Richards and Bergin's (2005) model to be helpful in evaluating the role that religiousness and spirituality may play in a client's case presentation (see Walker, Reese, Hughes, & Troskie, 2010, for several case presentations). We have also wondered why researchers have yet to apply this model to psychotherapy involving religiously committed children and teens and to conduct clinical research involving its application. To the extent that this assessment model is useful, we would expect several outcomes of such a research investigation. First and foremost, we would expect that applying the model would assist clinicians in developing clinically useful hypotheses about the role of clients' spirituality and religion in their presenting problems. Second, to the extent that religiously committed parents view the world through a religious lens, we would expect that engaging in the Richards and Bergin assessment model would also assist in the development of the working alliance in psychotherapy. These hypotheses remain to be empirically tested. In a related vein, little research has been done with children and teens to identify and describe clinically useful domains of spiritual and religious functioning. In addition to identifying these domains, the development of reliable, clinically useful instruments is needed. Also missing are developmentally sensitive instruments (particularly self-report inventories) tapping spiritual and religious functioning among children.

Quagliana et al. (Chapter 4) highlighted the vital importance of considering a client's developmental level across different domains when considering spiritual interventions with children and teens. Their chapter is among the emerging literature that we are aware of attempting to describe what children can understand about spirituality and religion at different ages. If spiritual interventions are to be truly effective with religiously committed children and adolescents, they must be developmentally sensitive. In these next sections, we consider the future of practice and research with spiritually oriented interventions.

Spiritual Interventions That Are Tied to Evidence-Based Secular Child Treatments

The bulk of these interventions involve using sacred texts and prayer in cognitive–behavioral treatment packages for a variety of presenting problems—empirically supported parenting programs for oppositional behavior, cognitive–behavioral therapy for depression and anxiety, and trauma-focused cognitive behavior therapy. We are excited at the prospects for addressing religious and spiritual diversity within these secular treatments. When referring to sacred writings or incorporating prayer within secular evidence-based treatments for childhood disorders, we are not attempting to supplant or otherwise weaken the effectiveness of the treatment in its purest form. Rather, we see an opportunity to help psychotherapists live out their ethical call to treat client religion and spirituality with sensitivity and respect. Our own experience in working with a religiously and spiritually diverse range of psychotherapists in a variety of practice settings has been that psychotherapists sometimes view spiritual issues with confusion or outright disdain. One benefit to practitioners of applying spiritual interventions within secular empirically supported treatments is that the secular forms of the treatments are familiar to a number of treatment providers, as is the process of attempting to be culturally sensitive in their application. This should make it easier to accept our recommendations for practice and to implement them with religiously and spiritually diverse clients.

However, in our view the primary advantage of using spiritual practices in secular evidence-based treatments is that highly religious clients and their families will feel more comfortable with the secular treatment. As a result, we believe that secular evidence-based treatments will be more effective with highly religious clients and their families when incorporating spiritual interventions as described in Chapters 7 and 8. These chapters provide anecdotal evidence with religiously diverse case studies indicating that this is the case. What is needed are randomized clinical trials that further support the efficacy of these approaches with highly religious clients.

One advantage to developing spiritual interventions building on secular evidence-based treatment protocols is that it will be relatively easy, in terms of design and analysis, to develop a research base in this area. Many of the secular treatment protocols that we referenced in Chapter 7 (including, for example, parent–child interaction therapy and trauma-focused cognitive–behavioral therapy) have received federal grant funding to support outcome studies and dissemination of the protocol. As a result, the secular forms of these treatments have a proven track record of effectiveness as well as a generally accepted standard for demonstrating treatment effectiveness.

If clinical research in the clinical child psychology of religion and spirituality is to advance, then outcome researchers must secure funding to conduct robust clinical trials and disseminate the information. To date, few clinical scientists of religion and spirituality have been willing to take up the call to conduct clinical trials involving spiritual interventions, particularly for childhood disorders. If the discipline is to advance, clinical researchers must be willing to undertake this task. It would seem that using spiritually oriented adaptations of proven secular treatments would make outcome research involving these protocols more attractive to potential funding sources. Scholars in the area are not starting from scratch but are instead building on accepted treatments. We look forward to the development of outcome research involving this category of spiritually oriented interventions with children and teens.

Spiritual Interventions That Are Independent of Evidence-Based Secular Child Treatments

The majority of spiritual interventions described in this book by the various chapter authors were developed without consideration of child and adolescent psychotherapy, at least initially. Interventions such as these, in particular, spiritual awareness, some uses of prayer, consideration of God images, and forgiveness (Chapters 6, and 8–10, respectively) have been used with adult psychotherapy clients for some time and are only now being adapted for use with children and teens. All of the spiritual interventions described in this book that are independent of evidence-based secular child treatments are adaptable for use with a variety of theoretical orientations, as discussed in their respective chapters. Some of these interventions are more easily integrated into humanistic, psychodynamic, or even psychoanalytic psychotherapies (e.g., acceptance, spiritual awareness, God images), although some cut across theoretical perspectives (e.g., God images, forgiveness, prayer). We view the flexibility and adaptability of these various spiritual interventions as relative strengths.

It is interesting to note that using some of the spiritual interventions that fall in this second category allows psychotherapists to achieve different spiritual goals than those that are tied to a secular treatment protocol. Promoting spiritual awareness and inner acceptance, correcting God images, and deepening one's relationship with the Divine using prayer involve relational spiritual goals that are ends unto themselves. As such, the interventions look different from spiritual interventions that promote a primarily symptom-related goal, such as improving child behavior in a parenting program or reducing a teenager's level of anxiety using cognitive–behavioral psychotherapy. This is not to say that using these spiritual interventions will not also promote symptom relief. However, the mechanism by which they promote symptom relief may be through a secondary pathway in which clients' spiritual needs are addressed en route to relieving their mental health symptoms. We have no real empirical research on which to base this claim. However, we are encouraged by the case studies that have illustrated the effectiveness of these interventions and elucidated the mechanisms by which they appear to be effective.

As with other areas in this book, outcome research using this category of spiritually oriented interventions is sorely needed to further demonstrate their effectiveness. The pioneering work of Everett Worthington Jr. and his colleagues over the past 15 years has provided a template on which to build this evidence base. Before 1990, there were virtually no studies on the psychotherapeutic use of forgiveness. Worthington and DiBlasio (1990) advanced some initial considerations for promoting forgiveness in psychotherapy, and a recent PsycINFO search conducted by Donald F. Walker using the search term *forgiveness* yielded more than 11,000 citations. As part of this progression, a number of studies have demonstrated the effectiveness of Worthington's (2006) REACH model of forgiveness in helping people to forgive and improving their mental health (see Chapter 10 for a review). This sort of work is needed for each of the spiritual interventions described in this book that do not inherently belong to a specific theoretical orientation but have been adapted developmentally for children using different theoretical perspectives.

CONCLUSION

It is a difficult task to end a volume that, somewhat ironically, represents in many ways a beginning for the clinical child psychology of religion and spirituality. We are thrilled to be part of an exciting movement within psychology and counseling in which the very best empirically supported treatment methods for childhood disorders are being informed by the knowledge available from the psychology of religion and spirituality in service to religiously committed children, teens, and their families. Throughout this book, we have tried to temper our enthusiasm with our acknowledgment that, to a large extent, this particular area of psychotherapy remains behind other areas of child treatment.

As child psychotherapists, we are reminded as we conclude this book of Aesop's famous fable involving a tortoise and a hare. Like the tortoise in Aesop's story, we have seen other areas of psychology develop much more quickly. The field of clinical child psychology has progressed to the point at which psychotherapists have available to them dozens of funded empirical studies of treatment methods for various childhood disorders that speak to their effectiveness. In a similar, although less spectacular, fashion, the psychology of religion and spirituality has within the past 15 years seen a relative expanse in the scope of research related to religion and mental health, as well as the application of spiritually oriented interventions. Reminiscent of the tortoise in Aesop's fable, our particular area of interest—the intersection of both of these fields of practice—has moved much more slowly. We take heart in knowing that, with steadfast persistence, Aesop's tortoise eventually won his race. We are encouraged by the clinical case examples that have been presented throughout this book, and we look forward to the completion of additional basic clinical research with respect to assessment and case conceptualization, as well as randomized clinical trials for the spiritual interventions that have been presented.

REFERENCES

Hathaway, W. L. (2003). Clinically significant religious impairment. *Mental Health, Religion & Culture*, 6, 113–129.

Hathaway, W. L., & Barkley, R. (2003). Self-regulation, ADHD, and child religiousness. *Journal of Psychology and Christianity*, *22*, 101–114.

Marker, C., Weeks, M., & Kraegel, I. (2007). Integrating faith and treatment for children with high functioning autism spectrum disorders. *Journal of Psychology and Christianity*, *26*, 112–121.

Raiya, H. A., Pargament, K. I., & Magyar-Russell, G. (2010). When religion goes awry: Religious risk factors for poorer health and well-being. In P. J. Verhagen, H. M. van Praag, J. J. Lopez-Ibor Jr., & J. L. Cox (Eds.), *Religion and psychiatry: Beyond boundaries* (pp. 389–411). Chichester, England: Wiley.

Richards, P. S., & Bergin, A. E. (2005). *A spiritual strategy for counseling and psychotherapy* (2nd ed.). Washington, DC: American Psychological Association. doi:10.1037/11214-000

Walker, D. F., Reese, J., Hughes, J., & Troskie, M. (2010). Addressing religious and spiritual issues in trauma-focused cognitive behavior therapy. *Professional Psychology: Research and Practice*, *41*, 174–180. doi:10.1037/a0017782

Worthington, E. L., Jr. (2006). *Forgiveness and reconciliation: Theory and application.* New York, NY: Routledge.

Worthington, E. L., Jr., & DiBlasio, F. (1990). Promoting mutual forgiveness within the fractured relationship. *Psychotherapy: Theory, Research, Practice, Training*, *27*, 219–223. doi:10.1037/0033-3204.27.2.219

INDEX

ABOUT THE EDITORS

Donald F. Walker, PhD, directs the Child Trauma Institute, an interdisciplinary research center devoted to understanding the role of religious faith in recovery from childhood abuse, treating survivors of child abuse, and training professionals in addressing spiritual issues in treatment. Dr. Walker also teaches in the PsyD program in clinical psychology at Regent University. As a professor, he teaches courses on clinical child psychology and trauma and supervises students at all levels of the program. He is a member of the Society for the Psychology of Religion and Spirituality, the Society for Child and Family Policy and Practice, and the Division of Trauma Psychology (American Psychological Association Divisions 36, 37, and 56, respectively). A clinical child psychologist, he maintains a small private practice treating children, teens, and families at Genesis Counseling Center in Hampton, VA.

William L. Hathaway, PhD, currently serves as a dean and professor in the School of Psychology & Counseling at Regent University. He completed his postdoctoral fellowship in clinical child psychology with Russell Barkley at the University of Massachusetts Medical Center and has worked in both military and civilian child specialty clinics. His doctoral research focused on the psychology of religion and coping, and he has served in various governance roles, including president of the Society for the Psychology of Religion and Spirituality (Division 36) of the American Psychological Association. He has published on attention-deficit/hyperactivity disorder, the clinical psychology of religion, spirituality and self-regulation, and relevant clinical training issues.